D1527320

Management of Soft Tissue Sarcoma

Murray F. Brennan · Cristina R. Antonescu
Robert G. Maki

Management of Soft Tissue Sarcoma

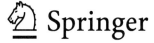 Springer

Murray F. Brennan
International Center & Department
  of Surgery
Memorial Sloan-Kettering Cancer Center
New York, NY, USA

Cristina R. Antonescu
Department of Pathology
Memorial Sloan-Kettering Cancer Center
New York, NY, USA

Robert G. Maki
Departments of Medicine
  Pediatrics, and Orthopaedics
Mount Sinai School of Medicine
New York, NY, USA

ISBN 978-1-4614-5003-0   ISBN 978-1-4614-5004-7 (eBook)
DOI 10.1007/978-1-4614-5004-7
Springer New York Heidelberg Dordrecht London

Library of Congress Control Number: 2012946193

Printed on acid-free paper

Springer is part of Springer Science+Business Media (www.springer.com)

Preface

The authors were approached some time ago to write a text regarding the management of soft tissue sarcomas. There are several existing texts in the literature, and before embarking on such a project it was necessary to identify what could be added that was unique to the existing literature.

We note that although there have been several texts that discuss management of sarcomas, there are few that discuss subtypes individually, given the rare nature of any one of these diagnoses. The prospectively accrued soft tissue sarcoma database initiated by Dr. Brennan in 1982 represents the largest single collection of individual soft tissue sarcoma patient data, allowing characterization of subtype by prevalence, age, and site. This is a unique resource for patient care and management and for outlining the clinical outcomes and management for each sarcoma subtype.

In addition, there are few data collected in one place regarding systemic therapy for different diagnoses. While there have been a large number of phase II studies and retrospective analyses of outcomes with specific agents, there has not been a consistent place to refer for subtype-specific data. Despite issues regarding recall bias and other well-recognized weaknesses of retrospective analyses, we have endeavored to collect at least some of those data herein, and to speculate based on anecdote and case reports possible treatments for rarer subtypes.

We stand on the cusp of a revolution in the diagnosis of cancer, with the emergence of genetic and other sophisticated tests of specific cancers now leading rapidly to the development and use of new agents to treat those cancers. One need not look beyond the success of imatinib in Gastrointestinal Stromal Tumors (GIST) or chronic myeloid leukemia (CML), vemurafenib in melanoma, or crizotinib in anaplastic lymphoma kinase (ALK)+lung cancer (and ALK+inflammatory myofibroblastic tumor) to realize that we will not diagnose or treat sarcomas the same way 10 years from now as we do today. We hope this contribution will serve as a cairn on a long and otherwise largely unmarked journey to best identify, characterize, treat, and hopefully eliminate these forms of cancer.

Acknowledgments

Limited author texts such as this are a great challenge. They cannot be completed without the help of many people. Over the 30 years of the Memorial Sloan-Kettering Cancer Center database, we have been fortunate to have outstanding support, particularly from our colleagues in pathology, medicine, surgery, and radiation therapy. The accumulation and maintenance of such a prospective database, reviewed and updated on a weekly basis, has been the province of many committed data managers. Most recently, Nicole Moraco has been responsible for the oversight and maintenance of the quality of the databases and production of the majority of the figures in this text.

As we review a database of more than 9,000 treated patients, it is hard to accept that each one is an individual patient with individual defining characteristics. We thank those individuals for the ability to use the data generated during their course of illness to create information valuable for the treatment of those yet undiagnosed patients.

The synthesis of the text would not have happened but for the efforts of Ms. Victoria Frohnhoefer. Her tireless commitment to the project and meticulous oversight of the authors are what brought this project to fruition. We cannot thank her enough.

Contents

Chapter 1
General Description

Introduction

Soft tissue sarcomas are an unusual group of tumors deriving their name from the Greek term for a fleshy excrescence. As early as Galen (130–200 CE), it was suggested they were a cancerous tumor and caution was advised against any surgical intervention [1]. Early reports of myxoid liposarcoma by Severinius (1580–1637) and retroperitoneal liposarcoma by Morgagni (1682–1771) have been recorded [2]. Wardrop (1782–1869), an Edinburgh surgeon who had studied in Vienna, introduced the term soft cancer. In his book *Surgical Observations*, published in 1816, Charles Bell (1772–1842) has been credited with the utilization of the term soft tissue sarcoma to differentiate them from carcinoma [3]. The first classification of sarcoma has been attributed to Abernethy in 1804. Johannes Müller (1801–1858) has been credited with coining the term desmoid in 1838 [3]. Stout (1885–1967) published a seminal monograph in 1932 on the pathology and treatment of sarcomas [4].

Important contributions to the description and classification of sarcomas have been made at the Memorial Sloan-Kettering Cancer Center starting with Dr. James Ewing (1866–1943). Ewing was the first Professor of Pathology at Cornell University Medical College and the Clinical Director at Memorial Sloan-Kettering Cancer Center. He was Chief of Pathology at Memorial in 1899 at the age of 33 and published the first edition of his classic monograph, *Neoplastic Diseases*, in 1919. His original description of soft tissue sarcoma, "sarcoma is a malignant tumor composed of cells of the connective tissue type...," was based on the morphology of tumor cells and on their histogenesis. Ewing was one of the first to list benign and

M.F. Brennan et al., *Management of Soft Tissue Sarcoma*,
DOI 10.1007/978-1-4614-5004-7_1, © Springer Science+Business Media New York 2013

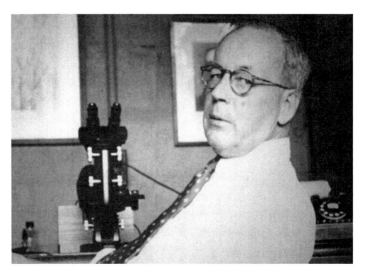

Fig. 1.1 Fred W. Stewart, M.D., Ph.D., 1894–1991, Pathologist, Memorial Sloan-Kettering Cancer Center (Used with permission from Brennan and Lewis [7])

malignant counterparts of tumors arising in the soft tissues. The most recognized contribution of Ewing was the description in 1920 of the tumor that bears his name [5].

Sarcoma has played a major contribution in the Memorial Sloan-Kettering Cancer Center's history. William Coley in 1889 treated the 17-year-old Elizabeth Dashiell at the hospital for an extremity sarcoma. This young woman, a friend of J.D. Rockefeller, Jr., died from her disease in June of 1890, and it was said to have influenced Coley's willingness to study sarcoma. Rockefeller contributed as a consequence of this experience with continued financial and endowment support of the Memorial Sloan-Kettering Cancer Center (MSKCC). Coley was recognized for his first attempts at what we would now call immunotherapy based on the utilization of Coley's toxins. He made the observation that a patient's sarcoma resolved after an episode of postoperative erysipelas infection, although it is not clear that the involved lesion was a sarcoma.

The first description of liposarcomas in 1944 has been attributed to Stout, also at Memorial Sloan-Kettering, as was the description with Ackerman of leiomyosarcoma of soft tissue in 1947. Dr. Stout's comprehensive listing of the sarcomas was described in an Armed Forces Institute of Pathology (AFIP) *Atlas of Tumor Pathology* in 1953 [6]. One of the classical sarcoma syndromes, the Stewart-Treves syndrome, was described by Fred W. Stewart and Norman Treves (Figs. 1.1 and 1.2) in the first issue of Cancer in 1948. Stewart, the Chairman of Pathology at MSKCC, and Treves, a member of the MSKCC Breast Service, described the highly malignant lymphangiosarcoma occurring in postmastectomy patients with chronic lymphedema [8].

Fig. 1.2 Norman Treves,
MD, 1894–1964, Breast
Surgeon, Memorial Sloan-
Kettering Cancer Center
(Used with permission from
Brennan and Lewis [7])

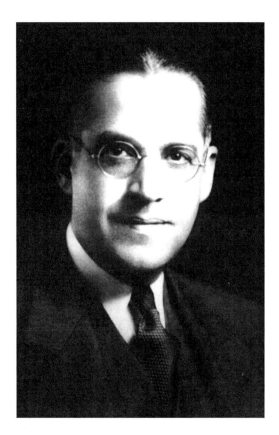

Incidence and Prevalence

It is difficult to determine the true incidence of soft tissue sarcoma in the United
States. It has previously been suggested to be between 10,000 and 14,000 new cases
a year, but difficulties in classification, the inclusion of metastasis from sarcoma
with other pathologies, and the relatively increased identification of gastrointestinal
stromal tumors suggest that this number is considerably higher.

Much of the data presented in this book is derived from a prospective database of
patients being admitted over the age of 16 to the Memorial Sloan-Kettering Cancer
Center beginning in July of 1982. A review from this database of over 8,000 patients
suggests that gender is equally distributed (Fig. 1.3). Distribution by site is shown
in Fig. 1.4, and distribution within the extremities is seen in Fig. 1.5. Distribution of
tumors by age and site is found for each relevant histology in individual chapters,
where sufficient numbers exist. The overall distribution by histology is in Fig. 1.6.
The distribution of dominant histology type by site is in Fig. 1.7.

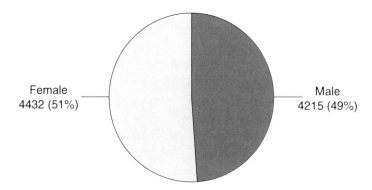

Fig. 1.3 Distribution by gender for adult patients with soft tissue sarcoma, all sites. MSKCC 7/1/1982-6/30/2010 n = 8,647

Fig. 1.4 Distribution by site for adult patients with soft tissue sarcoma. MSKCC 7/1/1982-6/30/2010 n = 8,647

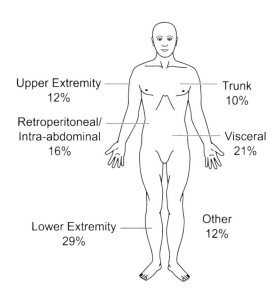

Grade (Fig. 1.8), depth (Fig. 1.9), and primary size (Fig. 1.10) are covered and their relevance to prognosis suggested in the appropriate sections.

The breakdown of site within extremity is included for lower and upper limbs (Figs. 1.11 and 1.12). Size of extremity primary tumors, a widely recognized variable for outcome, is included in Fig. 1.13.

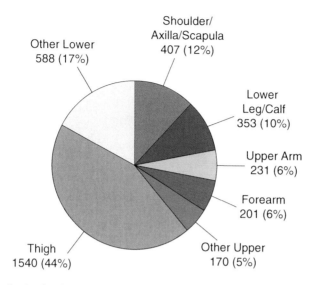

Fig. 1.5 Distribution by site within the extremities for adult patients with soft tissue sarcoma. MSKCC 7/1/1982-6/30/2010 n = 3,490

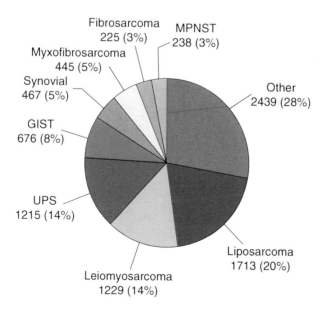

Fig. 1.6 Distribution by histology for adult patients with soft tissue sarcoma, all sites. MSKCC 7/1/1982-6/30/2010 n = 8,647. *GIST* gastrointestinal stromal tumor, *UPS* undifferentiated pleomorphic sarcoma, *MPNST* malignant peripheral nerve sheath tumor

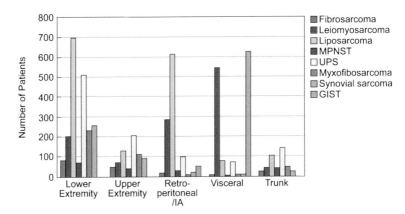

Fig. 1.7 Predominant histopathology by site for adult patients with soft tissue sarcoma. MSKCC 7/1/1982-6/30/2010 n = 5,653. *MPNST* malignant peripheral nerve sheath tumor, *GIST* gastrointestinal stromal tumor, *UPS* undifferentiated pleomorphic sarcoma, *IA* intra-abdominal

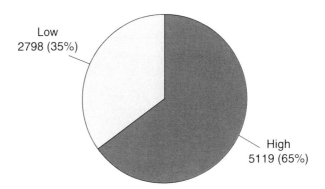

Fig. 1.8 Distribution by grade for adult patients with soft tissue sarcoma (excludes GIST), all sites. MSKCC 7/1/1982-6/30/2010 n = 7,917

Fig. 1.9 Distribution of primary lesion by depth for adult patients with soft tissue sarcoma. MSKCC 7/1/1982-6/30/2010 n = 8,578

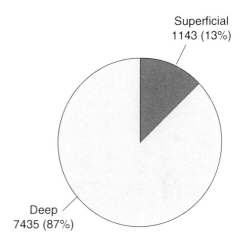

Fig. 1.10 Distribution by size for adult patients with soft tissue sarcoma, all primary sites. MSKCC 7/1/1982-6/30/2010 n = 7,988

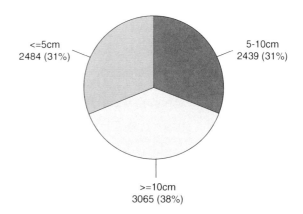

Fig. 1.11 Distribution within the lower extremity by site for adult patients with soft tissue sarcoma. MSKCC 7/1/1982-6/30/2010 n = 2,481

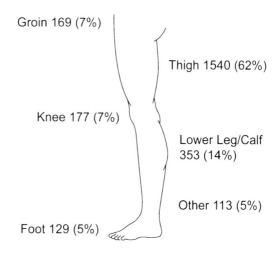

Fig. 1.12 Distribution within the upper extremity by site for adult patients with soft tissue sarcoma. MSKCC 7/1/1982-6/30/2010 n = 1,109

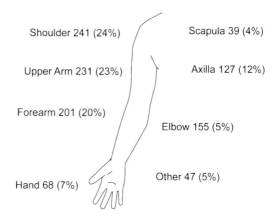

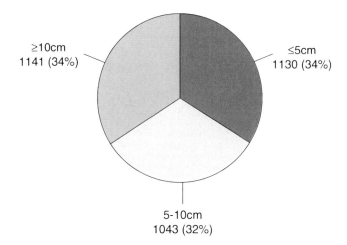

≥10cm
1141 (34%)

≤5cm
1130 (34%)

5-10cm
1043 (32%)

Fig. 1.13 Distribution within extremities by size for adult patients with soft tissue sarcoma. MSKCC 7/1/1982-6/30/2010 n = 3,314

Predisposing and Genetic Factors

Predisposing and genetic factors have been identified and include the genetic predisposition in the patient with neurofibromatosis (Fig. 1.14), familial adenomatous polyposis (FAP) coli, Li-Fraumeni syndrome, and retinoblastoma, although the majority of soft tissue sarcomas have no clear identified cause. There are two separate types: one that contains specific genetic alterations (Table 1.1), including variable gene rearrangements, fusion genes, reciprocal translocations, and specific mutations, such as those seen for *KIT* or *PDGFRA* in gastrointestinal stromal tumors and the *APC* loss or *CTNNB1* mutations seen in desmoid tumors. Although advances in molecular characterization are changing our view of the genetics of many cancers, including sarcomas, most sarcomas have nonspecific genetic alterations, which are often complex and multiple and represent variable chromosomal gains or losses. This latter group often has a high prevalence of *TP53* and *RB1* mutations or deletion. *TP53* mutations have been associated with the Li-Fraumeni syndrome [83]. In addition to *TP53*, various genes that modulate the activity of p53, such as *CDKN2A* and *HDM2*, are also observed to be altered in some way in sarcomas. These cell cycle-regulating genes have been incriminated in the high incidence of germ line mutation as is seen in hereditary retinoblastoma and suggested to be casually associated to the genetic predisposition to soft tissue sarcoma as has been seen in neurofibromatosis [84] and familial adenomatous polyposis [85]. These genetic aberrations have been suggested to be responsible for the increased susceptibility to second malignancy in such patients undergoing radiation therapy.

In neurofibromatosis, there is a high prevalence of malignant tumors, with almost 45% of such patients developing malignant tumor in a lifetime [86]. Patients who

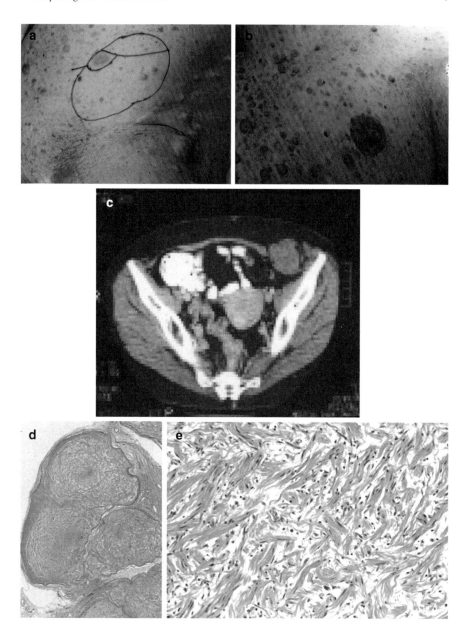

Fig. 1.14 Neurofibromatosis – neurofibroma left abdominal wall: (**a**, **b**) gross appearance of multiple neurofibromas and café au lait spots; (**c**) contrast-enhanced CT scan of the pelvis showing a soft tissue neurofibroma; (**d**) whole mount low-power microscopic appearance (H&E) and (**e**) high-power (200×)

Table 1.1 Cytogenetic table

Sarcoma subtype	Genetic alteration	Affected gene(s)	Frequency	References
Alveolar rhabdomyosarcoma	t(2;13)(q35;q14)	PAX3-FOXO1A	70%	[9–11]
	t(1;13)(p36;q14)	PAX7-FOXO1A	15%	
Alveolar soft part sarcoma	t(X;17)(p11.2;q25)	ASPSCR1-TFE3	>95%	[12]
Angiomatoid fibrous histiocytoma	t(2;22)(q34;q12)	EWSR1-CREB1	>90%	[13, 14]
	t(12;22)(q13;q12)	EWSR1-ATF1	<5%	
Clear-cell sarcoma (melanoma of soft parts)	t(12;22)(q13;q12)	EWSR1-ATF1	>90%	[15–19]
	t(2;22)(q34;q12)	EWSR1-CREB1	<5%	
Atypical Ewing sarcoma	t(4;19)(q35;q13.1)	CIC-DUX4	unk	[20–24]
	t(10;19)(q26.3;q13.1)			
	inv(X)(p11.4;p11.22)			
Congenital (infantile) fibrosarcoma	t(12;15)(p13;q25)	ETV6-NTRK3	>80%	[25, 26]
Dermatofibrosarcoma protuberans	t(17;22)(q22;q13)	COL1A1-PDGFB	>60%	[27–29]
Desmoplastic round cell tumor	t(11;22)(p13;q12)	WT1-EWSR1	>90%	[30–33]
Endometrial stromal sarcoma	t(7;17)(p15;q11)	JAZF1-SUZI2	>65%	[34–36]
	t(6;7)(p21;p15)	JAZF1-PHF1	unk	
	t(6;10)(p21;p11)	EPC1-PHF1	unk	
Undifferentiated endometrial sarcoma/"high-grade endometrial stromal sarcoma"	t(10;17)(q22;p13); others	YWHAE-FAM22A/B, other partners	unk	[37]
Epithelioid hemangioendothelioma	t(1;3)(p36.3;q25)	WWTR1-CAMTA1	>90%	[38]
Epithelioid sarcoma	INI1 inactivation [22(q11.2)]	hSNF5/INI1	>80%	[39–43]
Extraskeletal myxoid chondrosarcoma	t(9;22)(q22;q12)	EWSR1-NR4A3	>80%	[44–46]
	t(9;17)(q22;q11)	TAF15-NR4A3	unk	
	t(9;15)(q22;q21)	TCF12-NR4A3	unk	
Ewing sarcoma/PNET[a]	t(11;22)(q24;q12)	EWSR1-FLI1	85%	[47, 48]
	t(21;22)(q22;q12)	EWSR1-ERG	5–10%	
Fibromyxoid sarcoma (Evans' tumor)	t(7;16)(q33;p11)	FUS-CREB3L2	>70%	[49–51]
	t(11;16)(p11;p11)	FUS-CREB3L1	<20%	
Gastrointestinal stromal tumor	4q	KIT exon 11 mut	65%	[52–57]

	Cytogenetic abnormality	Molecular genetics	Frequency	References
	4q	KIT exon 9 mut	15%	
	4q	PDGFRA mut	<5%	
Giant cell tumor of tendon sheath	t(1;2)(p13;q37)	COL6A3-CSF1	>75%	[58]
Inflammatory myofibroblastic tumor[a]	t(2;19)(p23;p13.1)	TPM4-ALK	unk	[59–61]
	t(1;2)(q22-23;p23)	TPM3-ALK	unk	
Myoepithelial tumors	t(6;22)(p21;q12)	EWSR1-POU5F1	10%	[62]
	t(1;22)(q23;q12)	EWSR1-PBX1	10%	[61]
		Other fusion partners		
Myxoid-round cell liposarcoma	t(12;16)(q13;p11)	FUS-DDIT3	>90%	[63–65]
	t(12;22)(q13;q12)	EWSR1-DDIT3	<5%	
Pericytoma with t(7;12)	t(7;12)(p22;q13)	ACTB-GLI	unk	[66, 67]
(Extrarenal) rhabdoid tumor	del 22(q11.2)	hSNF5/INI1	~50%	[68–70]
Synovial sarcoma	t(X;18)(p11;q11)	SS18-SSX1/SSX2	>95%	[71–76]
		SS18-SSX4	<5%	
Well-differentiated/dedifferentiated liposarcoma	12q amplification	CDK4, MDM2, others	>80%	[77–82]

[a]Other fusion partners or alterations are known

mut mutation, unk unknown

have had retinoblastoma have an increased risk of development of non-ocular tumors [87]. A review of the data suggests that 211 of 1,506 patients with retinoblastoma developed a second tumor, 142 died before any malignancy developed, and 28 developed a third tumor at a median of 5–8 years. This is an important finding as pertains to this book, since the predominant tumors were soft tissue sarcomas. The relative risk of developing a second tumor after treatment for retinoblastoma is dose-dependent and has spurred the rise of intra-arterial chemotherapy as primary treatment for retinoblastoma [88].

Patients with familial adenomatous polyposis (FAP) often develop desmoid tumors which are intra-abdominal or in the abdominal wall. Although debate exists as to whether desmoid tumors are benign or malignant, they behave as low-grade soft tissue sarcomas, with invasion of local structures and significant potential for morbidity and mortality.

Radiation therapy is a causative agent for soft tissue sarcoma, although the mechanism is unknown. Patients undergoing radiation therapy for common diseases such as breast, prostate, lymphoma, and cervical cancer are at increased risk of subsequent soft tissue sarcoma and other cancers. Often these soft tissue sarcomas develop at the edge of the radiation field, suggesting incomplete repair of normal tissue that ultimately results in malignant transformation. Whether it is radiation that is causative alone or requires the underlying genetic defect that initiated the initial tumor is unclear. Almost 20 years ago, we reviewed our experience with radiation-associated sarcomas [89] suggesting that these tumors usually have a poor prognosis as they are often high grade and large at the time of diagnosis. Common soft tissue sarcomas that develop following radiation are osteogenic sarcoma, angiosarcoma, and what used to be termed "malignant fibrous histiocytoma," now seen more commonly as undifferentiated pleomorphic sarcoma (UPS) or myxofibrosarcoma (see below). It is rare for these patients to have low-grade tumors or translocation-associated sarcomas. We have great concern that as use of radiation therapy as a primary treatment for ductal carcinoma in situ or early-stage breast cancer increases, we can expect a greater prevalence of lethal radiation-induced sarcomas. Many studies have examined this risk, and it would appear that the risk of developing soft tissue sarcoma approaches 5 in 1,000 at 15 years [90]. This risk appears to continue to increase with time. Studies performed from the Scandinavian datasets show a greater prevalence of sarcoma following radiation than would be expected in the absence of radiation therapy. An updated review of our experience has recently been reported [91]. Radiation-associated sarcomas are described more fully under Chap. 16.

We have had a long-standing interest in the association of lymphedema with the development of soft tissue sarcoma since the earliest report by Stewart and Treves from our institution [8]. While often the lymphedema is associated with extent of operation and radiation therapy, it is not a radiation-induced sarcoma per se, as the sarcoma develops in the lymphedematous extremity outside the radiation field. Such (lymph)angiosarcomas also develop after chronic lymphedema, such as that seen with filarial infection [92].

Various chemical agents have long been utilized in the laboratory to develop sarcomas in murine models and have been implicated in the etiology of soft tissue sarcoma. The relationship between phenoxyacetic acids found in various herbicides is controversial and was highlighted because of the concern that dioxins were the active agents in "Agent Orange" utilized during the Vietnam War. While not proved, these data are suggestive of chemical association. Chemical carcinogens are known to be associated with the development of hepatic angiosarcoma although rare. Thorotrast, vinyl chloride, and arsenic have all been incriminated, but more vigilant avoidance of these agents makes this diagnosis much less likely at the present time.

It is difficult to identify whether trauma is a causative agent in soft tissue sarcoma as often an antecedent injury draws attention to the presence of a mass rather than being causative of the mass. This remains unproven although it does appear that the development of the desmoid tumor, which may be considered a fibroblastic hyper-proliferation in response to injury, is more common in athletes.

References

1. Long ER. History of pathology. Baltimore: Williams & Wilkins; 1928.
2. Morgagni JB. The seats and causes of disease investigated by anatomy, vol. 2. London: Millen & Cadell; 1769.
3. Hajdu SI. Differential diagnosis of soft tissue and bone tumors. Philadelphia: Lea & Febiger; 1986.
4. Stout AP. Human cancer: etiologic factors, precancerous lesions, growth, spread, symptoms, diagnosis, prognosis, principles of treatment. Philadelphia: Lea & Febiger; 1932.
5. Ewing J. Further report on endothelial myeloma of bone. Proc NY Pathol Soc. 1924;24:93–101.
6. Stout AP. Tumors of the soft tissues. In: Atlas of tumor pathology. Washington, DC: Armed Forces Institute of Pathology; 1953.
7. Brennan MF, Lewis JJ. Diagnosis and management of soft tissue sarcoma. London: Martin Dunitz; 1998.
8. Stewart FW, Treves N. Lymphangiosarcoma in postmastectomy lymphedema: a report of six cases of elephantiasis chirurgica. Cancer. 1948;1:64–81.
9. Turc-Carel C, Lizard-Nacol S, Justrabo E, et al. Consistent chromosomal translocation in alveolar rhabdomyosarcoma. Cancer Genet Cytogenet. 1986;19(3–4):361–2.
10. Seidal T, Mark J, Hagmar B, et al. Alveolar rhabdomyosarcoma: a cytogenetic and correlated cytological and histological study. Acta Pathol Microbiol Immunol Scand A. 1982; 90(5):345–54.
11. Douglass EC, Valentine M, Etcubanas E, et al. A specific chromosomal abnormality in rhab-domyosarcoma. Cytogenet Cell Genet. 1987;45(3–4):148–55.
12. Ladanyi M, Lui MY, Antonescu CR, et al. The der(17)t(X;17)(p11;q25) of human alveolar soft part sarcoma fuses the TFE3 transcription factor gene to ASPL, a novel gene at 17q25. Oncogene. 2001;20(1):48–57.
13. Antonescu CR, Dal Cin P, Nafa K, et al. EWSR1-CREB1 is the predominant gene fusion in angiomatoid fibrous histiocytoma. Genes Chromosomes Cancer. 2007;46(12):1051–60.
14. Tanas MR, Rubin BP, Montgomery EA, et al. Utility of FISH in the diagnosis of angiomatoid fibrous histiocytoma: a series of 18 cases. Mod Pathol. 2010;23(1):93–7.
15. Peulve P, Michot C, Vannier JP, et al. Clear cell sarcoma with t(12;22) (q13-14;q12). Genes Chromosomes Cancer. 1991;3(5):400–2.
16. Fletcher JA. Translocation (12;22)(q13-14;q12) is a nonrandom aberration in soft-tissue clear-cell sarcoma. Genes Chromosomes Cancer. 1992;5(2):184.

17. Stenman G, Kindblom LG, Angervall L. Reciprocal translocation t(12;22)(q13;q13) in clear-cell sarcoma of tendons and aponeuroses. Genes Chromosomes Cancer. 1992;4(2):122–7.
18. Antonescu CR, Nafa K, Segal NH, et al. EWS-CREB1: a recurrent variant fusion in clear cell sarcoma–association with gastrointestinal location and absence of melanocytic differentiation. Clin Cancer Res. 2006;12(18):5356–62.
19. Hisaoka M, Ishida T, Kuo TT, et al. Clear cell sarcoma of soft tissue: a clinicopathologic, immunohistochemical, and molecular analysis of 33 cases. Am J Surg Pathol. 2008;32(3):452–60.
20. Italiano A, Sung YS, Zhang L, et al. High prevalence of CIC fusion with double-homeobox (DUX4) transcription factors in EWSR1-negative undifferentiated small blue round cell sarcomas. Genes Chromosomes Cancer. 2012;51(3):207–18.
21. Graham C, Chilton-Macneill S, Zielenska M, et al. The CIC-DUX4 fusion transcript is present in a subgroup of pediatric primitive round cell sarcomas. Hum Pathol. 2012;43(2):180–9.
22. Yoshimoto M, Graham C, Chilton-MacNeill S, et al. Detailed cytogenetic and array analysis of pediatric primitive sarcomas reveals a recurrent CIC-DUX4 fusion gene event. Cancer Genet Cytogenet. 2009;195(1):1–11.
23. Kawamura-Saito M, Yamazaki Y, Kaneko K, et al. Fusion between CIC and DUX4 up-regulates PEA3 family genes in Ewing-like sarcomas with t(4;19)(q35;q13) translocation. Hum Mol Genet. 2006;15(13):2125–37.
24. Pierron G, Tirode F, Lucchesi C, et al. A new subtype of bone sarcoma defined by BCOR-CCNB3 gene fusion. Nat Genet. 2012;44(4):461–6.
25. Knezevich SR, McFadden DE, Tao W, et al. A novel ETV6-NTRK3 gene fusion in congenital fibrosarcoma. Nat Genet. 1998;18(2):184–7.
26. Rubin BP, Chen CJ, Morgan TW, et al. Congenital mesoblastic nephroma t(12;15) is associated with ETV6-NTRK3 gene fusion: cytogenetic and molecular relationship to congenital (infantile) fibrosarcoma. Am J Pathol. 1998;153(5):1451–8.
27. Pedeutour F, Coindre JM, Sozzi G, et al. Supernumerary ring chromosomes containing chromosome 17 sequences. A specific feature of dermatofibrosarcoma protuberans? Cancer Genet Cytogenet. 1994;76(1):1–9.
28. Dal Cin P, Sciot R, de Wever I, et al. Cytogenetic and immunohistochemical evidence that giant cell fibroblastoma is related to dermatofibrosarcoma protuberans. Genes Chromosomes Cancer. 1996;15(1):73–5.
29. Linn SC, West RB, Pollack JR, et al. Gene expression patterns and gene copy number changes in dermatofibrosarcoma protuberans. Am J Pathol. 2003;163(6):2383–95.
30. Sawyer JR, Tryka AF, Lewis JM. A novel reciprocal chromosome translocation t(11;22) (p13;q12) in an intraabdominal desmoplastic small round-cell tumor. Am J Surg Pathol. 1992;16(4):411–6.
31. Gerald WL, Rosai J, Ladanyi M. Characterization of the genomic breakpoint and chimeric transcripts in the EWS-WT1 gene fusion of desmoplastic small round cell tumor. Proc Natl Acad Sci USA. 1995;92(4):1028–32.
32. Gerald WL, Ladanyi M, de Alava E, et al. Clinical, pathologic, and molecular spectrum of tumors associated with t(11;22)(p13;q12): desmoplastic small round-cell tumor and its variants. J Clin Oncol. 1998;16(9):3028–36.
33. Shimizu Y, Mitsui T, Kawakami T, et al. Novel breakpoints of the EWS gene and the WT1 gene in a desmoplastic small round cell tumor. Cancer Genet Cytogenet. 1998;106(2):156–8.
34. Dal Cin P, Aly MS, De Wever I, et al. Endometrial stromal sarcoma t(7;17)(p15-21;q12-21) is a nonrandom chromosome change. Cancer Genet Cytogenet. 1992;63(1):43–6.
35. Koontz JI, Soreng AL, Nucci M, et al. Frequent fusion of the JAZF1 and JJAZ1 genes in endometrial stromal tumors. Proc Natl Acad Sci USA. 2001;98(11):6348–53.
36. Nucci MR, Harburger D, Koontz J, et al. Molecular analysis of the JAZF1-JJAZ1 gene fusion by RT-PCR and fluorescence in situ hybridization in endometrial stromal neoplasms. Am J Surg Pathol. 2007;31(1):65–70.
37. Lee CH, Ou WB, Marino-Enriquez A, et al. 14-3-3 fusion oncogenes in high-grade endometrial stromal sarcoma. Proc Natl Acad Sci USA. 2012;109(3):929–34.

38. Errani C, Zhang L, Sung YS, et al. A novel WWTR1-CAMTA1 gene fusion is a consistent abnormality in epithelioid hemangioendothelioma of different anatomic sites. Genes Chromosomes Cancer. 2011;50(8):644–53.
39. Chbani L, Guillou L, Terrier P, et al. Epithelioid sarcoma: a clinicopathologic and immunohistochemical analysis of 106 cases from the French sarcoma group. Am J Clin Pathol. 2009; 131(2):222–7.
40. Hornick JL, Dal Cin P, Fletcher CD. Loss of INI1 expression is characteristic of both conventional and proximal-type epithelioid sarcoma. Am J Surg Pathol. 2009;33(4):542–50.
41. Modena P, Lualdi E, Facchinetti F, et al. SMARCB1/INI1 tumor suppressor gene is frequently inactivated in epithelioid sarcomas. Cancer Res. 2005;65(10):4012–9.
42. Lee MW, Jee KJ, Han SS, et al. Comparative genomic hybridization in epithelioid sarcoma. Br J Dermatol. 2004;151(5):1054–9.
43. Quezado MM, Middleton LP, Bryant B, et al. Allelic loss on chromosome 22q in epithelioid sarcomas. Hum Pathol. 1998;29(6):604–8.
44. Orndal C, Carlen B, Akerman M, et al. Chromosomal abnormality t(9;22)(q22;q12) in an extraskeletal myxoid chondrosarcoma characterized by fine needle aspiration cytology, electron microscopy, immunohistochemistry and DNA flow cytometry. Cytopathology. 1991;2(5):261–70.
45. Kleinfinger P, Labelle Y, Melot T, et al. Localization of TEC to 9q22.3-q31 by fluorescence in situ hybridization. Ann Genet. 1996;39(4):233–5.
46. Wang WL, Mayordomo E, Czerniak BA, et al. Fluorescence in situ hybridization is a useful ancillary diagnostic tool for extraskeletal myxoid chondrosarcoma. Mod Pathol. 2008; 21(11):1303–10.
47. Turc-Carel C, Philip I, Berger MP, et al. Chromosomal translocation (11; 22) in cell lines of Ewing's sarcoma. C R Seances Acad Sci III. 1983;296(23):1101–3.
48. Turc-Carel C, Philip I, Berger MP, et al. Chromosome study of Ewing's sarcoma (ES) cell lines. Consistency of a reciprocal translocation t(11;22)(q24;q12). Cancer Genet Cytogenet. 1984;12(1):1–19.
49. Panagopoulos I, Storlazzi CT, Fletcher CD, et al. The chimeric FUS/CREB3l2 gene is specific for low-grade fibromyxoid sarcoma. Genes Chromosomes Cancer. 2004;40(3):218–28.
50. Mertens F, Fletcher CD, Antonescu CR, et al. Clinicopathologic and molecular genetic characterization of low-grade fibromyxoid sarcoma, and cloning of a novel FUS/CREB3L1 fusion gene. Lab Invest. 2005;85(3):408–15.
51. Guillou L, Benhattar J, Gengler C, et al. Translocation-positive low-grade fibromyxoid sarcoma: clinicopathologic and molecular analysis of a series expanding the morphologic spectrum and suggesting potential relationship to sclerosing epithelioid fibrosarcoma: a study from the French Sarcoma Group. Am J Surg Pathol. 2007;31(9):1387–402.
52. Hirota S, Isozaki K, Moriyama Y, et al. Gain-of-function mutations of c-kit in human gastrointestinal stromal tumors. Science. 1998;279(5350):577–80.
53. Nishida T, Hirota S, Taniguchi M, et al. Familial gastrointestinal stromal tumours with germline mutation of the KIT gene. Nat Genet. 1998;19(4):323–4.
54. Sakurai S, Fukasawa T, Chong JM, et al. C-kit gene abnormalities in gastrointestinal stromal tumors (tumors of interstitial cells of Cajal). Jpn J Cancer Res. 1999;90(12):1321–8.
55. Hirota S, Isozaki K, Nishida T, et al. Effects of loss-of-function and gain-of-function mutations of c-kit on the gastrointestinal tract. J Gastroenterol. 2000;35 Suppl 12:75–9.
56. Miettinen M, Lasota J. Gastrointestinal stromal tumors–definition, clinical, histological, immunohistochemical, and molecular genetic features and differential diagnosis. Virchows Arch. 2001;438(1):1–12.
57. Heinrich MC, Corless CL, Demetri GD, et al. Kinase mutations and imatinib response in patients with metastatic gastrointestinal stromal tumor. J Clin Oncol. 2003;21(23):4342–9.
58. Nilsson M, Hoglund M, Panagopoulos I, et al. Molecular cytogenetic mapping of recurrent chromosomal breakpoints in tenosynovial giant cell tumors. Virchows Arch. 2002;441(5):475–80.
59. Bridge JA, Kanamori M, Ma Z, et al. Fusion of the ALK gene to the clathrin heavy chain gene, CLTC, in inflammatory myofibroblastic tumor. Am J Pathol. 2001;159(2):411–5.

60. Griffin CA, Hawkins AL, Dvorak C, et al. Recurrent involvement of 2p23 in inflammatory myofibroblastic tumors. Cancer Res. 1999;59(12):2776–80.
61. Coffin CM, Hornick JL, Fletcher CD. Inflammatory myofibroblastic tumor: comparison of clinicopathologic, histologic, and immunohistochemical features including ALK expression in atypical and aggressive cases. Am J Surg Pathol. 2007;31(4):509–20.
62. Antonescu CR, Zhang L, Chang NE, et al. EWSR1-POU5F1 fusion in soft tissue myoepithelial tumors. A molecular analysis of sixty-six cases, including soft tissue, bone, and visceral lesions, showing common involvement of the EWSR1 gene. Genes Chromosomes Cancer. 2010;49(12):1114–24.
63. Tallini G, Akerman M, Dal Cin P, et al. Combined morphologic and karyotypic study of 28 myxoid liposarcomas. Implications for a revised morphologic typing, (a report from the CHAMP Group). Am J Surg Pathol. 1996;20(9):1047–55.
64. Knight JC, Renwick PJ, Dal Cin P, et al. Translocation t(12;16)(q13;p11) in myxoid liposarcoma and round cell liposarcoma: molecular and cytogenetic analysis. Cancer Res. 1995;55(1):24–7.
65. Turc-Carel C, Limon J, Dal Cin P, et al. Cytogenetic studies of adipose tissue tumors. II. Recurrent reciprocal translocation t(12;16)(q13;p11) in myxoid liposarcomas. Cancer Genet Cytogenet. 1986;23(4):291–9.
66. Dahlen A, Mertens F, Mandahl N, et al. Molecular genetic characterization of the genomic ACTB-GLI fusion in pericytoma with t(7;12). Biochem Biophys Res Commun. 2004;325(4):1318–23.
67. Dahlen A, Fletcher CD, Mertens F, et al. Activation of the GLI oncogene through fusion with the beta-actin gene (ACTB) in a group of distinctive pericytic neoplasms: pericytoma with t(7;12). Am J Pathol. 2004;164(5):1645–53.
68. Biegel JA, Zhou JY, Rorke LB, et al. Germ-line and acquired mutations of INI1 in atypical teratoid and rhabdoid tumors. Cancer Res. 1999;59(1):74–9.
69. Raisanen J, Biegel JA, Hatanpaa KJ, et al. Chromosome 22q deletions in atypical teratoid/ rhabdoid tumors in adults. Brain Pathol. 2005;15(1):23–8.
70. Versteege I, Sevenet N, Lange J, et al. Truncating mutations of hSNF5/INI1 in aggressive paediatric cancer. Nature. 1998;394(6689):203–6.
71. Turc-Carel C, Dal Cin P, Limon J, et al. Translocation X;18 in synovial sarcoma. Cancer Genet Cytogenet. 1986;23(1):93.
72. Kawai A, Woodruff J, Healey JH, et al. SYT-SSX gene fusion as a determinant of morphology and prognosis in synovial sarcoma. N Engl J Med. 1998;338(3):153–60.
73. Clark J, Rocques PJ, Crew AJ, et al. Identification of novel genes, SYT and SSX, involved in the t(X;18)(p11.2;q11.2) translocation found in human synovial sarcoma. Nat Genet. 1994; 7(4):502–8.
74. Shipley JM, Clark J, Crew AJ, et al. The t(X;18)(p11.2;q11.2) translocation found in human synovial sarcomas involves two distinct loci on the X chromosome. Oncogene. 1994;9(5): 1447–53.
75. de Leeuw B, Balemans M, Weghuis DO, et al. Molecular cloning of the synovial sarcoma-specific translocation (X;18)(p11.2;q11.2) breakpoint. Hum Mol Genet. 1994;3(5):745–9.
76. Smith S, Reeves BR, Wong L, et al. A consistent chromosome translocation in synovial sarcoma. Cancer Genet Cytogenet. 1987;26(1):179–80.
77. Pedeutour F, Forus A, Coindre JM, et al. Structure of the supernumerary ring and giant rod chromosomes in adipose tissue tumors. Genes Chromosomes Cancer. 1999;24(1):30–41.
78. Dei Tos AP, Doglioni C, Piccinin S, et al. Coordinated expression and amplification of the MDM2, CDK4, and HMGI-C genes in atypical lipomatous tumours. J Pathol. 2000; 190(5):531–6.
79. Micci F, Teixeira MR, Bjerkehagen B, et al. Characterization of supernumerary rings and giant marker chromosomes in well-differentiated lipomatous tumors by a combination of G-banding, CGH, M-FISH, and chromosome- and locus-specific FISH. Cytogenet Genome Res. 2002;97(1–2):13–9.

80. Italiano A, Bianchini L, Keslair F, et al. HMGA2 is the partner of MDM2 in well-differentiated and dedifferentiated liposarcomas whereas CDK4 belongs to a distinct inconsistent amplicon. Int J Cancer. 2008;122(10):2233–41.
81. Weaver J, Downs-Kelly E, Goldblum JR, et al. Fluorescence in situ hybridization for MDM2 gene amplification as a diagnostic tool in lipomatous neoplasms. Mod Pathol. 2008;21(8):943–9.
82. Coindre JM, Pedeutour F, Aurias A. Well-differentiated and dedifferentiated liposarcomas. Virchows Arch. 2010;456(2):167–79.
83. Li FP, Fraumeni Jr JF. Soft-tissue sarcomas, breast cancer, and other neoplasms. A familial syndrome? Ann Intern Med. 1969;71(4):747–52.
84. D'Agostino AN, Soule EH, Miller RH. Sarcomas of the peripheral nerves and somatic soft tissues associated with multiple neurofibromatosis (Von Recklinghausen's Disease). Cancer. 1963;16:1015–27.
85. Fraumeni Jr JF, Vogel CL, Easton JM. Sarcomas and multiple polyposis in a kindred. A genetic variety of hereditary polyposis? Arch Intern Med. 1968;121(1):57–61.
86. Sorensen SA, Mulvihill JJ, Nielsen A. Long-term follow-up of von Recklinghausen neurofibromatosis. Survival and malignant neoplasms. N Engl J Med. 1986;314(16):1010–5.
87. Abramson DH, Melson MR, Dunkel IJ, et al. Third (fourth and fifth) nonocular tumors in survivors of retinoblastoma. Ophthalmology. 2001;108(10):1868–76.
88. Abramson DH, Dunkel IJ, Brodie SE, et al. A phase I/II study of direct intraarterial (ophthalmic artery) chemotherapy with melphalan for intraocular retinoblastoma initial results. Ophthalmology. 2008;115(8):1398–404. 1404 e1391.
89. Brady MS, Gaynor JJ, Brennan MF. Radiation-associated sarcoma of bone and soft tissue. Arch Surg. 1992;127(12):1379–85.
90. Kirova YM, Vilcoq JR, Asselain B, et al. Radiation-induced sarcomas after radiotherapy for breast carcinoma: a large-scale single-institution review. Cancer. 2005;104(4):856–63.
91. Gladdy RA, Qin LX, Moraco N, et al. Do radiation-associated soft tissue sarcomas have the same prognosis as sporadic soft tissue sarcomas? J Clin Oncol. 2010;28(12):2064–9.
92. Muller R, Hajdu SI, Brennan MF. Lymphangiosarcoma associated with chronic filarial lymphedema. Cancer. 1987;59(1):179–83.

Chapter 2
Natural History: Importance of Size, Site, and Histopathology

Natural History

The natural history of soft tissue sarcoma is highly influenced by the site of the primary lesion, tumor histopathology, and tumor size. Multiple approaches have been developed to define outcome variables based on these factors, and as data accumulate with sufficient numbers, progressively more refined staging or predictive systems can be provided for rare tumors with multiple variables.

Influence of Site

The anatomic site of the primary lesion is clearly a determinant of outcome. This is most dramatically illustrated when one looks at the risk of local recurrence at various sites (Fig. 2.1). Retroperitoneal and intra-abdominal lesions have a significant risk of local recurrence, whereas extremity lesions have a much lower risk. When one considers disease-specific survival (Fig. 2.2), it is clear that disease-specific survival in retroperitoneal lesions is associated with similar prevalence to local recurrence, whereas for visceral lesions, systemic disease is the cause of death as local recurrence is relatively infrequent. This emphasizes the value of prospective, long-term databases in determining aspects of biology as well as outcome.

Staging

Staging of soft tissue sarcoma continues to evolve. Most staging systems depend on the grade and presence or absence of metastasis. The original system was initially based on data from 1977 (Fig. 2.3). Stage was subdivided based on the primary size of the initial tumor, into categories of <5 cm and >5 cm (T1/T2). By 1992, the absence or presence of nodal metastasis was included (N0/N1).

M.F. Brennan et al., *Management of Soft Tissue Sarcoma*,
DOI 10.1007/978-1-4614-5004-7_2, © Springer Science+Business Media New York 2013

Fig. 2.1 All adult sarcomas, local disease-free survival by site. MSKCC 7/1/1982–6/30/2010 n = 8,647

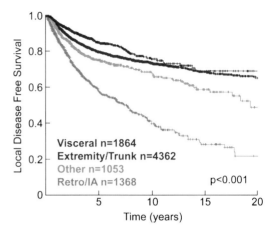

Fig. 2.2 All adult sarcomas, disease-specific survival by site. MSKCC 7/1/1982–6/30/2010 n = 8,647

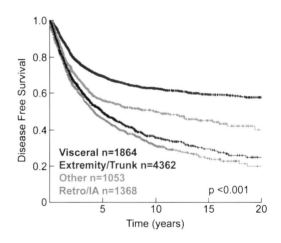

Fig. 2.3 1977 AJCC staging system (Used with permission from Russell et al. [1])

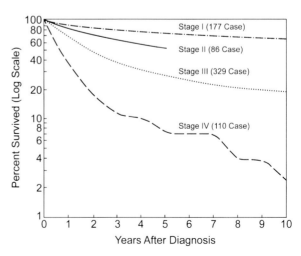

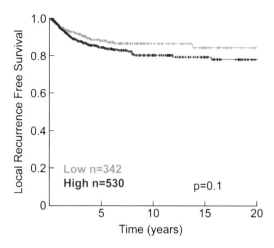

Fig. 2.4 Local recurrence-free survival, primary extremity ≤5 cm by grade. MSKCC 7/1/1982–6/30/2010 n = 872

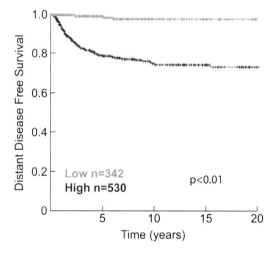

Fig. 2.5 Distant disease-free survival, primary extremity ≤5 cm by grade. MSKCC 7/1/1982–6/30/2010 n = 872

It has become progressively clear that tumors of very small size have a much better prognosis than was predicted by the initial American Joint Committee on Cancer (AJCC) staging system. Small (<5 cm) high-grade lesions (Fig. 2.4) have a favorable local recurrence-free survival similar to low-grade lesions. Small, low-grade tumors have a negligible risk of death from sarcoma, and small high-grade tumors have a 10-year disease-specific survival of approximately 80% (Fig. 2.5) [2]. We have shown that grade, depth, and size are independent predictors of outcome, and most systems base the risk of developing distant metastases giving each factor equal weight. However, tumor grade is dominant in the initial presentation where patients with high-grade lesions are more likely to have an early distant metastasis, whereas patients with lower grade but large tumors have progressive and prolonged risk of metastatic recurrence (Fig. 2.6) [3, 4]. Early metastatic disease is dominated by the grade of the tumor.

Fig. 2.6 Distant metastasis, extremity primary, and local recurrent by grade. MSKCC 7/1/1982–6/30/2010 n = 2,522

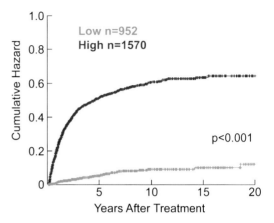

Fig. 2.7 Disease-specific survival by lymph node metastases alone or with other metastasis and other metastasis. MSKCC 7/1/1982–6/30/2010 n = 1,615

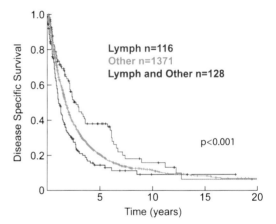

The outcome for patients with lymph node metastasis is similar, but not identical, to patients with other metastases (Fig. 2.7). It is important to emphasize that lymph node metastasis is infrequent in soft tissue sarcoma (Table 2.1) with an overall prevalence of <5% for all sarcomas and occurring predominantly in those having epithelioid features. There clearly are patients with limited nodal metastasis who are salvaged by resection, and such patients tend to do better than those with metastasis to other sites (Fig. 2.7).

A study comparing three different staging systems [6] was published in 2000. At that time, the authors found that depth, grade, and size were significant prognostic indicators and that inclusion of these criteria could better define patients who might benefit from systemic therapy. This was in contradistinction to the Musculoskeletal Tumor Society study [7] which employed a staging system based on extra compartmental extension (which is itself influenced by size).

The latest staging system by the AJCC (7th edition, 2010) [8] has made a number of changes to the prior edition of 2002 (Tables 2.2 and 2.3). Gastrointestinal stromal

Table 2.1 Histologic type of sarcomas and lymph node metastasis (Adapted with permission from Fong et al. [5])

Histologic findings	No. of nodal metastases/all sarcoma patients			% of all lesions		
	Weingrad[a]	Mazeron[b]	This study[c]	Weingrad	Mazeron	This study
Fibrosarcoma	55/1083	54/215	0/162	5.1	4.4	0
Malignant fibrous histiocytoma	1/30	84/823	8/316	3.3	10.2	2.6
Undifferentiated spindle cell	–	–	0/42	–	0	–
Rhabdomyosarcoma (all types)	108/888	201/1354	–	12.2	14.8	–
Rhabdomyosarcoma (non-embryonal)	–	–	1/35	–	–	2.9
Embryonal rhabdomyosarcoma	–	–	12/88	–	–	13.6
Leiomyosarcoma	10/94	21/524	9/328	10.6	4.0	2.7
Malignant peripheral nerve sheath tumor	0/60	3/476	2/96	0	0.6	2.1
Vascular	–	43/376	–	–	11.4	–
Angiosarcoma	–	–	5/37	–	–	13.5
Hemangiopericytoma	3/23	–	0/21	13.0	–	0
Lymphangiosarcoma	–	–	1/4	–	–	25.0
Osteosarcoma	20/327	–	0/11	6.1	–	0
Chondrosarcoma	–	–	1/46	–	–	2.2
Synovial sarcoma	91/535	117/851	2/145	19.1	13.7	1.4
Epithelioid sarcoma	–	14/70	2/12	–	20	16.7
Liposarcoma	15/288	16/504	3/403	5.7	3.2	0.7
Alveolar soft part sarcoma	6/62	3/24	0/13	9.7	12.5	0
Clear cell sarcoma	–	11/40	–	–	27.5	–
Other	11/125	–	0/27	8.8	–	0
Total	320/3515	567/5257	47/1772	9.1	10.8	2.6

[a]Adapted from a review by Weingrad and Rosenberg summary of 47 studies (Weingrad DN, et al. Surgery 1978; 84:231–40)
[b]Adapted from a review of Mazeron and Suit summary of 122 studies (Mazeron JJ, Suit HD. Cancer 1987; 60:1800–8)
[c]Database only includes extraskeletal osteo- and chondrosarcomas

tumors, desmoid tumors, Kaposi sarcoma, and infantile fibrosarcoma are now excluded from the staging system. New histopathologies including angiosarcoma, extraskeletal Ewing sarcoma, and dermatofibrosarcoma protuberans have been added. Nodal disease, included as stage IV previously, has been reclassified as stage III, although the differences in outcome between patients with nodal and other metastases are small (Fig. 2.7). This reclassification highlights the ability to rescue patients with lymph node metastasis alone by further treatment, usually surgical resection. Anatomic stage and prognostic groups are defined in Table 2.2. This

Table 2.2 Anatomic stage and prognostic groups from AJCC Cancer Staging Manual, 7th edition (Used with the permission of the American Joint Committee on Cancer (AJCC), Chicago, Illinois. The original source for this material is the AJCC Cancer Staging Manual, seventh edition (2010) published by Springer Science and Business Media LLC, www.springer.com)

Anatomic stage – prognostic groups									
Clinical					Pathologic				
Group	T	N	M		Group	T	N	M	
IA	T1a	N0	M0	G1, GX	IA	T1a	N0	M0	G1, GX
	T1b	N0	M0	G1, GX		T1b	N0	M0	G1, GX
IB	T2a	N0	M0	G1, GX	IB	T2a	N0	M0	G1, GX
	T2b	N0	M0	G1, GX		T2b	N0	M0	G1, GX
IIA	T1a	N0	M0	G2, G3	IIA	T1a	N0	M0	G2, G3
	T1b	N0	M0	G2, G3		T1b	N0	M0	G2, G3
IIB	T2a	N0	M0	G2	IIB	T2a	N0	M0	G2
	T2b	N0	M0	G2		T2b	N0	M0	G2
III	T2a, T2b	N0	M0	G3	III	T2a, T2b	N0	M0	G3
	Any T	N1	M0	Any G		Any T	N1	M0	Any G
IV	Any T	Any N	M1	Any G	IV	Any T	Any N	M1	Any G
Stage unknown					Stage unknown				

Table 2.3 Stage grouping from AJCC Cancer Manual, 6th edition (Used with the permission of the American Joint Committee on Cancer (AJCC), Chicago, Illinois. The original source for this material is the AJCC Cancer Staging Manual, seventh edition (2010) published by Springer Science and Business Media LLC, www.springer.com)

Stage grouping						
Stage I	T1a, 1b, 2a, 2b	N0	M0	G1–2	G1	Low
Stage II	T1a, 1b, 2a	N0	M0	G3–4	G2–3	High
Stage III	T2b	N0	M0	G3–4	G2–3	High
Stage IV	Any T	N1	M0	Any G	Any G	High or low
	Any T	N0	M1	Any G	Any G	High or low

defines T stage as less than or greater than 5 cm. We and others have shown that size is a continuous variable with increasing risk of death from high-grade sarcoma as size increases. Wherever possible, size should be recorded three dimensionally (Fig. 2.8).

In the AJCC Staging Manual, 7th edition, depth continues to be recorded relative to the investing fascia of the extremity and trunk, but has no meaning for retroperitoneal or visceral primary tumors. Because depth is an independent prognostic value, depth is included in relationship to tumor size. Thus, a superficial tumor <5 cm is classified T1A, while T1B is deep. Similarly, a primary superficial tumor >5 cm is superficial, while T2B is deep. Survival is however still influenced by both depth and size (Fig. 2.9 and Table 2.2). However, if we examine the staging table in the AJCC 7th edition, depth has functionally been discarded. It should be emphasized that superficial lesions >5 cm are rare (<1%) in the extremity.

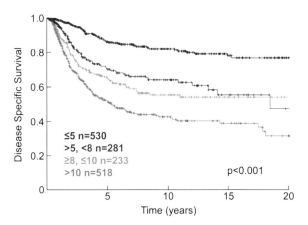

Fig. 2.8 Disease-specific survival, primary extremity high grade by size. MSKCC 7/1/1982–6/30/2010 n = 1,562

≤5 n=530
>5, <8 n=281
≥8, ≤10 n=233
>10 n=518
p<0.001

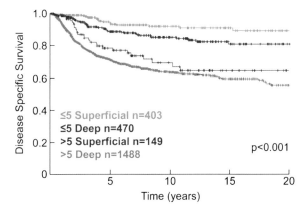

Fig. 2.9 Disease-specific survival, primary extremity high grade by size and depth. MSKCC 7/1/1982–6/30/2010 n = 2,510

≤5 Superficial n=403
≤5 Deep n=470
>5 Superficial n=149
>5 Deep n=1488
p<0.001

Grade has historically been a dominant factor in outcome for soft tissue sarcoma. Previous AJCC systems used four grade levels, but this has been effectively functioning as a two-grade system, i.e., grades I and II as low grade and grades III and IV as high grade. This was the system employed at Memorial Sloan-Kettering for many years with good discrimination. Grade is interpreted not only by differentiation but also by specific histological subtype, mitotic rate, and degree of necrosis. The new AJCC staging system has incorporated a 3-tier grading system, but the AJCC does have a dichotomy in that the grade 2 and 3 tumors are both considered high grade.

Where a three-tier system is utilized, i.e., the FNCLCC grading system (Fédération Nationale des Centres de Lutte Contre le Cancer), grade is determined by three different parameters, specifically differentiation, mitotic activity, and extent of necrosis. Each parameter is then scored, and the sum score used to assign grade. Specifically, differentiation is scored 1–3, mitotic activity scored 1–3, and necrosis scored 0–2. Summation then makes grade I (2 or 3 points), grade II (4 or 5 points), and grade III (6–8 points). Most encouraging is the attempt to place measurable

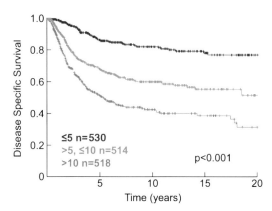

Fig. 2.10 Disease-specific survival, primary extremity high grade by size. MSKCC 7/1/1982–6/30/2010 n = 1,562

numbers on the mitotic count, i.e., a score of 1 for 0–9 mitoses per 10 high-powered fields, score of 2 for 10–19 mitoses per 10 high-powered fields, and score of 3 for 20 or more mitoses per 10 high-powered fields. A score of 2 is defined by histologic type, much as some sarcomas are automatically classified as high grade by their cellular subtype. The functional outcome of this grading system is that grade I–II tumors are tumors of defined histological types with less than 10 mitoses per 10 high-powered fields and no tumor necrosis, whereas grade III tumors require lack of differentiation and greater than 10 mitoses and some tumor necrosis. All others then become intermediate lesions.

We have previously shown that in high-grade lesions, size is better considered as a continuous variable or at least considered as three categories, i.e., <5, 5–10, and >10 (Fig. 2.10). Future staging systems will be aided by inclusion of at least a three-tier size system and a reevaluation of the value of depth and anatomic site. As more variables are added, staging systems become exponentially more complex, an argument that relies on new tools such as nomograms or Bayesian belief networks for risk estimation (see Prognostic Factors: Nomograms below).

Neurovascular and bone invasions are negative prognostic factors, but are not included in current staging systems. Molecular markers are currently being evaluated as determinants of outcome, and they are discussed in the histology-specific sections that follow.

Staging of Retroperitoneal Visceral Sarcoma

As noted immediately above, it is important to emphasize that no adequate staging system to date has specifically addressed retroperitoneal or visceral sarcomas. The historical components of size, grade, and depth become meaningless when the majority of retroperitoneal lesions are large and low grade, while visceral lesions may present as small, high-grade lesions. While death from local recurrence is possible with a large, low-grade tumor, death from visceral lesions is usually from

Table 2.4 Analysis of local recurrence-free survival in 231 primary retroperitoneal sarcoma patients with resectable disease (Used with permission from Lewis et al. [9])

	N	p-value[a] (univariate)	p-value (multivariate)	Relative risk[b] (95% CI)
Sex		0.06		
Male	140			
Female	91			
Age		0.9		
>50 years	156			
<50 years	75			
Grade		0.05		
High	134		0.01	2.1 (1.2–3.4)
Low	97			
Size		0.07		
>10 cm	170			
≤10 cm	59			
Histologic subtype		0.02		
Liposarcoma	109		0.01	2.6 (1.5–4.6)
Others	58			
Leiomyosarcoma	48			
Fibrosarcoma	16			
Surgical resection margins		0.2		
Negative micro and gross margins	136			
Positive micro and negative gross margins	49			
Positive micro and gross margins	46			

95% CI: 95 percent confidence interval
[a]Univariate *p* refers to log-rank test of no difference versus any difference between categories
[b]Relative risk to other categories of the same factor

systemic disease. This emphasizes the importance of approaches to therapy, as the predominant factor in outcome for retroperitoneal sarcoma is the adequacy of the initial resection. Without complete gross resection, essentially all patients recur regardless of grade. Only following complete resection does grade become a factor for outcome, i.e., high that are completely resected. This finding is consistent with the fact that many of the high-grade lesions have a risk of metastatic spread. This makes meaningful staging more difficult for these anatomic sites [9]. This is one reason for development of a specific AJCC version 7 staging system for GIST.

We described the factors that influence outcome for primary retroperitoneal patients [9]. Local recurrence-free survival for such lesions is summarized in Table 2.4 and for distant metastasis-free survival in Table 2.5. Important sites of metastasis include the lung and liver. Once metastasis develops, then survival is poor, at a median of 13 months (Fig. 2.11). It is important to emphasize that recurrence is common in retroperitoneal tumors, such primary sarcomas can occur late, and that many patients can undergo further resection, which is associated with prolonged survival (Figs. 2.1 and 2.2). The complete resection rate diminishes

Table 2.5 Analysis of distant metastasis-free survival in 231 primary retroperitoneal sarcoma patients with resectable disease (Used with permission from Lewis et al. [9])

	N	p-value[a] (univariate)	p-value (multivariate)	Relative risk[b] (95% CI)
Sex		0.8		
Male	140			
Female	91			
Age		0.8		
>50 years	156			
<50 years	75			
Grade		0.01		
High	134		0.01	5.0 (1.7–15)
Low	97			
Size		0.06		
>10 cm	170			
≤10 cm	59			
Histologic subtype		0.01		
Liposarcoma	109		0.01	0.2 (0.07–0.7)
Others	58			
Leiomyosarcoma	48			
Fibrosarcoma	16			
Surgical resection margins		0.01		
Negative micro and gross margins	136			
Positive micro and negative gross margins	49			
Positive micro and gross margins	46		0.01	3.9 (1.6–9.5)

95% CI: 95 percent confidence interval
[a]Univariate *p* refers to log-rank test of no difference versus any difference between categories
[b]Relative risk to other categories of the same factor

Fig. 2.11 Disease-specific survival for retroperitoneal sarcoma patients who had surgery at MSKCC (n = 745) and then developed metastases (n = 173). MSKCC 7/1/1982–6/30/2010

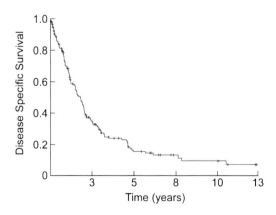

with each subsequent local recurrence (Fig. 2.12). If one looks at multivariate analysis of disease-specific survival of patients who undergo complete resection, the important factors for overall survival include grade and size, as emphasized previously (Table 2.6).

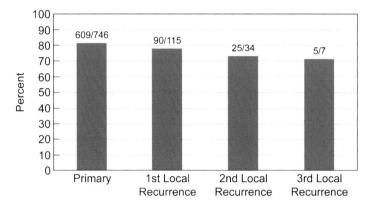

Fig. 2.12 Complete resection rate at primary operation and then following recurrence. MSKCC 7/1/1982–6/30/2010

Table 2.6 Analysis of disease-specific survival in 278 primary retroperitoneal sarcoma patients (Used with permission from Lewis et al. [9])

	N	p-value[a] (univariate)	p-value (multivariate)	Relative risk[b] (95% CI)
Sex		0.6		
Male	170			
Female	108			
Age		0.08		
>50 years	183			
<50 years	95			
Grade		0.001		
High	168			
Low	119		0.001	3.2 (2.0–5.0)
Size		0.2		
>10 cm	196			
≤10 cm	170		0.02	1.7 (1.1–2.7)
Histological subtype		0.08		
Liposarcoma	116			
Others	87			
Leiomyosarcoma	109			
Fibrosarcoma	22			
Surgical resection margins		0.001		
Negative micro and gross margins	136			
Positive micro and negative gross margins	49		0.001	4.7 (2.9–7.5)
Positive micro and gross margins	46		0.001	4.0 (2.5–6.5)

[a]Univariate p refers to log-rank test of no difference versus any difference between categories
[b]Relative risk to other categories of the same factor

Prognostic Factors for Extremity and Superficial Soft Tissue Sarcoma

We published [10] an analysis of a single-institution study of over 1,000 patients with extremity soft tissue sarcoma treated between 1982 and 1994. In this analysis, patient, tumor, and pathological factors were all analyzed by univariate and multivariate analysis to better define prognostic factors for local recurrence, metastatic recurrence, death from sarcoma, and post-metastasis survival. Prognostic factors identified are illustrated in Table 2.7. It was clear that age >50, recurrent presentation, positive initial microscopic margin, and the histopathological subtype of fibrosarcoma or malignant peripheral nerve tumor were all factors in multivariate analysis and were associated with a higher risk of local recurrence. Local recurrence is not grade dependent, and an analysis of extremity lesions is shown in Fig. 2.13. Local recurrence for all is approximately 25%. Local recurrence by size is illustrated (Fig. 2.14) emphasizing the progressive increase in local recurrence as the lesion increases in size, whether low grade (Fig. 2.15) or high grade (Fig. 2.16).

Table 2.7 Prognostic factors in extremity soft-tissue sarcoma – summary of significant adverse prognostic factors. MSKCC 1982–1994 n = 1,041 (Adapted from Pisters et al. [10]. Adapted with permission. © 2008 American Society of Clinical Oncology. All rights reserved)

Local recurrence	Distant recurrence	Post-metastasis survival	Disease-specific survival
LR at presentation	High grade	Size >10 cm	High grade
Positive margins	Size >5 cm		Size >10 cm
MPNST	Size >10 cm		Deep location
Age >50	Deep location		Positive margins
	LR at presentation		LR at presentation
			Lower extremity site
			MPNST
			Leiomyosarcoma

MPNST malignant peripheral nerve sheath tumor

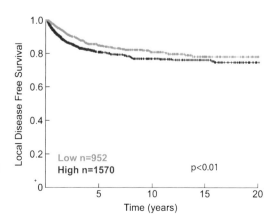

Fig. 2.13 Local disease-free survival for all primary extremity by grade. MSKCC 7/1/1982–6/30/2010 n = 2,522

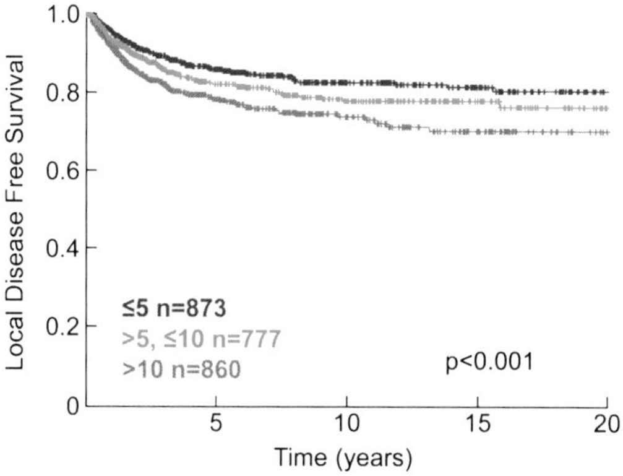

Fig. 2.14 Local disease-free survival for all primary extremity by size. MSKCC 7/1/1982-6/30/2010 n = 2,510

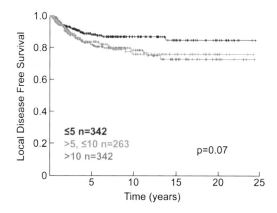

Fig. 2.15 Local recurrence-free survival primary extremity low grade, by size. MSKCC 7/1/1982–6/30/2010 n = 947

Fig. 2.16 Local recurrence-free survival for primary high-grade extremity, by size. MSKCC 7/1/1982–6/30/2010 n = 1,562

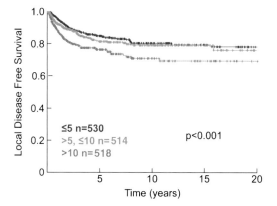

Disease-Specific Survival

Disease-specific survival or death from disease can be characterized by grade, size, and location; presence of positive margins; and local recurrence at presentation (Table 2.7). As with all of these issues, many of these factors are not arbitrary, but

Fig. 2.17 Disease-specific
survival all primary extremity
by size. MSKCC 7/1/1982–
6/30/2010 n = 2,510

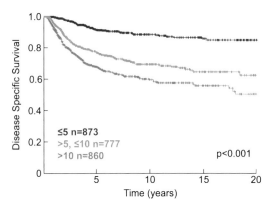

dependent and continuous. For example, in size, increase in size (Fig. 2.17) shows an increasing risk of disease-specific death.

Prognostic Factors for Survival Following Local Recurrence of Extremity Sarcoma

Prognostic factors for outcome after a patient has recurred have been defined [11]. We found that the median time to local recurrence was 19 months, 65% of patients had developed local recurrence by 2 years, and 90% of all patients who will recur will do so within 4 years. Transition from low to high grade is uncommon, and independent predictors for disease-specific survival after recurrence are high grade, the local recurrence tumor size, and the recurrence-free interval. Patients who developed a local recurrence >5 cm in less than 16 months had a 4-year disease-specific survival of 18% compared to 81% for patients who developed a local recurrence less than or equal to 5 cm in greater than 16 months. These data are reflected in Figs. 2.18 and 2.19.

Prognostic Factors: Nomograms

Nomograms can yield improved specificity of a given clinical outcome for an individual patient, but at the present time are available for a limited number of histological types and subtypes, e.g., liposarcoma and GIST.

Nomograms are graphical representations of statistical models that provide the probability of outcome based on patient-specific covariates following specific treatment. They are usually expressed as time to a specific event, such as local recurrence or survival. They require large datasets in which there are a significant number of both negative and positive events, and they require extended length of follow-up.

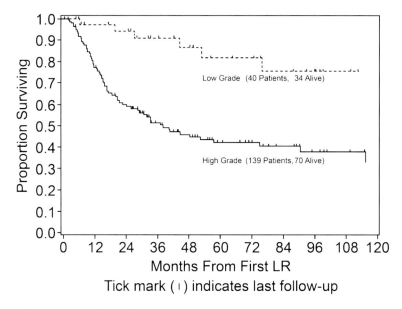

Fig. 2.18 Disease-specific survival extremity by primary tumor grade from time of local recurrence (Used with permission from Eilber et al. [11])

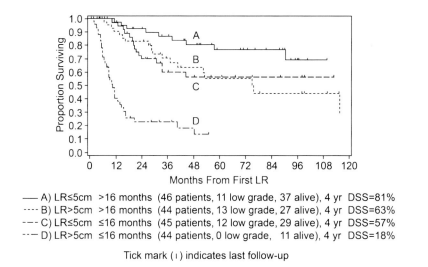

——— A) LR≤5cm >16 months (46 patients, 11 low grade, 37 alive), 4 yr DSS=81%
---- B) LR>5cm >16 months (44 patients, 13 low grade, 27 alive), 4 yr DSS=63%
--- C) LR≤5cm ≤16 months (45 patients, 12 low grade, 29 alive), 4 yr DSS=57%
--- D) LR>5cm ≤16 months (44 patients, 0 low grade, 11 alive), 4 yr DSS=18%

Tick mark (ı) indicates last follow-up

Fig. 2.19 Disease-specific survival extremity by local recurrence-free interval and size of local recurrence (Used with permission from Eilber et al. [11])

We have been actively involved in defining nomograms for prediction of sarcoma outcome. As we have a defined population with defined outcomes, known risk factors, and selected covariates, we are able to construct such nomograms in a meaningful way. Our initial attempt was a postoperative nomogram for 12-year sarcoma-specific death [12]. In that study, we are clearly able to utilize the known factors of our large dataset to predict outcome. As there were only sufficient data for six defined histologies, i.e., fibrosarcoma, liposarcoma, leiomyosarcoma, synovial sarcoma, undifferentiated pleomorphic sarcoma (UPS), and malignant peripheral nerve sheath tumor (MPNST), outcomes were only defined for these categories. Other barriers to defining outcomes better using nomograms include the knowledge that different liposarcoma subtypes each have distinct recurrence risk or chance of death and the definition of myxofibrosarcoma as a unique sarcoma subtype, differing from malignant fibrous histiocytoma, which is now itself called undifferentiated pleomorphic sarcoma (UPS) [12]. The original sarcoma nomogram subsequently has been validated using an independent dataset [13] and has been further validated by others [14].

Because of the multiple subtypes of liposarcoma, we developed a specific liposarcoma nomogram for disease-specific survival [15]. Such nomograms can then be developed to be site or histology specific; they can be considered to develop in time-altered sequence and have the potential to add biological variables. We further developed nomograms for probability of death from sarcoma following a local recurrence [16].

Nomograms have the potential to be utilized as a tool for evaluating the effects of treatment. While this requires validation by testing in a randomized trial, it has been suggestive [17] in our study of ifosfamide-based chemotherapy in adults with synovial sarcoma. Similar nomograms have been developed for predicting local recurrence both for all histologies and for desmoid tumors and can provide useful tools in patient management.

References

1. Russell WO, Cohen J, Enzinger F, Hajdu SI, Heise H, Martin RG, Meissner W, Miller WT, Schmitz RL, Suit HD. A clinical and pathological staging system for soft tissue sarcomas. Cancer. 1977;40:1562–70.
2. Geer RJ, Woodruff J, Casper ES, et al. Management of small soft-tissue sarcoma of the extremity in adults. Arch Surg. 1992;127(11):1285–9.
3. Grosso F, Sanfilippo R, Virdis E, et al. Trabectedin in myxoid liposarcomas (MLS): a long-term analysis of a single-institution series. Ann Oncol. 2009;20(8):1439–44.
4. De Wever I, Dal Cin P, Fletcher CD, et al. Cytogenetic, clinical, and morphologic correlations in 78 cases of fibromatosis: a report from the CHAMP study group. CHromosomes and morphology. Mod Pathol. 2000;13(10):1080–5.
5. Fong Y, Coit DG, Woodruff JM, Brennan MF. Lymph node metastasis from soft tissue sarcoma in adults. Analysis of data from a prospective database of 1772 sarcoma patients. Ann Surg. 1993;218:72–7.
6. Wunder JS, Healey JH, Davis AM, et al. A comparison of staging systems for localized extremity soft tissue sarcoma. Cancer. 2000;88(12):2721–30.
7. Wolf RE, Enneking WF. The staging and surgery of musculoskeletal neoplasms. Orthop Clin North Am. 1996;27(3):473–81.
8. AJCC. AJCC cancer staging manual. New York: Springer; 2009.
9. Lewis JJ, Leung D, Woodruff JM, Brennan MF. Retroperitoneal soft-tissue sarcoma: analysis of 500 patients treated and followed at a single institution. Ann Surg. 1998;228(3):355–65.

10. Pisters PW, Leung DH, Woodruff J, et al. Analysis of prognostic factors in 1,041 patients with localized soft tissue sarcomas of the extremities. J Clin Oncol. 1996;14(5):1679–89.
11. Eilber FC, Brennan MF, Riedel E, Alektiar KM, Antonescu C, Singer S. Prognostic factors for survival in patients with locally recurrent extremity soft tissue sarcomas. Ann Surg Oncol. 2005;12(3):228–36.
12. Kattan MW, Leung DH, Brennan MF. Postoperative nomogram for 12-year sarcoma-specific death. J Clin Oncol. 2002;20(3):791–6.
13. Eilber FC, Brennan MF, Eilber FR, et al. Validation of the postoperative nomogram for 12-year sarcoma-specific mortality. Cancer. 2004;101(10):2270–5.
14. Mariani L, Miceli R, Kattan MW, et al. Validation and adaptation of a nomogram for predicting the survival of patients with extremity soft tissue sarcoma using a three-grade system. Cancer. 2005;103(2):402–8.
15. Dalal KM, Kattan MW, Antonescu CR, et al. Subtype specific prognostic nomogram for patients with primary liposarcoma of the retroperitoneum, extremity, or trunk. Ann Surg. 2006;244(3):381–91.
16. Kattan MW, Heller G, Brennan MF. A competing-risks nomogram for sarcoma-specific death following local recurrence. Stat Med. 2003;22(22):3515–25.
17. Canter RJ, Qin LX, Maki RG, et al. A synovial sarcoma-specific preoperative nomogram supports a survival benefit to ifosfamide-based chemotherapy and improves risk stratification for patients. Clin Cancer Res. 2008;14(24):8191–7.

Chapter 3
General Statement as to Efficacy of Surgery/ Chemotherapy/Radiation Therapy

Extent of Primary Surgery

The principal management of primary soft tissue sarcoma is surgical resection. The clinical goal is resection with negative margins, preferably that extend 2 cm from the grossly determined border. This can be difficult to assess and is often limited by the presence of major neurovascular and bony structures. The majority of soft tissue sarcomas do not invade into bone unless there has been previous injury to bone or the lesion has an epitheloid component, such as synovial sarcoma.

When major arteries or nerves are involved, a decision must be made as to whether the morbidity of the procedure justifies the resection of an often negative vascular structure just because of proximity. We have been liberal in the resection of major veins, often not reconstructing them. The inferior vena cava can be resected without being replaced, and an excellent postoperative functional result obtained [1, 2]. The majority of soft tissue sarcomas do not invade into arterial structures but when they do, limited resection is possible. However, arterial invasion is rarely the primary determinant of outcome, and there is usually a secondary component that limits the adequacy of the procedure. In the retroperitoneum, vascular structures can be surrounded by low-grade liposarcoma (Fig. 3.1), often with ureteric encasement. When soft tissue tumors abut the periosteum, we have been liberal in removing the periosteum without further damage to the cortical bone. This can weaken the bone and increase the risk of subsequent fracture, especially in those receiving adjuvant radiation (Table 3.1).

The most extensive resection for extremity lesions is amputation. At present, this is only rarely indicated as the majority of extremity sarcomas can undergo a limb-sparing operation with or without radiation therapy. The experience of our institution is illustrated in Fig. 3.2 showing that the 50% amputation in the late 1960s and 1970s is now less than 10%. It is important to understand that on occasion, amputation is still indicated. In patients with large low-grade tumors with no evidence of metastasis who present with fungating or painful extremities, amputation can be lifesaving.

M.F. Brennan et al., *Management of Soft Tissue Sarcoma*,
DOI 10.1007/978-1-4614-5004-7_3, © Springer Science+Business Media New York 2013

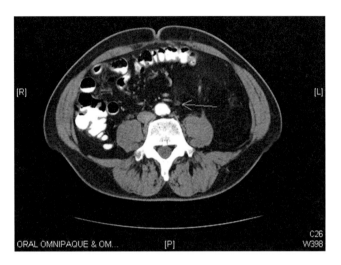

Fig. 3.1 CT of low-grade liposarcoma surrounding superior and inferior mesenteric vessels

Table 3.1 Risk of bone fracture in soft tissue sarcomas of the extremity after radiation therapy

	n	Radiation therapy type	% Fracture
MSKCC [71]	369	Brachytherapy	4%
University of Florida [52]	285	Preoperative	4%
National Cancer Institute [53]	145	Postoperative	6%
Princess Margaret Hospital [56]	364	Preoperative and postoperative	6%

MSKCC Memorial Sloan-Kettering Cancer Center

We have examined the benefit of extending resections to take further organs, particularly intra-abdominally. This has not proven to be of benefit as the kidney parenchyma is rarely invaded by soft tissue sarcoma unless there has been a prior operation. In those situations where adherence to the capsule is obtained, the capsule of the kidney can be resected to improve the margin [3]. The resection of an organ just because it approximates the lesion to improve margin in one direction when the defining margin is limited in another does not make sense, in particular in sarcomas where local regional recurrence risk is already very high. One should consider the concept of the least definitive margin as the margin that determines the ultimate outcome. Often in retroperitoneal tumors, the bowel is displaced and can be salvaged, but once an operation has taken place followed by recurrence, there is often serosal adherence and invasion, which is more difficult to manage without intestinal resection.

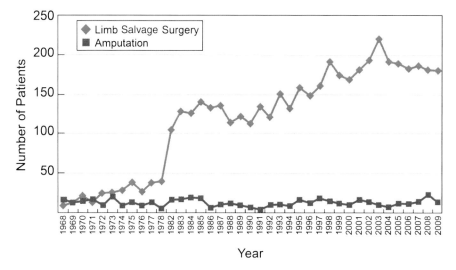

Fig. 3.2 Change in frequency of the need for amputation by time. MSKCC 1968–2009

The extent of surgical resection and the uncommon major ablative resection, such as forequarter amputation and hindquarter resection, are described in greater detail in dedicated surgical texts [4].

Surgical Treatment of Local Recurrence

The treatment of local recurrence after limb-sparing operation is often possible. Unfortunately, there is limited impact on long-term survival. We do know that early recurrence of a high-grade lesion is a very bad prognostic event. This is summarized in a paper from Eilber et al. [5]. Chapter 2, Fig. 2.19 shows the outcome of patients who have a late small recurrence versus those with a large high-grade recurrence. As anticipated, a large, high-grade recurrence is associated with poor survival.

Diagnostic Imaging

Diagnostic imaging is presented along with the definitive pathologies as they are discussed in turn. Imaging of the primary tumor is obtained from computerized tomography (CT) and magnetic resonance imaging (MRI). Both are most reliable and provide varying information. Comparative value of MRI versus CT was studied by the Radiological Diagnostic Oncology Group (RDOG), where 367 patients were examined with both modalities, less than 4 weeks from operation [6].

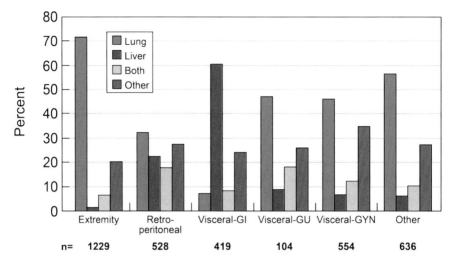

Fig. 3.3 Commonest sites of metastasis based on primary site. MSKCC 7/1/1982–6/30/2010 n = 3470. *GI* Gastrointestinal, *GU* genitourinary, *GYN* gynecologic

When comparing the imaging characteristics both prior to the operation and in alternate institutions, similar information was obtained. Not one modality was better than the other in determining whether or not the tumor involved bone, joint, or neurovascular structures. There was consistent but definite variability between individual reviewers. As this study was done in the early 1990s and CT and MRI imaging have markedly improved since then, one assumes the findings would be the same, although certainly the resolution in both modalities has markedly improved. Initially, MRI had the advantage of multiplanar imaging, but this result can now be achieved with CT reconstruction [6]. Currently, with the concerns over the radiation dose obtained from CT [7], many clinicians are moving progressively more to the utilization of MRI of the primary site.

Imaging is important in determining the extent of disease at primary presentation. We now know the sites of primary metastasis for most lesions. For example, 80% of people with extremity lesions develop metastasis in the lung, often as the only site of metastatic disease. On the other hand, visceral lesions commonly result in liver metastasis (Fig. 3.3). ^{18}F-fluorodeoxyglucose positron emission tomography (FDG-PET) is utilized, but has not been as valuable as one initially hoped. It is possible to differentiate high- versus low-grade primary sarcomas by FDG-PET, although there are false negatives and false positives in our experience [8]. FDG-PET may be used as a predictor of response to cytotoxic treatment in high-grade lesions [9, 10], but in terms of imaging distant metastatic disease, it has been less valuable. Much of this is due to the fact that low-grade liposarcoma has limited FDG-PET avidity, and so the distinction between a low-grade sarcoma and a lipoma is not able to be made. Conversely, high-grade sarcomas are usually FDG-PET avid and this can help evaluate the extent of the disease and the presence or absence of metastasis from a high-grade lesion.

Surgery for Metastatic Disease

Pulmonary Metastasis

The lung is the primary site of extremity sarcoma metastasis. It is much more common in high-grade lesions, and on occasion development can be most rapid. An example is given in Fig. 3.4a on the chest x-ray taken prior to resection of a high-grade leiomyosarcoma of the right groin. Within 6 weeks (Fig. 3.4b), pulmonary metastases are identifiable in a chest x-ray, and a CT scan (Fig. 3.5a, b) shows extensive pleural effusion and widespread metastasis with rapid progression and death within 6 weeks.

The Role of Pulmonary Metastatic Resection

Patients with high-grade soft tissue sarcoma are at risk of metastatic disease. The dominant and often only first site of metastasis from extremity lesions especially is the lung. It has been previously proposed [11] that pulmonary metastatic resection is a valuable modality. Early reports [12] emphasized the important role of pulmonary resection.

In our initial report of 716 adult patients admitted with primary or local recurrence of extremity soft tissue sarcoma, 135 (19%) patients had pulmonary metastasis as the initial or only site of distant recurrence [11]. At that time, the indications for pulmonary resection were (1) the absence of or presence of a controllable primary recurrence; (2) no known simultaneous distant metastases; (3) the ability, based on radiologic assessment, to anticipate complete removal of all metastasis; and (4) adequate pulmonary function to tolerate resection. Aggressive approaches with unilateral, bilateral, thoracotomy, and mediastinotomy were performed.

Of the 135 patients, 112 were admitted for pulmonary tumor management and 23 for local resection of recurrent disease. Thirty percent of the patients presented with synchronous disease. Primary histological types when contrasted to the overall database suggested that pulmonary metastases were more common than their initially presenting prevalence in synovial sarcoma, spindle cell sarcoma (i.e., leiomyosarcoma and undifferentiated pleomorphic sarcoma) and less common in liposarcoma. Pulmonary metastasis was more likely to develop from large, high-grade tumors. Of the 135 patients, 78 were treated with pulmonary resection, 65% or 83% could be completely resected. Resectability rate was not affected by age, sex, disease-free interval, presentation, size, or grade. The overall median survival for the 135 patients was 12 months with a 7% 3-year survival rate. Of the 65 patients who were completely resected, the median survival was 19 months, and the 3-year survival was 23%. However, two-thirds of the patients who had complete resection of pulmonary metastases had a second pulmonary recurrence with a median disease-free interval of 4 months. So if we consider the 135 patients who had pulmonary metastases as the initial and only identified site of recurrence, 86% of those were treated and 78 were treated surgically (58%). Of the 78, 65 (83%) underwent

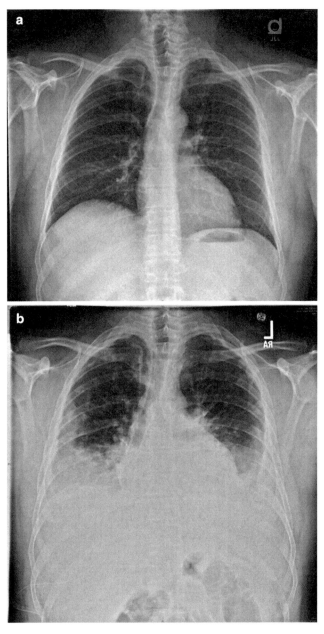

Fig. 3.4 Chest x-rays of rapid development of pulmonary metastases in a high-grade leiomyosarcoma of the left groin, (**a**) pre-resection, and (**b**) 6 weeks post-resection

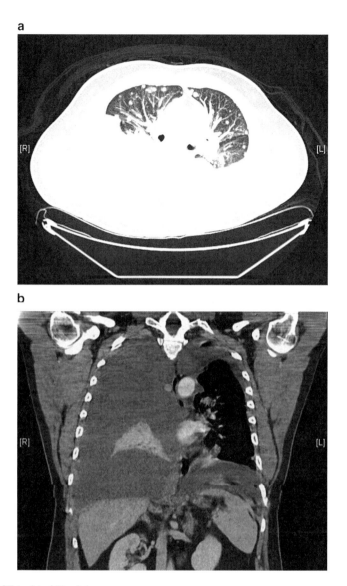

Fig. 3.5 CT (**a**, **b**) of Fig. 3.4

Table 3.2 Lung metastases from soft tissue sarcoma: incidence by primary site for all patients with pulmonary metastases (used with permission from Billingsley et al. [13])

Primary site	Total no. of patients (%)	Patients with lung metastases (% of total)	% of all lung metastases
Extremity/trunk	1,837 (58)	474 (26)	65
Retroperitoneal	466 (15)	63 (14)	9
Thoracic	193 (6)	44 (23)	6
Visceral-GI	206 (7)	12 (6)	2
Visceral-GYN	172 (6)	65 (38)	9
Visceral-GU	101 (3)	23 (23)	3
Head and neck	141 (5)	25 (18)	4
Skin/others	33 (1)	13 (36)	2
Total	3,149	719	100

a complete resection and of those 23% were alive at 3 years. So of the initial 135 patients, 15 (11%) of the original presenting cohort with pulmonary or lung disease were alive at 3 years.

A follow-up study [13] examined over 3,000 patients with soft tissue sarcoma admitted and treated at Memorial Sloan-Kettering Cancer Center, of which 719 developed or presented with lung metastases. The prevalence of lung metastasis from soft tissue sarcoma is highly dependent on the original site of the lesion. The most dominant site of metastasis is the extremity (Table 3.2). In addition, lung metastasis from soft tissue sarcoma varies according to the original histopathology with leiomyosarcoma and synovial sarcoma the most common (Table 3.3). Overall disease-specific survival has a median of 15 months. In 719 examined patients, the value of resection is outlined in Fig. 3.6. An aggressive approach to resection was taken. Median survival from diagnosis of pulmonary metastasis for all patients was 15 months with a 3-year actuarial survival of 25%. Patients treated with complete resection had a median survival of 33 months and 3-year actuarial survival of 46%. Negative factors for survival included liposarcoma, malignant peripheral nerve tumors, and patients over the age of 50. Patients who did not undergo a complete resection had only marginal survival benefit over those who did not have any resection. Of the 138 patients evaluable for 5-year survival, 14% were alive. That analysis showed disease-free interval greater than 12 months was a favorable factor for prolonged survival. Patients who underwent complete resection had a median survival of 33 months. However, of the total presenting with pulmonary metastasis, only 161 could undergo complete resection (22%).

Outcomes for patients who had more than one resection for metastatic disease have been examined [14]. Two hundred forty-eight patients were studied having undergone at least one resection of pulmonary metastasis, and 86 of those (35%) underwent re-exploration. Of those patients able to have complete re-resection, median disease-free survival was 51 months. Factors predicative of a poor outcome at the time of re-resection included greater than 3 nodules, any metastasis larger

Table 3.3 Lung metastases from soft tissue sarcoma: distribution by histologic type and grade (used with permission from Billingsley et al. [13])

Histology	Overall (% overall)	High-grade histology	% high-grade	Patients with lung metastases	% patients with lung metastases	% of all patients with lung metastases
Alveolar soft part sarcoma	22 (0.7)	22	100	13	59	2
Embryonal rhabdomyosarcoma	97 (3.0)	97	100	25	26	3
Synovial sarcoma	225 (7.0)	215	96	98	44	14
Epithelioid	21 (1.0)	20	95	8	38	1
Spindle cell (without specific lineage assigned)	56 (1.7)	51	91	20	36	3
Undifferentiated (sarcoma not otherwise specified)	25 (0.7)	22	88	15	60	2
Others[a]	221 (7.0)	190	86	65	29	9
Malignant peripheral nerve sheath tumor	130 (4.0)	111	85	36	28	5
Leiomyosarcoma	590 (18.7)	492	83	149	25	21
Angiosarcoma	124 (3.9)	97	78	33	27	5
Undifferentiated pleomorphic sarcoma	559 (18.0)	376	67	132	24	18
Extraskeletal chondrosarcoma	57 (2.0)	32	56	18	32	2
Liposarcoma	657 (20.8)	329	50	86	13	12
Fibrosarcoma	314 (10.0)	15	16	19	6	3
Gastrointestinal stromal tumor	51 (2.0)	5	10	2	4	<1

[a]Includes adenosarcoma, anaplastic sarcoma, clear cell sarcoma, cystosarcoma phyllodes, and desmoplastic sarcoma

Fig. 3.6 Disease-specific survival for patients with pulmonary metastases undergoing thoracotomy by treatment. Incomplete gross resection is only minimally better than operation with no resection (used with permission from Billingsley et al. [13])

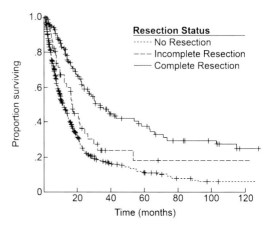

than 2 cm and high-grade tumor histology. Patients with three of these prognostic factors had a median disease-specific survival of 10 months, whereas patients with zero or one of these risk factors had a median disease specific survival of greater than 65 months. The role of metastasis surgery has been summarized [15].

The use of perioperative chemotherapy in patients undergoing pulmonary resection for metastatic disease was examined in a study reviewing the MSKCC database [16]. The study was comprised of 508 patients (27% of 1,897 patients) with extremity soft tissue sarcoma who developed lung metastasis as the first site of distant disease. Of those, 138 (27%) patients underwent pulmonary resection. Of those 138, 53 (38%) received perioperative chemotherapy. While some factors were similar, i.e., sex, grade, size, primary tumor, depth, histology, and number and size of lung metastasis, there was a significant difference between the patients who received perioperative chemotherapy in terms of disease-free interval. The rate of complete resection was the same. Complete resection was the only factor shown to be associated with prolonged survival. Those data suggested that the median postmetastasis disease-specific survival was 24 months in those patients treated with surgery and chemotherapy compared to 33 months in patients who were treated with surgery alone. Treatment outcome is highly influenced by patient selection, and it is thus not possible to evaluate the benefit of chemotherapy directly. Given the lack of substantial benefit in patients who were treated with chemotherapy, systemic chemotherapy before or after pulmonary resection appears to be of limited value. A randomized clinical trial to test this hypothesis has failed for lack of accrual.

Surgery and the Management of Sarcoma Liver Metastasis

The liver is a rare site of metastasis from extremity soft tissue sarcoma, but more common for gastrointestinal primary sarcomas such as gastrointestinal stromal

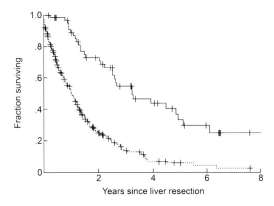

Fig. 3.7 Disease-specific survival for patients with liver metastases who had complete gross resection (n = 56) (*upper line*) of all metastases were associated with improved survival compared to similar patients (275) treated without gross complete resection (*lower line*) of all liver lesions (used with permission from DeMatteo et al. [17])

tumor (GIST). Standard treatment for sarcomas other than gastrointestinal stromal tumor (GIST) metastatic to the liver usually entails chemotherapy or supportive care. Very few reports of resection exist for metastatic sarcoma, whereas hepatectomy for other types of metastatic disease is well established. From a database of 4,270 we analyzed 331 (8%) patients who developed liver metastases. Of those 331 patients, 56 (17%) underwent complete resection of all gross liver disease. There was considerable patient selection based on the absence of disease elsewhere, the physical status of the patient, and the distribution of the metastases. Of the patients who had metastases to the liver from sarcoma, 40% were patients with gastrointestinal stromal tumors [17]. Prior to 1993, GISTs were often considered leiomyosarcoma, and approximately one-fourth had extraintestinal leiomyosarcoma. Many of these patients would now be treated with imatinib, but even these patients may come to liver resection. Of the group studied, the ability to undergo a liver resection was associated with improved survival (Fig. 3.7). This association with a survival benefit was histology independent. The only factor predicting improved survival was a disease-free interval of greater than two years. In those patients undergoing resection, there was no perioperative death. However, there were three perioperative deaths in patients who had incomplete resection. Given the ability to perform liver resection with low morbidity and mortality, this should be considered in selected patients with apparent liver-only disease, with reasonable possibility for complete gross resection, although recurrence is common Fig. 3.8. With present imaging techniques, the likelihood of complete resection can now be much more adequately predicted; however, on rare occasions, palliative resection is performed for the seriously symptomatic patient (Fig. 3.9). The role of liver resection for GIST in the age of imatinib remains investigational.

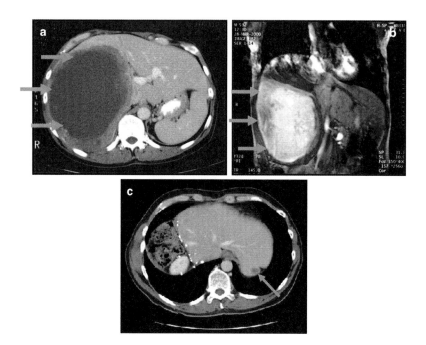

Fig. 3.8 Preoperative CT scan of liver metastases from GIST (**a, b**). Contralateral recurrence at 6 months (**c**)

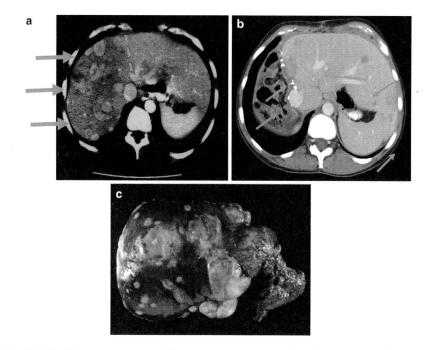

Fig. 3.9 CT of large symptomatic GIST, asymptomatic progression: (**a**) preoperative, (**b**) postoperative, (**c**) gross specimen

Radiation Therapy

Radiation therapy may be given in the adjuvant setting following surgical resection or on occasions for primary treatment of inoperable lesions.

Adjuvant Radiation Therapy

The goal of utilizing adjuvant radiation therapy is to limit local recurrence, avoid amputation, and contribute to tissue preservation by limiting the extent of resection. In the absence of an adequate margin of 1–2 cm following a surgical procedure, or the presence of microscopic wound positivity, local recurrence is increased. This local recurrence can be limited by the judicious use of radiation therapy. Two randomized trials have examined the benefit of adjuvant radiation therapy to limit local control following conservative, especially limb-sparing surgical resection. One trial used external beam radiation therapy and the other brachytherapy [18, 19]. An update of the brachytherapy trial performed at our institution sustained the long-term ability to improve local control by adjuvant radiation therapy (Fig. 3.10). This benefit is most marked for high-grade lesions (Fig. 3.11). Unfortunately, this is not translated into a survival benefit and does not limit metastasis (Fig. 3.12). There are limited, if any, local control benefits using brachytherapy for low-grade tumors but marked increase in local control with external beam radiation therapy [19].

Exact indications for external beam radiation therapy remain uncertain and are often arbitrary. The majority of surgeons prefer to avoid radiation therapy particularly for lesions that are less than 5 cm who have adequate tissue margins, following complete resection.

Fig. 3.10 Local disease-free survival for adult patients with extremity soft tissue sarcoma excluding desmoids: a prospective randomized trial of adjuvant brachytherapy versus observation. MSKCC 7/1/1982–6/30/1992, follow-up to 6/30/2010 n = 164

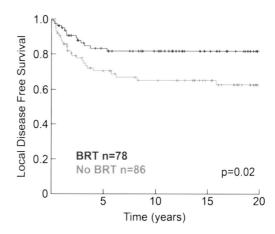

Fig. 3.11 Local disease-free survival for adult patients with extremity soft tissue sarcoma, high grade only, excluding desmoids: a prospective randomized trial of adjuvant brachytherapy versus observation. MSKCC 7/1/1982–6/30/1992, follow-up to 6/30/2010 n = 112

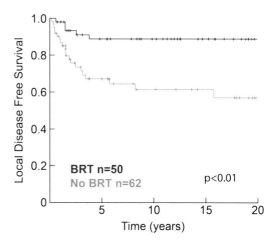

Fig. 3.12 Disease-specific survival for adult patients with extremity soft tissue sarcoma excluding desmoids: a prospective randomized trial of adjuvant brachytherapy versus observation. MSKCC 7/1/1982–6/30/1992, follow-up to 6/30/2010 n = 158

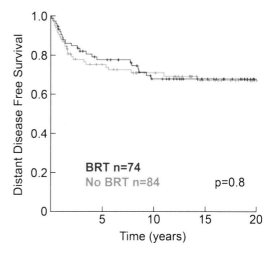

External beam radiation therapy is the most widely used adjuvant approach without requiring the sophistication of catheter replacement for brachytherapy. The issue of whether it is preferable to use preoperative radiation therapy or postoperative radiation therapy is also uncertain. A prospective randomized control trial [20] demonstrated equivalence in terms of local control by either preoperative and postoperative radiation therapy but with a greater complication rate in terms of wound healing and early postoperative diminution of function with the preoperative treatment. As radiation therapy and techniques improve and intensity-modulated radiation therapy is more widely utilized, complications and side effects can be expected to continue to diminish. Certainly advances have been achieved with the utilization of intensity-modulated radiation therapy (IMRT) [21]. In a nonrandomized comparison of brachytherapy and IMRT, IMRT appeared to be associated with superior local control despite higher risk factors (close margins, larger size, and nerve stripping) [22]. Attempts at performing evaluable trials of preoperative radiation therapy for large abdominal lesions, an approach favored by many, have unfortunately not been possible.

Postoperative radiation therapy is also accompanied by late tissue complications such as lymphedema, fibrosis, and scarring. Five-year results of the Canadian trial have been reported [23]. Local control with radiation therapy was identical at 92% and 93%. A disadvantage of postoperative radiation therapy is the increase in volume required to encompass all the "at-risk" tissue, whereas preoperatively, the focus can be made on the primary lesion with an extension of 2–4 cm either longitudinally or axially to define the clinical target volume.

Dose of Radiation Therapy

Clear definition of the necessary dose of radiation therapy for soft tissue sarcoma is relatively imprecise. Preoperative doses of 50 Gy in daily fractions of 1.8–2 Gy over 5 weeks are commonly utilized. The patient receives preoperative radiation therapy with a postoperative boost administered only if the surgical margins remain positive after resection. Proof of this strategy is unclear. Postoperative radiation therapy is often arbitrary with doses usually used to 50 Gy with some data to suggest that doses less than this, e.g., 45 Gy, have less of an impact on local control. The utilization of high-dose intensity-modulated radiation therapy (IMRT) [21] appears to limit damage to normal tissue or to lesser quantities of normal tissue. Such approaches are essential when anatomical barriers such as the spinal cord or a remnant kidney are close to or part of the intended field. The role of high-dose IMRT (1–3 fractions total) remains unevaluated in the setting of primary disease.

Adjuvant Brachytherapy

Brachytherapy (BRT) is an attractive approach which we have utilized over many years, although with the advent of IMRT that utilization is diminishing. The attractiveness of brachytherapy is that a completed course can be delivered in 5–7 days as opposed to the 5–6 weeks required for external beam radiation therapy. The other attraction for BRT is that less normal tissue is damaged or more normal tissue is protected. Usual doses are 45 Gy given over 4–6 days, and we have shown that it is very important that this dose will not begin before the sixth postoperative day to avoid potential wound problems [24, 25]. The majority utilize ^{192}Ir although ^{125}I has been utilized in lesions that are close to reproductive structures. Our original trial of adjuvant brachytherapy showed a clear benefit in local control to the group receiving radiation therapy. This has been maintained over years (Fig. 3.10). It does appear that external beam radiation therapy is preferable to brachytherapy for patients with low-grade lesions [19]. As the local control in the external beam randomized trial was much improved over the local control in low-grade lesions with the brachytherapy technique. On rare occasions, both external beam radiation therapy and brachytherapy can be combined, usually when there are issues about the geometry of the BRT implant or difficulties with surgical margins. Importantly, brachytherapy can be given to patients who have received previous external beam radiation therapy providing that reconstructive techniques are taken to preserve tissue coverage [26].

Radiation Therapy in the Presence of Positive Microscopic Margins

This is a topic of great debate. One might imagine that this would be the perfect situation for the utilization of an adjunct known to limit local recurrence when applied. Studies do suggest that the addition of radiation therapy limits recurrence in the presence of a positive margin [27]. The problem with these nonrandomized studies is patient selection. We know that at least two-thirds of patients who have a positive microscopic margin do not recur locally, even in the absence of adjuvant therapy. Radiation therapy can be particularly well utilized when crucial function is required, e.g., in the preservation of function in the hands and feet. In situations where the bone is at greater risk in terms of function preservation, radiation therapy should always be considered prior to moving to an amputation. This becomes a crucial consideration when we realize that amputation is not going to improve survival, so attempts at function conservation even risking a subsequent local recurrence are certainly justified.

Definitive Radiation Therapy

Definitive radiation therapy is occasionally utilized in patients with unresectable disease or severe medical comorbidities preventing operation [28]. In one study, 112 patients underwent radiation therapy for gross residual primary disease. Local control was achieved at the 50% level at 5 years for small lesions and less than 10% for large, greater than 10 cm lesions. Complications increase as dose increased, but there does appear to be a range, i.e., 63–68 Gy where complications are minimized and local control maximized. Treatment with high-dose limited fraction IMRT remains a topic of investigation in this clinical setting.

Radiation to Patients with Neurovascular Involvement

There is debate concerning the tolerance of neurovascular structures to external beam radiation therapy, and there are no real data that examine tolerance of such tissues to local interstitial radiation therapy. We have previously reported a review of 299 patients undergoing limb-sparing surgery [29] and tumor bed iridium-192 interstitial implants. Of these patients, 45 (15%) had locally advanced tumors invading major neurovascular structures, 64% were high grade, 11% had gross residual disease, and 58% had positive microscopic disease following resection. Utilizing a median dose of 44 Gy including patients who had previous radiation, 5-year disease-free survival of 69% was obtained, and the freedom from infield failure was 79%. Most importantly, 84% of the patients maintained long-term preservation of limb function without the need for amputation. Radiation neuritis was seen in four patients (9%) in a time interval of 6–20 months following therapy. All of these patients were patients who had received accumulative doses exceeding 90 Gy. Therefore, it is possible to preserve limbs in the presence of neurovascular function with selective use of precise local radiation therapy.

Wound Complications of Radiation Therapy

Previous studies have been performed [30], and a further study looking at the morbidity of adjuvant radiation therapy has been described [31]. A review of our morbidity contained within the randomized trial of brachytherapy versus no brachytherapy suggested significant increase in wound complications in those undergoing brachytherapy requiring reoperation. It is clear based on prior wound-healing studies [24, 25] that there is a definitive point following placement of catheters at which time radiation can be loaded. Any interval less than 5 days from the time of operation results in increase in wound complications such that we load brachytherapy catheters more than 5 days from the time of operation.

Adjuvant and Neoadjuvant Chemotherapy for Soft Tissue Sarcomas

The question of adjuvant chemotherapy for soft tissue sarcomas remains important since up to half of high-risk, predominantly high-grade patients with adequate local control of disease develop distant metastasis, usually to the lungs (extremity, trunk, and uterus primaries) and/or liver (gastrointestinal stromal tumors [GIST], other abdominal primaries). Given the increasing appreciation of the different biologies of each type of sarcoma, a blanket discussion of adjuvant chemotherapy for soft tissue sarcomas is difficult. The development of imatinib for GIST is the best example of the importance of choosing a therapy appropriate to a specific soft tissue sarcoma histology. Nonetheless, a number of principles are germane to adjuvant therapy and can be grouped into discussions of GIST, sarcomas more common in pediatric populations, and sarcomas more common in adult populations.

Sarcomas More Common in Adults

Nearly 20 studies of adjuvant therapy for soft tissue sarcoma have been performed. Because anthracyclines are the most active agents in sarcoma therapy in the metastatic setting, they have been used in nearly all of the adjuvant trials, alone or in combination. More recent studies have included ifosfamide in the treatment regimen. Most of the studies have been small and lack statistical power to detect small changes in overall survival. Meta-analyses have been performed on the randomized trials for adjuvant chemotherapy in soft tissue sarcoma. After the Sarcoma Meta-analysis Collaboration (SMAC) of 1997 [32], five studies involving ifosfamide have been performed, one of which is positive. All but the largest of these studies were included as part of a new meta-analysis, which did not examine individual patient data like the SMAC meta-analysis, but now shows a survival advantage for adjuvant chemotherapy, not observed in prior meta-analyses (or in most randomized clinical trials). Some of the data of the individual trials involved are discussed below, followed by a discussion of the meta-analyses of 1997 and 2008.

Larger Randomized Studies

The Gynecologic Oncology Group (GOG) performed one of the only adjuvant studies for patients with non-extremity (specifically uterine) sarcomas [33]. Two hundred and twenty-five patients with stage I or II uterine sarcomas (any subtype) were treated with surgery for local control, adding radiation at the discretion of the treating physician. Patients were randomly assigned to receive doxorubicin 60 mg/m^2 every 3 weeks for eight cycles or to observation. For the 156 evaluable patients, disease-free survival was no different between the two groups, nor was there a statistically significant difference in overall survival (73.7 months [doxorubicin] vs. 55.0 months [control]). The addition of radiation therapy did not affect survival, although there was a lower rate of vaginal relapse in the radiation group. The GOG and SARC (Sarcoma Alliance for Research through Collaboration) have followed up on these data with phase II studies of 4 cycles of adjuvant gemcitabine-docetaxel (GOG) [34] or 4 cycles of adjuvant gemcitabine-docetaxel followed by 4 cycles of doxorubicin (SARC) [35] in patients with uterine leiomyosarcoma. Results of these studies may prompt a new randomized clinical trial to determine the efficacy of gemcitabine-docetaxel-based adjuvant therapy.

The Scandinavian Sarcoma Group performed the largest adjuvant study of doxorubicin [36]. After surgery and optional radiation, 240 patients were randomly assigned to receive doxorubicin 60 mg/m^2 every 4 weeks for nine cycles or no chemotherapy. One hundred eighty-one patients were evaluable. With a median 40 months of follow-up, there was no difference in local control, disease-free survival, or overall survival. Survival data were also assessed for the entire 240-patient cohort; there was no difference among treatment groups in disease-free or overall survival.

The largest single study of adjuvant combination chemotherapy in soft tissue sarcoma was performed by the European Organisation for Research and Treatment of Cancer (EORTC) [37]. Four hundred sixty-eight patients (excluding those with "very low-grade" sarcomas) were treated with surgery for their primary sarcoma and adjuvant radiation if surgical margins were under 1 cm. Patients then randomly assigned combination chemotherapy with cyclophosphamide, vincristine, doxorubicin, and dacarbazine (CyVADIC) given every four weeks for eight cycles. While disease-free survival and local control were both better in the chemotherapy arm, overall survival was not significantly different between the two arms. Criticism has been raised as to the 11-year accrual time, the inability of nearly half the patients to complete all 8 cycles, and the relatively large number of patients ineligible for analysis, most commonly due to radiation therapy outside that defined by the study.

The first large study to incorporate ifosfamide as part of adjuvant therapy for truncal and extremity soft tissue sarcomas is that from the Italian Sarcoma Study Group [38]. After surgery with or without local radiation, 104 patients received either no chemotherapy or received ifosfamide (9 g/m^2 split over 5 days) and epirubicin (120 mg/m^2 split over 2 days), with filgrastim. Interim analysis in 1996 led to early termination of the trial for meeting the primary endpoint of improved disease-free survival. With median 36-month follow-up, overall survival in the chemotherapy arm was 72% versus 55% in the control arm ($p = 0.002$). Interpretation of the study is made somewhat more difficult by the finding of equal rates of distant or local recurrence or both at 4 years as well as by subtle imbalances in the distribution of patients on the control and treatment arms of the study. With longer follow-up, overall and disease-free survival no longer reach a statistical significance level of $p = 0.05$, but 5-year overall survival was still significantly better with chemotherapy. These data indicate that chemotherapy may delay, but may not ultimately eliminate, metastatic disease for most patients but is the first study with a survival advantage for chemotherapy with modern ifosfamide-anthracycline-based therapy. Three smaller studies of adjuvant or neoadjuvant chemotherapy were negative, but were underpowered to determine small differences in overall survival [39, 40].

The largest randomized study of adjuvant ifosfamide and an anthracycline (doxorubicin) was performed by the EORTC (study 62029). A total of 351 patients were recruited over 8 years. Patient characteristics were evenly distributed between the two arms with 47% of patients older than 50; 54% were male. Histologies included leiomyosarcoma, 15%; liposarcoma, 13%; MFH, 11%; synovial, 11%; with 60% of grade III tumors; and two-thirds with an extremity primary. 88% of patients received radiation. An interim analysis for futility was performed as survival in the observation arm was better than expected and presented at American Society of Surgical Oncology (ASCO) in 2007. Estimated 5-year relapse-free survival was 52% in both arms, and overall survival was 69% (observation) and 64% (chemotherapy) [41].

Selected Meta-analyses of Randomized Trials of Adjuvant Chemotherapy

Given the lack of statistical power of many of the existing randomized trials, it was hoped that combining data from individual studies of adjuvant chemotherapy would reveal improvement in overall survival undetectable in smaller studies. Arguably, the most rigorous meta-analysis regarding adjuvant chemotherapy for soft tissue sarcoma was published in 1997 [42]. In this analysis, 23 potential studies were considered and 14 ultimately included. Tumor histology for each patient was recorded, but pathology review was not centralized. Median follow-up was 9.4 years. Analyses were stratified by trial, and hazard ratios were calculated for each trial and combined, which allowed for an assessment of the risk of death or recurrence in comparison to control patients. Disease-free survival at 10 years was superior with chemotherapy (55% vs. 45%, $p=0.0001$). Local disease-free survival at 10 years also favored chemotherapy, 81% versus 75%, $p=0.016$. Although overall survival was superior with chemotherapy at 10 years (54% vs. 50%), this difference was not statistically significant ($p = 0.12$). Notably, the largest difference in overall survival was found in a subgroup analysis of the 886 patients with extremity sarcomas; overall survival was 46% for patients receiving chemotherapy versus 39% for those who did not ($p=0.029$).

Five recent studies using ifosfamide as part of adjuvant or neoadjuvant therapy were added to the SMAC meta-analysis in a 2008 meta-analysis [43]. Approximately 95% of the patients had had primary sites in the extremity or trunk, patients in whom adequate surgical margins are most likely achieved. Considering the ifosfamide-anthracycline-containing studies alone or in combination with the older doxorubicin-based studies (without ifosfamide) yielded similar results. Local, distant, and overall recurrence risks were lower with chemotherapy, and survival was statistically improved for patients receiving chemotherapy versus those who did not. Considering all trials together, there was an absolute risk reduction of death of 6% (95% CI 2–11%; $p=0.003$), or 5-year survival of 46% for patients receiving chemotherapy and 40% for those who did not.

As has been seen with large studies of patients receiving chemotherapy for non-small cell lung cancer, the large size of the recent meta-analysis supports the use of chemotherapy in the adjuvant setting for patients with soft tissue sarcoma, with some caveats. Most individual clinical trials of adjuvant chemotherapy are negative, though most are small by modern standards. One is thus left to balance the individual studies (such as the two large negative EORTC studies of adjuvant chemotherapy) with the meta-analysis data. Further analysis is hampered to some degree by the quality of the data reported in individual studies [44]. It is safe to say that if there is a benefit to chemotherapy, it remains a small one and that new agents are needed to improve the lot of patients with a large primary adult extremity soft tissue sarcoma.

The issue of histological sensitivity is also lost in meta-analyses and individual trials alike since no subtype represents a majority in any of these studies. Since synovial sarcoma and myxoid-round cell liposarcoma are more sensitive to chemotherapy in the metastatic setting than other subtypes, perhaps these are the best potential candidates for adjuvant therapy, though there have not been subset analyses by histology to examine this issue. We consider adjuvant chemotherapy most seriously for patients with these histologies, noting that the benefit, if any, is a small one, with significant short-term and potential long-term toxicity to face for anyone who receives such treatment. It is also worth noting that the retroperitoneal, visceral, and head/neck locations are often those in which a good margin cannot be achieved and that it is less likely that chemotherapy itself will provide a survival advantage, borne out to some degree from the negative data from multiple studies with doxorubicin that included patients with retroperitoneal, abdominal, and visceral disease (noting that some of these sarcomas would be today called GIST). Uterine leiomyosarcoma is one example of active research in an organ- and histology-specific manner and hopefully will yield results that can be applied to other sites with the same histology.

The data regarding the 2008 meta-analysis parallel data from non-small cell lung cancer where it has taken large randomized trials to demonstrate a modest difference in survival for the use of adjuvant chemotherapy. It will be difficult to proceed with adjuvant studies given negative randomized trials and positive meta-analysis; using one set of data or the other physicians will decide whether or not they believe there is a role for chemotherapy. What is certain is that like GIST, better agents are needed for specific sarcoma subtypes, and may be here for some diagnoses, in the form of trabectedin for myxoid-round cell liposarcoma. Given the rare nature of any given subtype of sarcoma, it will likely prove extremely difficult to conduct a clinical trial of chemotherapy in the adjuvant setting for individual histopathologies.

Adjuvant Therapy for GIST

While GIST is impervious to standard cytotoxic chemotherapy, it is very sensitive to imatinib, begging the question of the utility of imatinib in the adjuvant setting. With the improvement in disease-free survival observed in the American College of Surgeons Oncology Group (ACOSOG) Z9001 randomized study described below [45], the FDA (Food and Drug Administration) and EMA (European Medicines Agency) approved imatinib in the adjuvant setting. As of now, there are no data that indicate imatinib improves the cure rate of patients with resection of primary disease.

The first study examining adjuvant imatinib for high-risk GIST (i.e., > 10 cm disease, ruptured tumor, or satellite implants near a primary tumor) was completed by the American College of Surgeons Oncology Group (ACOSOG) [45]. More than 100 evaluable patients were accrued on study Z9000 from September 2001 to September 2003. Patients received imatinib at a starting dose of 400 mg orally daily for 48 weeks and were then followed for recurrence. The data of Z9000 are consistent with the high-risk cohort of Z9001 discussed below.

The Z9000 study was followed by ACOSOG study Z9001, examining imatinib 400 mg daily versus placebo for 48 weeks for any GIST more than 3 cm in greatest dimension [45]. This study completed accrual in 2007 and showed a very significant difference in Progression-Free Survival (PFS) at the end of 1 year of therapy (3% vs. 17% for those on or not on imatinib). This difference did not translate to a survival advantage, although median follow-up was brief, less than 2 years at the time of publication. A delay in the progression-free survival curve of patients who received imatinib for one year toward that of the patients receiving placebo alone suggests that the cure rate is not improved with 1 year of imatinib [45]. Furthermore, of over 700 patients on study, only seven had died of progressive disease as of the time of the release of the initial data of the study. Thus, it appears at this early stage that (1) overall survival was not improved with 1 year of imatinib and (2) imatinib is an effective salvage therapy for people with recurrent GIST. Furthermore, like hormonal therapy for breast cancer, (3) if imatinib is to be curative, a longer course of adjuvant therapy may be necessary.

To this point, similar adjuvant studies in Europe are underway to examine some of these questions. A study of the EORTC is examining no therapy versus 2 years of imatinib, and a second study from the SSG and AIO examined 1 versus 3 years of imatinib. PFS and OS are superior on 3 years adjuvant therapy, and thus a standard of care for higher risk GIST as of 2011.

As noted in the GIST chapter (Chap. 4), and incorporating the SSG XVII data with data from Corless et al. at ASCO 2010 [46], the authors suggest that if adjuvant therapy be used, it should be employed for patients with higher risk tumors (≥5 cm *and* >5/50 HPF mitoses [gastric]; ≥5 cm *or* >5/50 HPF mitoses [non-gastric that can be assumed to have a high risk of metastasis]). These include high-risk tumors with *KIT* exon 11 mutations or *PDGFRA* mutations other than D842V. Initial data indicate patients with *KIT* exon 9 and "wild-type" GIST will not benefit from adjuvant therapy [46]. For the time being, the author suggests therapy for 3 years, the longest exposure employed in a randomized study. A study of imatinib for 5 years of adjuvant therapy for high-risk patients is now underway.

Sarcomas More Common in the Pediatric Setting

Without reviewing the positive studies performed in the past, the present standard of care for Ewing sarcoma is 9–15 weeks of systemic chemotherapy before local control (surgery, radiation, or both). A consensus standard of care in the United States, based on a large randomized clinical trial (more details can be found in Chap. 15 on pediatric sarcomas), is 5-drug therapy with ifosfamide and etoposide (IE) alternating with vincristine, doxorubicin, and cyclophosphamide (VAdrC), which is superior to 3-drug VAdrC therapy for patients with localized tumors [47]. A four-drug regimen, VIDE (vincristine, ifosfamide, doxorubicin, etoposide) is more commonly employed in Europe. A recent study has shown that treatment for pediatric patients given at compressed intervals (q2 week) for patients treated with "standard-dosing" 5-drug regimens is superior to patients treated q3 weeks [48]. Interestingly, increasing the dose per cycle of chemotherapy, while maintaining the same total cumulative dose of drugs administered, did not lead to an improvement in survival [49].

The most recent randomized data from randomized studies (IRS-IV) for most aggressive rhabdomyosarcomas indicate that the combination of vincristine, dactinomycin, and cyclophosphamide is as active as two other combinations (vincristine, dactinomycin, ifosfamide and vincristine, ifosfamide, etoposide) and less myelotoxic than the other two regimens, and thus a good standard of care [50]. Notably, the vincristine dosing needed in pediatric patients with rhabdomyosarcoma cannot be delivered to most adults. Also in rhabdomyosarcomas in adults, the cure rate is lower than in children, even on a histology-by-histology basis (embryonal, alveolar, and pleomorphic rhabdomyosarcomas). As a result, some physicians opt for the same VAC/IE chemotherapy employed in Ewing sarcoma. Other centers have used the MAID combination effectively in metastatic disease, raising it as a possible treatment for primary disease as well. However, there are no adjuvant data to support its use [51].

Brief Comments Regarding Chemotherapy for Metastatic Soft Tissue Sarcoma

It is well appreciated that different sarcoma subtypes have different patterns of sensitivity to a cytotoxic chemotherapy. We have attempted to address the histology specific issues in each subtype-specific section of this book. It is worth noting that agents not used in the adjuvant setting, namely, doxorubicin or ifosfamide, remain the best agents for a number of the sarcomas that require treatment. Certain systemic agents or combinations show predilection for one or more subtypes as well, such as dacarbazine or temozolomide in leiomyosarcoma [52–54] (and perhaps in solitary fibrous tumor), taxanes for angiosarcoma [55–57], or ifosfamide for synovial sarcoma [58, 59]. To date, few agents have achieved positive results in randomized clinical trials to be considered good drugs in a generic sense for metastatic sarcoma. Gemcitabine and docetaxel are active in leiomyosarcoma and undifferentiated pleomorphic sarcoma, as well as pleomorphic liposarcoma [60, 61]. Trabectedin, shown active in a 3-week schedule in comparison to a weekly schedule, was approved in Europe but not in the United States based largely on a single randomized phase II study [62]. Pazopanib was approved in 2012 for advanced sarcomas, but was found to have a progression-free survival advantage only in its pivotal phase III randomized study, and did not meet statistical significance for overall or disease-specific survival [63]. A TOR inhibitor was tested in a large phase III study in the maintenance setting, but the PFS benefit was too small for regulatory agencies to consider appropriate for approval. As a result, we remain in need of new agents with both generic activity in sarcomas as well as those agents with specificity for particular sarcoma subtypes. Given the breadth of biology encompassed by this family of cancers, it is expected to be quite some time before we have good first- and second-line options for all specific sarcoma subtypes.

Special Techniques for Primary and Locally Recurrent Disease

Intra-arterial Chemotherapy

A number of studies have examined the role of intra-arterial chemotherapy with doxorubicin, cisplatin, or both (among other drugs) for primary sarcomas [64]. The infusional approach is to be differentiated from local limb perfusion [65, 66]. Intra-arterial chemotherapy has the potential benefit of providing higher doses of chemotherapy to the limb in a first-pass effect. It remains a technique used at some centers and not used at others, perhaps due to the lack of compelling randomized data to support its use. Intra-arterial chemotherapy has been used in conjunction with radiation. In these studies, some patients have been able to avoid amputation. Infusional chemotherapy has its attendant complications, including arterial thromboembolism, infection, gangrene, and problems with wound healing, requiring amputation. Pathologic fractures have been reported in patients receiving chemotherapy and relatively large doses of radiation. Although there are situations in which such therapy could be considered, intra-arterial chemotherapy has a limited role at most institutions in the treatment of extremity sarcomas, given the technical expertise required, and the questionable benefits.

Limb Perfusion and Hyperthermia

In contrast to systemic intra-arterial chemotherapy infusion as noted above, perfusion of limbs requires isolating the arterial and venous system of the limb by means of a tourniquet, obtaining access to arteries and veins supplying the limb [65, 66]. The arterial and venous supply of the limb is connected to an external circulator to isolate the limb from the rest of the body. Blood from the limb is reoxygenated using a heart-lung machine. Radioactively tagged albumin is injected into the circuit, and a probe is used to insure isolation of the bypass circuit. Because mild hyperthermia may make chemotherapy more effective in some clinical settings (as mentioned later in this section), the blood of the circuit is often warmed to 39–40°C.

A number of chemotherapeutic agents have been used for limb perfusion, such as doxorubicin, melphalan, and dactinomycin. The most effective agent to date has been melphalan when given with tumor necrosis factor (TNF). The greatest experience with this technique comes from Eggermont et al. [65, 66]. After isolation of the extremity, 246 patients with unresectable sarcomas had melphalan perfused into the limb with TNF under mild hyperthermic conditions. Both components of the regimen appeared important; the omission of TNF led to a decrease in tissue dose of melphalan, probably from its effects on the tumor vasculature. Surgery to remove residual tumor was performed 2–4 months after limb perfusion. With a median follow-up of 3 years, 71% of patients had successful limb salvage. TNF remains unavailable in the United States, but is approved for use in Europe and elsewhere for this setting. It is important to note that isolated limb perfusion requires substantial expertise and specialized dedicated equipment, which has led to a decrease in the incidence and severity of complications over time. Isolated limb perfusion does appear to hold promise for at least a subset of patients who would otherwise require amputation for local control and has been approved for such patients in Europe.

Hyperthermia can potentially enhance the effects of chemotherapy in patients with locally advanced disease. Regional hyperthermia provided through an external electromagnetic field (phased array) has been examined in combination with ifosfamide and etoposide, as well as other combinations of chemotherapy [67–69]. In a series of studies, partial and complete responses in patients with locally advanced and metastatic soft tissue sarcoma have been noted. Randomized data also support the superior local control rate with chemotherapy given with hyperthermia versus chemotherapy [70], which has led to the approval of hyperthermia in Germany in this setting. Hyperthermia with chemotherapy remains investigational in the United States. The recent publications in melanoma, of the use of infusion rather than perfusion, suggest that the former technique may well be preferable and with less technical challenge in the absence of a need for a recirculation circuit.

References

1. Suzman MS, Smith AJ, Brennan MF. Fascio-peritoneal patch repair of the IVC: a workhorse in search of work? J Am Coll Surg. 2000;191(2):218–20.
2. Hollenbeck ST, Grobmyer SR, Kent KC, et al. Surgical treatment and outcomes of patients with primary inferior vena cava leiomyosarcoma. J Am Coll Surg. 2003;197(4):575–9.
3. Russo P, Kim Y, Ravindran S, et al. Nephrectomy during operative management of retroperitoneal sarcoma. Ann Surg Oncol. 1997;4(5):421–4.
4. Brennan MF, Lewis JJ. Diagnosis and management of soft tissue sarcoma. London: Martin Dunitz Ltd; 2002.
5. Eilber FC, Brennan MF, Riedel E, et al. Prognostic factors for survival in patients with locally recurrent extremity soft tissue sarcomas. Ann Surg Oncol. 2005;12(3):228–36.
6. Panicek DM, Gatsonis C, Rosenthal DI, et al. CT and MR imaging in the local staging of primary malignant musculoskeletal neoplasms: report of the Radiology Diagnostic Oncology Group. Radiology. 1997;202(1):237–46.
7. Fazel R, Krumholz HM, Wang Y, et al. Exposure to low-dose ionizing radiation from medical imaging procedures. N Engl J Med. 2009;361(9):849–57.
8. Benz MR, Dry SM, Eilber FC, et al. Correlation between glycolytic phenotype and tumor grade in soft-tissue sarcomas by 18F-FDG PET. J Nucl Med. 2010;51(8):1174–81.
9. Eary JF, Conrad EU. PET imaging: update on sarcomas. Oncology (Williston Park). 2007;21(2):249–52.
10. Schuetze SM. Utility of positron emission tomography in sarcomas. Curr Opin Oncol. 2006;18(4):369–73.
11. Gadd MA, Casper ES, Woodruff JM, et al. Development and treatment of pulmonary metastases in adult patients with extremity soft tissue sarcoma. Ann Surg. 1993;218(6):705–12.
12. Mountain CF, McMurtrey MJ, Hermes KE. Surgery for pulmonary metastasis: a 20-year experience. Ann Thorac Surg. 1984;38(4):323–30.
13. Billingsley KG, Burt ME, Jara E, et al. Pulmonary metastases from soft tissue sarcoma: analysis of patterns of diseases and postmetastasis survival. Ann Surg. 1999;229(5):602–10. discussion 610–602.

14. Weiser MR, Downey RJ, Leung DH, et al. Repeat resection of pulmonary metastases in patients with soft-tissue sarcoma. J Am Coll Surg. 2000;191(2):184–90. discussion 190–181.
15. Temple LK, Brennan MF. The role of pulmonary metastasectomy in soft tissue sarcoma. Semin Thorac Cardiovasc Surg. 2002;14(1):35–44.
16. Canter RJ, Qin LX, Downey RJ, et al. Perioperative chemotherapy in patients undergoing pulmonary resection for metastatic soft-tissue sarcoma of the extremity: a retrospective analysis. Cancer. 2007;110(9):2050–60.
17. DeMatteo RP, Shah A, Fong Y, et al. Results of hepatic resection for sarcoma metastatic to liver. Ann Surg. 2001;234(4):540–7. discussion 547–548.
18. Pisters PW, Harrison LB, Leung DH, et al. Long-term results of a prospective randomized trial of adjuvant brachytherapy in soft tissue sarcoma. J Clin Oncol. 1996;14(3):859–68.
19. Yang JC, Chang AE, Baker AR, et al. Randomized prospective study of the benefit of adjuvant radiation therapy in the treatment of soft tissue sarcomas of the extremity. J Clin Oncol. 1998;16(1):197–203.
20. O'Sullivan B, Davis AM, Turcotte R, et al. Preoperative versus postoperative radiotherapy in soft-tissue sarcoma of the limbs: a randomised trial. Lancet. 2002;359(9325):2235–41.
21. Alektiar KM, Hong L, Brennan MF, et al. Intensity modulated radiation therapy for primary soft tissue sarcoma of the extremity: preliminary results. Int J Radiat Oncol Biol Phys. 2007;68(2):458–64.
22. Alektiar KM, Brennan MF, Singer S. Local control comparison of adjuvant brachytherapy to intensity-modulated radiotherapy in primary high-grade sarcoma of the extremity. Cancer. 2011;117(14):3229–34.
23. Davis AM, O'Sullivan B, Turcotte R, et al. Late radiation morbidity following randomization to preoperative versus postoperative radiotherapy in extremity soft tissue sarcoma. Radiother Oncol. 2005;75(1):48–53.
24. Ormsby MV, Hilaris BS, Nori D, et al. Wound complications of adjuvant radiation therapy in patients with soft-tissue sarcomas. Ann Surg. 1989;210(1):93–9.
25. Arbeit JM, Hilaris BS, Brennan MF. Wound complications in the multimodality treatment of extremity and superficial truncal sarcomas. J Clin Oncol. 1987;5(3):480–8.
26. Alekhteyar KM, Leung DH, Brennan MF, et al. The effect of combined external beam radiotherapy and brachytherapy on local control and wound complications in patients with high-grade soft tissue sarcomas of the extremity with positive microscopic margin. Int J Radiat Oncol Biol Phys. 1996;36(2):321–4.
27. Alektiar KM, Velasco J, Zelefsky MJ, et al. Adjuvant radiotherapy for margin-positive high-grade soft tissue sarcoma of the extremity. Int J Radiat Oncol Biol Phys. 2000;48(4):1051–8.
28. Kepka L, DeLaney TF, Suit HD, et al. Results of radiation therapy for unresected soft-tissue sarcomas. Int J Radiat Oncol Biol Phys. 2005;63(3):852–9.
29. Zelefsky MJ, Nori D, Shiu MH, et al. Limb salvage in soft tissue sarcomas involving neurovascular structures using combined surgical resection and brachytherapy. Int J Radiat Oncol Biol Phys. 1990;19(4):913–8.
30. Shiu MH, Collin C, Hilaris BS, et al. Limb preservation and tumor control in the treatment of popliteal and antecubital soft tissue sarcomas. Cancer. 1986;57(8):1632–9.
31. Alektiar KM, Zelefsky MJ, Brennan MF. Morbidity of adjuvant brachytherapy in soft tissue sarcoma of the extremity and superficial trunk. Int J Radiat Oncol Biol Phys. 2000;47(5):1273–9.
32. Sarcoma Meta-Analysis Collaboration. Adjuvant chemotherapy for localised resectable soft-tissue sarcoma of adults: meta-analysis of individual data. Lancet. 1997;350(9092):1647–54.
33. Omura GA, Blessing JA, Major F, et al. A randomized clinical trial of adjuvant adriamycin in uterine sarcomas: a Gynecologic Oncology Group Study. J Clin Oncol. 1985;3(9):1240–5.
34. Hensley ML, Ishill N, Soslow R, et al. Adjuvant gemcitabine plus docetaxel for completely resected stages I-IV high grade uterine leiomyosarcoma: results of a prospective study. Gynecol Oncol. 2009;112(3):563–7.
35. Clinicaltrials.gov. Study NCT00282087 (2009). Accessed 15 July 2009.

36. Alvegard TA, Sigurdsson H, Mouridsen H, et al. Adjuvant chemotherapy with doxorubicin in high-grade soft tissue sarcoma: a randomized trial of the Scandinavian Sarcoma group. J Clin Oncol. 1989;7(10):1504–13.
37. Bramwell V, Rouesse J, Steward W, et al. Adjuvant CYVADIC chemotherapy for adult soft tissue sarcoma–reduced local recurrence but no improvement in survival: a study of the European Organization for Research and Treatment of Cancer Soft Tissue and Bone Sarcoma Group. J Clin Oncol. 1994;12(6):1137–49.
38. Frustaci S, Gherlinzoni F, De Paoli A, et al. Adjuvant chemotherapy for adult soft tissue sarcomas of the extremities and girdles: results of the Italian randomized cooperative trial. J Clin Oncol. 2001;19(5):1238–47.
39. Gortzak E, Azzarelli A, Buesa J, et al. A randomised phase II study on neo-adjuvant chemotherapy for 'high-risk' adult soft-tissue sarcoma. Eur J Cancer. 2001;37(9):1096–103.
40. Brodowicz T, Schwameis E, Widder J, et al. Intensified adjuvant IFADIC chemotherapy for adult soft tissue sarcoma: a prospective randomized feasibility trial. Sarcoma. 2000;4(4):151–60.
41. Woll PJ, van Glabbeke M, Hohenberger P, et al. Adjuvant chemotherapy (CT) with doxorubicin and ifosfamide in resected soft tissue sarcoma (STS): Interim analysis of a randomised phase III trial. J Clin Oncol (Meeting Abstr). 2007;25 Suppl 18:10008.
42. Collaboration SM-A. Adjuvant chemotherapy for localised resectable soft-tissue sarcoma of adults: meta-analysis of individual data. Lancet. 1997;350(9092):1647–54.
43. Pervaiz N, Colterjohn N, Farrokhyar F, et al. A systematic meta-analysis of randomized controlled trials of adjuvant chemotherapy for localized resectable soft-tissue sarcoma. Cancer. 2008;113(3):573–81.
44. Toulmonde M, Bellera C, Mathoulin-Pelissier S, et al. Quality of randomized controlled trials reporting in the treatment of sarcomas. J Clin Oncol. 2011;29(9):1204–9.
45. Dematteo RP, Ballman KV, Antonescu CR, et al. Adjuvant imatinib mesylate after resection of localised, primary gastrointestinal stromal tumour: a randomised, double-blind, placebo-controlled trial. Lancet. 2009;373(9669):1097–104.
46. Corless CL, Ballman KV, Antonescu C, et al. Relation of tumor pathologic and molecular features to outcome after surgical resection of localized primary gastrointestinal stromal tumor (GIST): Results of the intergroup phase III trial ACOSOG Z9001. J Clin Oncol. 2010;28 Suppl 15:10006.
47. Grier HE, Krailo MD, Tarbell NJ, et al. Addition of ifosfamide and etoposide to standard chemotherapy for Ewing's sarcoma and primitive neuroectodermal tumor of bone. N Engl J Med. 2003;348(8):694–701.
48. Balamuth NJ, Womer RB. Ewing's sarcoma. Lancet Oncol. 2010;11(2):184–92.
49. Granowetter L, Womer R, Devidas M, et al. Dose-intensified compared with standard chemotherapy for nonmetastatic Ewing sarcoma family of tumors: a Children's Oncology Group Study. J Clin Oncol. 2009;27(15):2536–41.
50. Crist WM, Anderson JR, Meza JL, et al. Intergroup rhabdomyosarcoma study-IV: results for patients with nonmetastatic disease. J Clin Oncol. 2001;19(12):3091–102.
51. Antman K, Crowley J, Balcerzak SP, et al. A Southwest Oncology Group and Cancer and Leukemia Group B phase II study of doxorubicin, dacarbazine, ifosfamide, and mesna in adults with advanced osteosarcoma, Ewing's sarcoma, and rhabdomyosarcoma. Cancer. 1998; 82(7):1288–95.
52. Talbot SM, Keohan ML, Hesdorffer M, et al. A phase II trial of temozolomide in patients with unresectable or metastatic soft tissue sarcoma. Cancer. 2003;98(9):1942–6.
53. del Garcia MX, Lopez-Pousa A, Martin J, et al. A phase II trial of temozolomide as a 6-week, continuous, oral schedule in patients with advanced soft tissue sarcoma: a study by the Spanish Group for Research on Sarcomas. Cancer. 2005;104(8):1706–12.
54. Boyar MS, Hesdorffer M, Keohan ML, et al. Phase II Study of temozolomide and thalidomide in patients with unresectable or metastatic leiomyosarcoma. Sarcoma. 2008;2008:412503.
55. Fury MG, Antonescu CR, Van Zee KJ, et al. A 14-year retrospective review of angiosarcoma: clinical characteristics, prognostic factors, and treatment outcomes with surgery and chemotherapy. Cancer J. 2005;11(3):241–7.

56. Penel N, Italiano A, Ray-Coquard I, et al. Metastatic angiosarcomas: doxorubicin-based regimens, weekly paclitaxel and metastasectomy significantly improve the outcome. Ann Oncol. 2012;23(2):517–23.
57. Italiano A, Cioffi A, Penel N, et al. Comparison of doxorubicin and weekly paclitaxel efficacy in metastatic angiosarcomas. Cancer. 2012;118(13):3330–6.
58. Bramwell VH, Mouridsen HT, Santoro A, et al. Cyclophosphamide versus ifosfamide: final report of a randomized phase II trial in adult soft tissue sarcomas. Eur J Cancer Clin Oncol. 1987;23(3):311–21.
59. Rosen G, Forscher C, Lowenbraun S, et al. Synovial sarcoma. Uniform response of metastases to high dose ifosfamide. Cancer. 1994;73(10):2506–11.
60. Hensley ML, Maki R, Venkatraman E, et al. Gemcitabine and docetaxel in patients with unresectable leiomyosarcoma: results of a phase II trial. J Clin Oncol. 2002;20(12):2824–31.
61. Maki RG, Wathen JK, Patel SR, et al. Randomized phase II study of gemcitabine and docetaxel compared with gemcitabine alone in patients with metastatic soft tissue sarcomas: results of sarcoma alliance for research through collaboration study 002 [corrected]. J Clin Oncol. 2007;25(19):2755–63.
62. Demetri GD, Chawla SP, von Mehren M, et al. Efficacy and safety of trabectedin in patients with advanced or metastatic liposarcoma or leiomyosarcoma after failure of prior anthracyclines and ifosfamide: results of a randomized phase II study of two different schedules. J Clin Oncol. 2009;27(25):4188–96.
63. van der Graaf WT, Blay JY, Chawla SP, et al. Pazopanib for metastatic soft-tissue sarcoma (PALETTE): a randomised, double-blind, placebo-controlled phase 3 trial. Lancet. 2012;379(9829):1879–86.
64. Mason M, Robinson M, Harmer C, et al. Intra-arterial adriamycin, conventionally fractionated radiotherapy and conservative surgery for soft tissue sarcomas. Clin Oncol (R Coll Radiol). 1992;4(1):32–5.
65. Eggermont AM, Schraffordt Koops H, Lienard D, et al. Isolated limb perfusion with high-dose tumor necrosis factor-alpha in combination with interferon-gamma and melphalan for nonresectable extremity soft tissue sarcomas: a multicenter trial. J Clin Oncol. 1996;14(10):2653–65.
66. Eggermont AM, de Wilt JH, ten Hagen TL. Current uses of isolated limb perfusion in the clinic and a model system for new strategies. Lancet Oncol. 2003;4(7):429–37.
67. Wiedemann GJ, D'Oleire F, Knop E, et al. Ifosfamide and carboplatin combined with 41.8 degrees C whole-body hyperthermia in patients with refractory sarcoma and malignant teratoma. Cancer Res. 1994;54(20):5346–50.
68. Wendtner CM, Abdel-Rahman S, Krych M, et al. Response to neoadjuvant chemotherapy combined with regional hyperthermia predicts long-term survival for adult patients with retroperitoneal and visceral high-risk soft tissue sarcomas. J Clin Oncol. 2002;20(14):3156–64.
69. Issels RD, Abdel-Rahman S, Wendtner C, et al. Neoadjuvant chemotherapy combined with regional hyperthermia (RHT) for locally advanced primary or recurrent high-risk adult soft-tissue sarcomas (STS) of adults: long-term results of a phase II study. Eur J Cancer. 2001;37(13):1599–608.
70. Issels RD, Lindner LH, Verweij J, et al. Neo-adjuvant chemotherapy alone or with regional hyperthermia for localised high-risk soft-tissue sarcoma: a randomised phase 3 multicentre study. Lancet Oncol. 2010;11(6):561–70.
71. Alektiar KM, Leung D, Zelefsky MJ, et al. Adjuvant brachytherapy for primary high-grade soft tissue sarcoma of the extremity. Ann Surg Oncol. 2002;9(1):48–56.

Part I
Management by Histopathology: Introduction

Having addressed some of the general issues regarding the characteristics of soft tissue sarcomas and their effects in people, in the next series of sections we attempt to address many of the diagnoses that comprise this family of rare tumors. We have included a discussion of deep fibromatoses/desmoids in Chap. 10, since these are relatively common, and can cause substantial morbidity, if not frequent mortality for patients. A chapter on sarcomas arising in specific anatomic sites represents the end of this series of chapters. Thereafter, for completeness, brief mention is made in Part II of tumors that are mostly benign or only rarely metastasizing. Some extremely rare subtypes of soft tissue tumors are not discussed here, and reference can be made to the published literature or pathology texts for some of these diagnoses.

We have arranged the chapters to describe the more common sarcomas first, followed by less common diagnoses. In each chapter, we endeavor to briefly describe the pathology, genetic and other biological features of each subtype (or groups of subtypes), and follow with a description of salient points in the diagnosis and treatment of each subtype. While trying to minimize repetition, we have tried to comment in each chapter on surgery, radiation therapy, and chemotherapy for each diagnosis, including a suggestion for systemic therapy for each subtype in the primary and metastatic setting, understanding that these data are out of date as soon as they are printed. We will endeavor to update these data in a separate forum. Furthermore, the recommendations regarding systemic therapy are based largely on experience and anecdote, given the lack of randomized data for specific subtypes. It is hoped that the chemotherapy suggestions will serve as a starting point for discussion of therapeutic options or possible bases for clinical trials in the future.

Liberal use is made of the Memorial Sloan-Kettering Cancer Center (MSKCC) sarcoma database to highlight the rarity or frequency of various subtypes. It must be noted that the database only includes patients admitted to MSKCC, and not all patients seen for consultations and second opinions. As a result, these data may not reflect the incidence of each diagnosis, but instead reflect the bias seen in a referral center. We invite readers to review the excellent summaries of the pathology of each diagnosis as are available from any one of a number of texts for details of subtypes they encounter, in order to develop a better understanding of the differential diagnosis and characteristics of this complicated but interesting family of tumors.

Chapter 4
Gastrointestinal Stromal Tumors (GISTs)

Gastrointestinal stromal tumors (GISTs) have been recognized as a distinct biological entity since 1998. Previously GISTs were considered to be smooth muscle neoplasms often classified as leiomyosarcoma or gastrointestinal autonomic nerve tumors (GANT) or combinations of both. Definition and cellular origin are suggested to be the interstitial cell of Cajal [1]. They commonly present as mass lesions, intra-abdominally, often of large size and with rupture and/or metastatic disease. Gastrointestinal stromal tumors make up one-third of all visceral sarcomas (Fig. 4.1). Our original report [2] described 200 gastrointestinal stromal tumors, which was approximately 6% of the 3,500 patients with sarcoma admitted to our institution. Age and sex distribution are shown in Fig. 4.2, and lesions are distributed in the stomach, more than in the small intestine and more than in other sites (Fig. 4.3). An example of a GIST of the stomach is demonstrated in Fig. 4.4.

Imaging

Imaging is usually by computed tomography or Magnetic Resonance Imaging (MRI), designed to examine the primary lesion (Fig. 4.5), site of origin, as well as the presence or absence of metastasis (Figs. 4.6 and 4.7).

Familial GIST

Familial GIST is a rare hereditary predisposition to develop GIST due to a germline mutation. Various kinds have been described, and the majority of patients have multiple tumors involving both stomach and jejunum and occasionally develop bowel diverticula. In familial GIST, the mean age at diagnosis was 53 [3]. The majority of tumors tend to have a low mitotic rate. Mutations may affect exons in *KIT* or rarely *PDGFRA*. Altered pigmentation patterns are common, with increased pigment on

M.F. Brennan et al., *Management of Soft Tissue Sarcoma*,
DOI 10.1007/978-1-4614-5004-7_4, © Springer Science+Business Media New York 2013

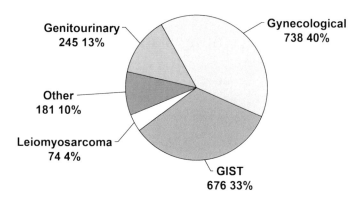

Fig. 4.1 Distribution by site for adult patients with visceral sarcomas. MSKCC 7/1/1982–6/30/2010 n = 1864 GIST = gastrointestinal stromal tumor

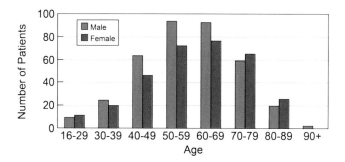

Fig. 4.2 Distribution by age and gender for adult patients with gastrointestinal stromal tumors (GIST). MSKCC 7/1/1982–6/30/2010 n = 676

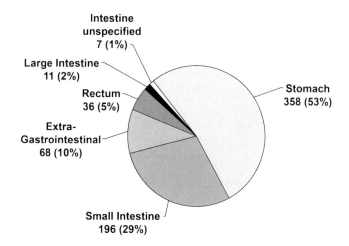

Fig. 4.3 Distribution by visceral site of adult patients with GIST. MSKCC 7/1/1982–6/30/2010 n = 676

Fig. 4.4 Contrast-enhanced axial CT of a primary large gastric GIST arising from the greater curvature, showing a large gastric wall mass, likely hypodense to spleen owing to central tumor necrosis

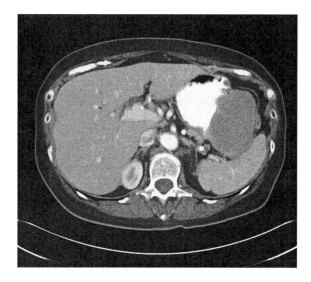

Fig. 4.5 Sagittal T2-weighted MRI of large primary rectal GIST

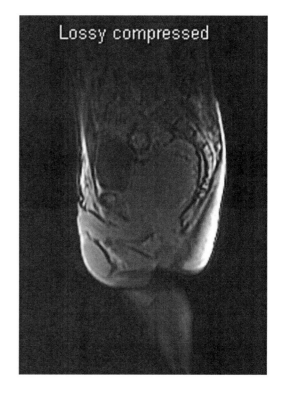

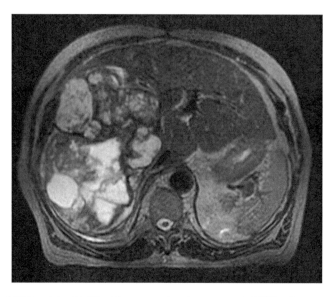

Fig. 4.6 Axial T2-weighted MRI with contrast showing metastatic GIST to liver

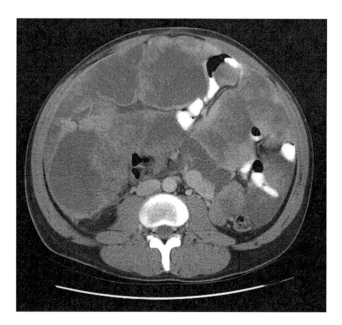

Fig. 4.7 Axial contrast-enhanced CT of extensive peritoneal metastases from GIST

the hands, feet, axilla areas, or groin (Fig. 4.8), and symptoms similar to irritable bowel syndrome from GI dysmotility are common, from hypertrophy of their myenteric plexus. The observation that *KIT* mutations may be inherited was used

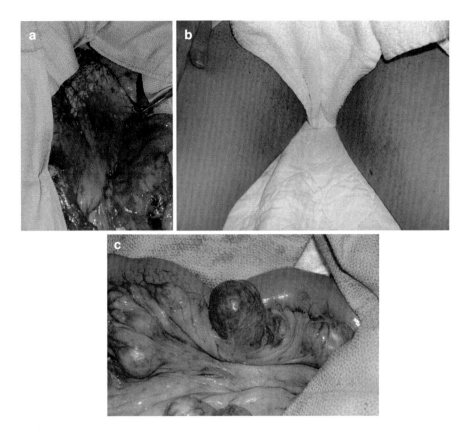

Fig. 4.8 Familial GIST with multifocal gastric and small bowel lesions (**a**), with characteristic inner thigh pigmentation (**b**) and small bowel diverticula (**c**)

to develop murine models harboring a germline gain-of-function mutation [4]. Interestingly, multiple GISTs also have been observed in patients with type I neurofibromatosis [5]; however, they often lack the presence of *KIT* or *PDGFRA* mutations. GIST is also characteristic of Carney-Stratakis syndrome (along with paragangliomas), and these tumors characteristically harbor loss-of-function mutations in succinate dehydrogenase (SDHB) associated with lack of expression of subunit B of the citric acid cycle enzyme SDHB.

Treatment of familial GIST is directed at removal of the lesion when feasible, with the understanding that metastatic disease can occur and often the source of metastasis may be indeterminate. Resection should be as conservative as possible since all sites along the GI (gastrointestinal) tract are at risk for development of GIST. Continuous long-term follow-up with symptomatic treatment appears appropriate. Imatinib is an effective treatment for unresectable or metastatic disease; however, long-term therapy in a preventative other than in an adjuvant setting is unlikely to be tested.

Natural History

Prior to the availability of tyrosine kinase inhibitors (TKI) [6], GIST had a two-year survival of 40% and a <25% five-year survival. Outcome for primary completely resected tumors was more favorable, especially for stomach and small intestine rather than for colon and rectum (Fig. 4.9) [7]. Primary tumor site, size, mitotic rate <5 mitosis per 50 high-powered fields, disease-free interval, and surgical resection were all independent predictors of improved survival. Mutational status did not predict outcome independently. It is recognized that *KIT* genetic alterations, such as deletion in exons 557–558, is a poor prognostic marker for recurrence.

With the advent of TKI, improvement in survival was clear for patients with metastatic disease. In an effort to define the role of adjuvant tyrosine kinase inhibitor, we developed a nomogram to predict relapse-free survival after operation in the absence of adjuvant therapy. This was based on the examination of 127 patients and validated utilizing an additional independent cohort. This nomogram had a concordance probability of 0.78 in the Memorial Sloan-Kettering Cancer Center dataset and 0.80 in the validation cohort. We were not able to show that inclusion of mutation status in the nomogram improved discriminatory ability of the nomogram. Utilizing this pre-tyrosine kinase dataset, we were able to show that mitotic rate, size, and location all independently predicted recurrence after resection of primary GIST. Newer versions of GIST nomograms have improved discrimination of outcome based on mitotic rate, which is a binary variable in the original nomogram [8]. In terms of risk stratification, gene expression profiling, examining for genes involved in cell checkpoints and chromosomal instability, seems to show a substantial ability to discern between people who will fare well versus those who do not [9].

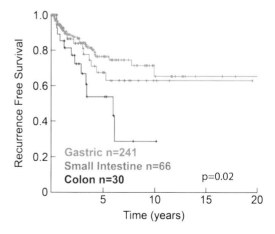

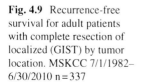
Fig. 4.9 Recurrence-free survival for adult patients with complete resection of localized (GIST) by tumor location. MSKCC 7/1/1982–6/30/2010 n = 337

Diagnosis, Molecular Pathology

Based on autopsy series, GIST is the most common sarcoma if "sarcomalets," such as microscopic GIST and incidentally noted GIST, are included, and without such caveats, GIST is the most common mesenchymal neoplasm of the gastrointestinal tract. Nearly all GISTs express the receptor tyrosine kinase KIT, and most have a mutation in the *KIT* gene. Microscopic imaging of an epithelioid GIST with KIT staining is shown in Fig. 4.10. Chi et al. demonstrated that oncogene *ETV1* is over-expressed in GIST and also characteristic of its neoplastic phenotype [10]. Much less commonly, GIST bears mutations in *PDGFRA*. Five to seven percent of GISTs do not have detectable *KIT* or *PDGFRA* and are generally termed "wild-type" (WT) GIST, although rare mutations seen in *BRAF* are the exception to the rule. Many wild-type GISTs express insulin-like growth factor 1 (IGF1) receptor (IGF1R) [11], and some of these show loss of expression of the subunit B of succinate dehydrogenase (SDHB) [12]. SDHB expression is also lost in patients with Carney-Stratakis syndrome, in whom paragangliomas are the defining tumor, due to mutations in one of the subunits of the SDH complex [13]. These two tumors and pulmonary chondromas are observed in Carney triad which has a less clear genetic etiology [14]. *IGF1R* is not mutated in GIST. It is important to be aware that there are other sarcomas that may show weak reactivity for KIT, such as leiomyosarcoma, while other tumors such as Ewing sarcoma and small cell carcinomas are often KIT positive, but such tumors do not carry activating *KIT* mutations and do not respond to imatinib. When other markers are needed to discern GIST from other tumors, *DOG1*, immunohistochemistry can be applied for a more definitive diagnosis [15, 16].

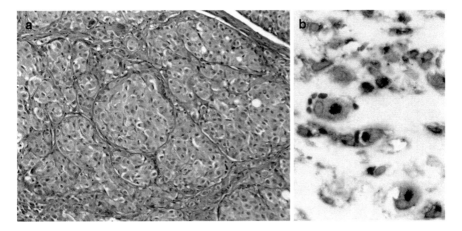

Fig. 4.10 Small bowel epithelioid GIST (**a**) with KIT positivity (**b**)

Treatment

The primary modality for higher risk tumors is surgical resection followed by 3-year adjuvant imatinib as standard of care (see below). Complete resection without encroachment of the pseudocapsule is a dominant factor in survival. The presence of metastatic disease and/or high-risk tumors is a clear indication for tyrosine kinase inhibitor treatment. Radiation has a limited role in the management of these tumors largely due to anatomic constraints and its relative radioresistance.

Adjuvant Imatinib for Primary GIST

The issue of adjuvant TKI in the treatment of GIST post-resection has been examined in prospective randomized trials. The first was designed under the aegis of the American College of Surgeons Oncology Group (ACOSOG). Patients with primary gastrointestinal stromal tumors ≥3 cm were randomized following complete gross resection and confirmation of KIT positivity to receive a placebo or imatinib for one year. This was a double-blind trial with crossover allowed if recurrence was identified. Three hundred twenty-five patients were randomized to imatinib and 319 to placebo, and there were 21 events in the imatinib group and 62 in the placebo group. This trial was positive (Fig. 4.11) with a highly significant recurrence-free survival identified and a hazard ratio of 0.33. Overall survival (Fig. 4.12) has not reached statistical significance [17]. The most dramatic effect was seen in patients

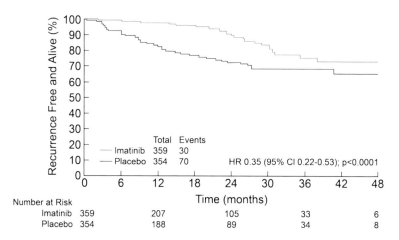

Fig. 4.11 Recurrence-free survival, randomized controlled trial of adjuvant imatinib versus placebo (Reprinted from The Lancet, Vol. 373, DeMatteo RP, Ballman KV, Antonescu CR, et al., Adjuvant imatinib mesylate after resection of localised, primary gastrointestinal stromal tumour: a randomised, double-blind, placebo-controlled trial, 1097–104, Copyright (2009), with permission from Elsevier)

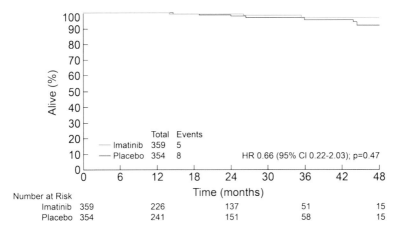

Fig. 4.12 Overall survival, randomized controlled trial of adjuvant imatinib versus placebo, size ≤5 cm (Reprinted from The Lancet, Vol. 373, DeMatteo RP, Ballman KV, Antonescu CR, et al. Adjuvant imatinib mesylate after resection of localised, primary gastrointestinal stromal tumour: a randomised, double-blind, placebo-controlled trial, 1097–104, Copyright (2009), with permission from Elsevier)

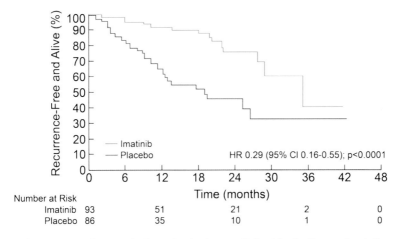

Fig. 4.13 Recurrence-free survival, randomized controlled trial of adjuvant imatinib versus placebo, size >10 cm (Reprinted from The Lancet, Vol. 373, DeMatteo RP, Ballman KV, Antonescu CR, et al. Adjuvant imatinib mesylate after resection of localised, primary gastrointestinal stromal tumour: a randomised, double-blind, placebo-controlled trial, 1097–104, Copyright (2009), with permission from Elsevier)

with tumor size >10 cm (Fig. 4.13). However, one year of imatinib does not appear sufficient to eliminate microscopic metastatic disease in most patients.

Recurrence-free survival by type of mutation was also examined [18] showing that patients with *KIT* exon 11 mutant GIST had improved recurrence-free survival over those patients with *KIT* exon 9 and *KIT* exon 11 with a deletion affecting amino acids 557 or 558 (Fig. 4.14). These initial data suggest that one year of adjuvant

Fig. 4.14 Recurrence-free survival in 127 patients with completely resected localized gastrointestinal stromal tumor (GIST) based on the type of mutation (Used with permission from DeMatteo, R.P., et al., Tumor mitotic rate, size, and location independently predict recurrence after resection of primary gastrointestinal stromal tumor (GIST). Cancer 2008. **112**(3): p. 608–15)

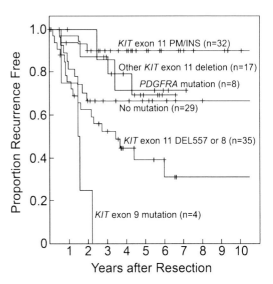

imatinib only delays recurrence but does not prevent it. The Federal Drug Administration and European Medicines Agency approved use of imatinib in the adjuvant setting. While as of 2012 the EORTC 0 versus 2 years adjuvant study data are immature, adjuvant imatinib for 3 years improved recurrence-free survival (RFS) and overall survival (OS) compared with 1 year of adjuvant treatment for GIST patients who had a high risk of recurrence after survey. RFS was longer in the 3-year group compared with the 1-year group. The 5-year RFS was 66% for the 3-year group versus 48% for the 1-year group.

The OS results were surprising. Patients assigned to 3 years of imatinib had improved 5-year OS (92%) compared to patients in the 1-year group (5-year OS = 82%). This finding had not been observed in the 1-year study of adjuvant imatinib nor in the BFR 14 study from France, in which patients with metastatic GIST stopped or continued imatinib after 1, 3, or 5 years of stable disease or better. In the latter case, there was improved PFS for those patients who continued imatinib versus those who interrupted imatinib therapy. However, OS was identical in both groups, indicating that even in the setting of metastatic disease one is not penalized by a break in therapy in terms of survival. The disparity between these three studies' overall survival outcomes is difficult to reconcile. It is noteworthy that the improvement in survival appears relatively late in the PFS and OS curves. Longer follow-up may be necessary to see if there is a true long-term difference in survival and if extenuating circumstances such as deaths from non-cancer causes or an imbalance in KIT mutation status between arms can account for some of the difference in OS observed in the SSGXVII/AIO study [19]. A subsequent phase II trial looking at 5 years of imatinib has been initiated.

Further mutation data have become available regarding adjuvant therapy from the ACOSOG Z9000 and Z9001 studies. These data will help discriminate which patients should receive therapy [20]. These data suggest that one can consider at least 1 year of therapy for patients with exon 11 *KIT* mutant gastric GIST >5 cm *and*

>5 mitoses per 50 hpf (high-power fields), or for exon 11 *KIT* mutant GIST from other sites >5 cm *or* >5 mitoses per 50 hpf. The use of imatinib in patients with GIST bearing exon 9 *KIT* mutations is controversial since 800 mg daily appear to yield a better outcome than 400 mg oral daily for such patients with metastatic disease, but was not clearly beneficial in the adjuvant setting. Patients with wild-type *KIT* and *PDGFRA* did not appear to benefit, but there appeared to be PFS benefit for patients with *PDGFRA* gene mutations other than D842V.

Neoadjuvant Therapy for Primary Disease Not Amenable to Surgery

Patients with clinically unresectable primary GIST provide an opportunity for neoadjuvant therapy prior to consideration of resection. In such a case, an unresectable or marginally resectable tumor can be rendered resectable in difficult anatomical locations such as the rectum [21]. It is generally advocated that patients continue imatinib after such surgery, given the high frequency of relapse off imatinib in such patients. In the setting of resectable disease, it is not clear at this time whether it will be better to consider imatinib with surgery as an "adjuvant" to imatinib, or imatinib as an adjuvant to surgery [22, 23]. Two studies of neoadjuvant imatinib for resectable disease indicate that such an approach is both feasible and effective [22, 23]. The long-term implications of such therapy will require longer follow-up.

Treatment of Recurrence

The primary management remains tyrosine kinase inhibitors, and the role of surgery in the treatment of recurrent disease is unclear. It does appear that there is a role for surgery or other interventions, such as radiofrequency ablation (RFA) or cryotherapy, particularly in the presence of nonresponding lesions or lesions that develop resistance to tyrosine kinase inhibitor therapy. Clinical trials are open or planned regarding the timing of surgery for recurrent disease.

Systemic Targeted Therapy for Metastatic GIST

The initial demonstration of imatinib-induced KIT inhibition and apoptosis in a GIST cell line [24] led to the first treatment of a patient with GIST with imatinib [25]. The activity of imatinib was most remarkable given the resistance of GIST to standard cytotoxic chemotherapy. The response of the first patient rapidly led to phase I [26], randomized phase II [27], and confirmatory phase II studies [28], demonstrating activity of imatinib in successively larger cohorts of patients.

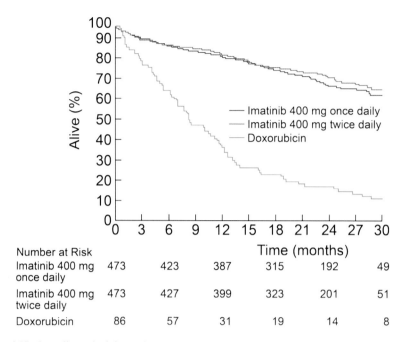

Fig. 4.15 Overall survival for patients receiving imatinib for metastatic GIST, 400 mg versus 800 mg oral daily, European/Australasian randomized study, n = 946 (Reprinted from The Lancet, Vol. 364, Verweij J, Casali PG, Zalcberg J, et al., Progression-free survival in gastrointestinal stromal tumours with high-dose imatinib: randomised trial, 1127–1134, Copyright (2004), with permission from Elsevier)

Patients with bulky disease showed improved symptoms within days of starting therapy, eventually prompting two randomized studies of 400 mg daily versus 400 mg twice daily imatinib in patients with metastatic GIST [29, 30]. The studies showed consistent ~50% RECIST (Response Evaluation Criteria In Solid Tumors) response rates in patients with metastatic disease, with survival being no different in the 400 mg and 800 mg arms, and allowed registration of imatinib at 400 mg oral daily as a first-line standard of care for metastatic GIST.

Overall survival of patients with metastatic GIST in the first published phase III study of imatinib (n = 946) is shown (Fig. 4.15). The third, nonrandomized comparator arm was a group of patients with gastrointestinal leiomyosarcoma/GIST treated with doxorubicin in older clinical trials, giving a sense of the improvement in survival achieved in patients with metastatic disease. The United States randomized study B2222 gave similar results, with median overall survival 58 months for all patients treated in this 746 patient study [29]. Patients with RECIST-stable disease survived just as long as patients with an overt RECIST partial or complete response, confirming that RECIST is inadequate for determining clinical outcomes for patients receiving imatinib for GIST [31, 32]. The lack of progression thus is the most important radiologic finding suggesting clinical benefit. PET scans can also

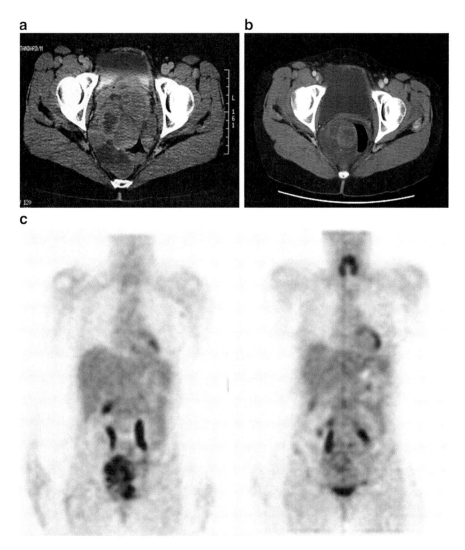

Fig. 4.16 CT and PET scan showing response to imatinib (exon 11 KIT mutation) (**a, b**) CT at 0 and 2 months, (**c**) PET at 0 and 2 weeks

track response of GIST to imatinib and other TKI but add little to CT-enhanced CT scans (Figs. 4.16 and 4.17).

Data from France indicated that patients with metastatic disease need to be treated on a lifelong basis. The basis of this recommendation is the French BFR14 study, in which patients received 12 months of imatinib. Patients doing well were randomized to continue or stop imatinib. Those stopping imatinib progressed with a median time of 6 months, compared to 28 months for those who continued imatinib [33]. Nearly all patients responded again when rechallenged with imatinib.

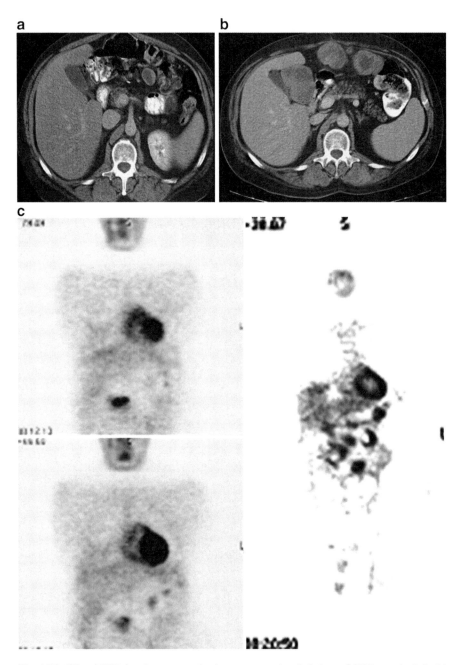

Fig. 4.17 CT and PET showing progression in response to imatinib (exon 9 KIT mutation), (**a, b**) CT at 0 and 2 mo, and (**c**) PET at 0 and 6 weeks

Overall survival for the two groups was not different. These data show imatinib can be interrupted for periods of time without a negative impact on survival. Nonetheless, as in patients with Human Immunodeficiency Virus (HIV) receiving antiretroviral therapy, the general consensus among medical oncologists is that patients tolerating imatinib well should continue imatinib unless there is intolerance despite dose reduction or disease progression. These data were confirmed in a similar study, in this case using 3 years of imatinib before randomization. A 5-year follow-up study has also been reported [34].

Although the overall survival was not different between patients receiving 400 versus 800 mg imatinib daily for metastatic disease, progression-free survival (PFS) was superior for patients taking 800 mg daily, with a hazard ratio of 0.89 at 3 years in favor of the higher dose, $p = 0.04$ [35]. It has become clear that the group of patients with largest difference in PFS by dose is that with exon 9 KIT mutations [35]. In this group, PFS was 6 months at the 400 mg daily dose versus 17 months for those taking 800 mg oral daily ($p = 0.017$). There is also a trend to improved survival for patients receiving the higher dose. Because of this subset analysis, NCCN (National Comprehensive Cancer Network) and ESMO (European Society for Medical Oncology) guidelines for GIST incorporate imatinib dose based on mutation status, specifically 400 mg oral BID for people with exon 9 KIT mutations and 400 mg oral daily for other patients [34]. KIT mutation testing is now commercially available and can also be used to guide this decision.

Who should have KIT mutation testing? Given the superior progression-free survival of patients with exon 9 mutations on higher rather than lower doses of imatinib, it would be useful to identify such patients. Notably, the vast majority of exon 9 KIT mutation GISTs arise in the small bowel; thus, consideration can be given to testing this subgroup. Of note, exon 9 KIT mutation GISTs are still the minority, even in the small bowel. Similarly, $PDGFRA$ mutations are most commonly found in the stomach, so in patients not responding to imatinib with a gastric GIST, $PDGFRA$ mutation testing can be entertained. However, since there has not been an overall survival advantage demonstrated for people who have mutation testing versus those who do not, in the era in which imatinib remains first-line therapy for treatment of GIST in the metastatic and adjuvant setting, the clinical value of such testing remains undefined.

We are also skeptical of the use of higher dose imatinib for patients with KIT exon 9 mutations since the benefit is so modest in the existing randomized clinical trials data. In the two large randomized studies of metastatic disease, at time of crossover from 400 to 800 mg oral daily imatinib, there is only modest benefit [29, 36]. Specifically, the response rate after increasing the imatinib dose is 2–3% and disease stabilization rate is 27–28% in the two randomized studies, with a median PFS of 2.5–5 months, and a 1-year PFS of ~20%.

After progression on imatinib, sunitinib was shown to be active in a phase I–II study. In comparison to placebo, sunitinib demonstrated superior PFS and overall survival in a phase III study [37]. It was approved by regulatory agencies with an 8% response rate for patients with GIST resistant or intolerant to imatinib (Fig. 4.18). In retrospect, an appropriate control group may have been to continue imatinib. It is now clear to medical oncologists that there can be an acceleration of symptoms for patients with metastatic disease when tyrosine kinase inhibitors are stopped.

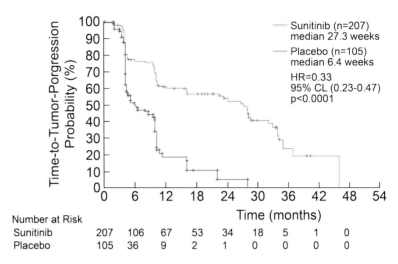

Fig. 4.18 Time to progression on sunitinib versus placebo in GIST patients failing or intolerant of imatinib (Reprinted from The Lancet, Vol. 368., Demetri GD, van Oosterom AT, Garrett CR, et al., Efficacy and safety of sunitinib in patients with advanced gastrointestinal stromal tumour after failure of imatinib: a randomised controlled trial, 1329–1338, Copyright (2006), with permission from Elsevier)

These data contribute to the concept that imatinib or sunitinib should be continued even in the setting of radiological or clinical progression since treatment may still limit tumor growth and be associated with longer survival.

Dose Intensity over Time

The first patient with GIST being treated with imatinib was in March 2000 [25]. It is worthwhile reviewing the dosing of this remarkable drug. Specifically, why is a flat dose of imatinib typically given to GIST patients, i.e., 400 mg oral daily? To a first approximation, in the five phase I-II-III studies, there appears to be no improvement in RECIST response rate or survival in patient who receive 400, 600, or 800 mg oral daily [26–30, 38]. What we do not know with this patient population is whether there will be long-term survival benefits in patients who receive lower or higher doses of imatinib. A more detailed analysis of data from the EORTC 62005 inter-group study of 400 versus 800 mg imatinib daily for patients with metastatic GIST [28] showed that a higher dose of imatinib was associated with improved response rate and survival in metastatic GIST patients who had exon 9 mutations in the *KIT* gene in their GIST [39]. Patients with exon 9 mutations fared poorly overall compared to other patients on this study.

A variety of factors that lead to imatinib resistance may be a function of dose, while others are not. Compliance, treatment interruptions, and variability of the pharmacokinetics of imatinib distribution in the body all affect the dose intensity of imatinib. However, secondary *KIT* mutations, *KIT* amplification, loss of *KIT* expression, or other factors such as OCT-1 or ABCB1 channel proteins responsible for influx and efflux of imatinib into the tumor cell are not likely so affected by dose intensity.

Reanalysis of the first large-scale randomized phase II data of patients treated with 400 versus 600 mg oral imatinib daily for GIST (B2222) showed that those patients in the lowest quartile of plasma drug concentration had the shortest time to progression, in comparison to all other patients [40]. These data are consistent with data from chronic myelogenous leukemia (CML), in which those patients with major molecular responses to therapy had a higher median trough level in comparison to patient who did not have a major molecular response; [41] however, other data do not support this contention [42].

The assessment of plasma levels of imatinib in patients with hematological malignancies is becoming a standard of care, and imatinib trough level testing should be considered in GIST in at least some clinical scenarios, though data are limited. For example, a 120-kg patient without side effects who has radiological progression on imatinib 400 mg daily could have trough level testing to indicate if dose escalation is appropriate to try and achieve a better result. These data also highlight a problem with oral therapy. It is difficult to monitor treatment on an ongoing basis when administering oral therapy, while it is much easier to document treatment compliance with intravenous agents. In examining patients with CML on imatinib, only lack of compliance was associated with failure to achieve a major molecular response [43].

Actual dose (as opposed to assigned dose) received can thus be an important indicator of benefit of imatinib therapy. In the EORTC 62005 400 versus 800 mg phase III study, patients with lower actual administered dose fared less well than those maintaining the full assigned dose. Furthermore, those patients crossed over in the 62005 study and the S0033 (USA 400 vs 800 mg) study showed that about one-third of patients had benefit when their dose was increased, i.e., stable disease or partial response as best outcome [36]. While some of this effect could be due to the well-recognized increased clearance of imatinib over time, a compliance effect was likely also important with more patients continuing the higher dose of therapy, understanding their tumor was getting worse.

Does surgery impact upon time to progression? Patients with resectable disease after imatinib therapy have a longer time to progression than those who did not have surgery. While these data are not randomized, these data suggest that resection for remaining residual disease is a way to eliminate potentially resistant disease [44–47]. Studies in Europe and the USA will help delineate this question in greater detail.

Imatinib Pharmacokinetics

Regarding imatinib pharmacokinetics, imatinib has an excellent oral bioavailability exceeding 95%, unaffected by food intake [48]. It is thought that ATP-binding cassette (ABC) pumps such as P-glycoprotein and breast cancer resistance protein

(BCP) mediate absorption of imatinib from the lining of the bowel into the circulation. ABC pumps, which are expressed in the gastrointestinal tract, are thought to pump imatinib back to the gastrointestinal lumen, thereby decreasing the absorption of imatinib [49]. As only the unbound fraction of imatinib is active, binding of imatinib to blood components also plays a major role in the activity of imatinib. The most important blood protein to which imatinib binds is alpha1-acid glycoprotein (AAG) [50].

Imatinib is converted into several metabolites. CPG74588, an N-demethylated piperazine derivate, is the most important. CPG74588 exhibits similar antitumor activity as imatinib *in vitro* and has an area under the curve (AUC) approximately 10% of that of imatinib [48]. The main metabolizing enzymes include the cytochrome P450 isoenzymes CYP3A4 and CYP3A5, though others contribute [48]. Elimination of imatinib and its metabolites occurs mainly via the bile. ABC transporters are also involved in this process, pumping imatinib and the metabolites into the bile. The remaining 15–20% is excreted by the kidneys [48]. Surprisingly, imatinib pharmacokinetics is not affected by severe hepatic dysfunction [51], and no dose modifications are required even in the case of moderate renal impairment (creatinine clearance of 20–39 mL/min) [52].

It appears that there are decreased imatinib plasma levels over time. In patients who used imatinib over approximately 12 months, the AUC after prolonged imatinib use was approximately 40% of that shortly after treatment initiation [53]. Two mechanisms have been suggested to underlie this phenomenon of decreasing imatinib levels over time. The first is increased expression of ABC transporters in the gut wall causing decreased absorption [49]; the other is increased uptake by erythrocytes [54]. Compliance and other factors may be involved.

One expects that there is a certain threshold blood level required for imatinib activity against GIST. Given the IC50 of different *KIT* isoforms, this threshold appears to differ by *KIT* or *PDGFRA* mutation status, with the highest levels required for *KIT* exon 9 mutated tumors and the lowest levels for patients with *KIT* exon 11 mutated tumors, consistent with the observed clinical data. Imatinib trough level testing may eventually become important in this setting as a result.

Second-Line Sunitinib for Imatinib-Resistant Metastatic GIST

Sunitinib was given regulatory approval based on a single phase III study, where imatinib-resistant (400 mg daily) or imatinib-intolerant patients were randomized (2:1) to sunitinib (50 mg, 4 on, 2 off) or placebo with an option to crossover at progression. In this trial, 310 patients were randomized and received sunitinib (n = 205) or placebo (n = 105). Partial responses and stable disease was seen in 7% and 58% of patients in the sunitinib arm, and no responses were seen with placebo. Median PFS in the treatment arm was 6.3 months and 1.5 months on placebo (Fig. 4.18) [37]. Interestingly, changes in serum KIT levels and other correlates of KIT and VEGF receptor blockade were observed in the sunitinib arm when compared to placebo [55, 56]. Specifically, a rising serum KIT level after 12 weeks of treatment was correlated with inferior outcome compared to those without such a rise. Responding patients tended to have either exon 9 mutations in GIST or wild-type GIST. Those patients with imatinib resistance and exon 11 mutations in KIT often had secondary mutations that rendered the masses resistant to imatinib [57].

More recently, 60 patients were treated on a phase II trial with imatinib-resistant or imatinib-intolerant GIST with daily continuous dosing of sunitinib at 37.5 mg; PFS and OS were 8.5 and 28 months, respectively [58]. This study indicated that with treatment, serum VEGF levels increased, while soluble KIT and VEGFR2 and VEGFR3 decreased. While there was a trend toward improvement in PFS and OS in patients whose serum KIT levels dropped from baseline, this was not significant until cycle 6 of treatment or later.

Other Tyrosine Kinase Inhibitors for Metastatic GIST Failing Imatinib and Sunitinib

Of the other existing tyrosine kinase inhibitors, sorafenib, nilotinib [59], vatalanib [60], and regorafenib [61] appear to have activity greater than observation alone; a phase III study of regorafenib vs placebo in patients with imatinib and sunitinib refractory GIST showed a significant difference in progression free survival, and is likely to become a de facto third line of therapy. Masitinib has activity in 1st-line metastatic GIST patients [62] and thus may be useful in later lines as well, as may be pazopanib. Dasatinib appears to have activity specifically in *PDGFRA* D842V mutation-positive GIST [63]. Activity of these agents in later lines of therapy [59] suggests examination of these drugs as an earlier line of treatment during a patient's clinical course.

Newer Agents

It appears that at least three-quarters of *KIT* mutant GIST patients progressing on imatinib develop secondary mutations in *KIT* that render the molecule insensitive to imatinib and often to other tyrosine kinase inhibitors. The heterogeneity of secondary mutations in one tumor limits the utility of tyrosine kinase inhibitors in this setting. How can these multiple resistant clones be managed medically? After imatinib and sunitinib, sorafenib and other TKI appear [64] to have some activity, as noted above, but by and large responses are limited, as is the duration of response.

It is clear that resistant GISTs are genetically heterogeneous, even within one tumor or anatomical site [44, 57, 65–68]. Resistant clones can be identified by polymerase chain reaction, indicating selection of clones as a reason for imatinib resistance [69]. Other than differences in mitotic rate, it is not at all clear why some patients develop resistance more rapidly than others. Regardless, patients need a therapy with a different mechanism for activity against a wide spectrum of evolving mutations.

One approach to imatinib- and/or sunitinib-refractory GIST is to "vertically" target multiple steps in *KIT* signaling. The recent availability of new inhibitors of downstream target TOR (target of rapamycin) and more recently the PI3K (phosphatidylinositol 3-kinase) family of proteins makes combinations with receptor tyrosine kinase inhibitors natural combinations to examine [70].

Drugs targeting the molecular chaperone hsp90 (heat shock protein of 90-kD molecular mass) may provide an avenue to pursue for tyrosine kinase inhibitor-resistant GIST. The hsp90 family of proteins (two proteins in humans, termed hsp84 and hsp86) are "chaperone" proteins, in that they are responsible for proper folding and function of oncogenic and normal proteins alike. It is hypothesized that proteins expressed from mutated genes are more structurally unstable and thus more dependent upon the refolding function of hsp90 family members than their wild-type counterparts [71]. Interestingly, both imatinib-sensitive and imatinib-resistant GIST cell lines are sensitive to the effects of hsp90 inhibitors such as retaspimycin (IPI504), a more soluble version of the classic geldanamycin analogue 17-AAG. It is also notable that a *PDGFRA* mutant GIST cell line is sensitive to IPI504.

These translational data informed a clinical trial of retaspimycin in patients with GIST. Decreased activity by PET (positron emission tomography) scan was observed in 16 of 22 evaluable patients, although only 1 of 36 had a RECIST response to therapy (as did 1 of 11 patients with other sarcomas treated with retaspimycin) [72]. Thus, like in CML and BCR-ABL, these findings provide some support for the contention that GIST remains dependent upon *KIT* expression and signaling even after the development of multiple mutations. However, a phase III study of retaspimycin against best supportive care was stopped early, owing to early deaths on the treatment arm. These data will be important in planning future studies of other agents in third and greater line of treatment.

The biology of GIST continues to fascinate biologists and clinicians alike, looking for a means to treat patients with this difficult clinical problem. Rational combinations of existing agents and new drugs targeted against non-kinase portions of *KIT* or components of the downstream signaling cascade may become increasingly important, and it will be important to rigorously prove benefit so that GIST remains an effective proof-of-concept disease for innovative drug development. For example, IGF1R (insulin-like growth factor 1 receptor) antagonists may be active in GIST that lack *KIT* mutations [73, 74]. Perhaps *KIT* inhibitors will have to be administered with IGF1R, EGFR (epidermal growth factor), or other inhibitors to block activation of parallel kinase pathways usurped by GIST to maintain AKT signaling. This example is one in which horizontal blockade of signaling pathways may prove as important as the vertical blockade of one pathway at different steps. Thanks to new basic and translational science, the near future will be exciting for GIST research, in particular as the signaling pathway and dependence of GIST upon *KIT* signaling are unraveled (Table 4.1).

Table 4.1 Recommendations for systemic therapy for patients with GIST[a]

Clinical scenario		Comments
Adjuvant setting		PFS and overall survival are improved with 3 years of imatinib in the adjuvant setting for higher risk tumors. An easy rule of thumb includes treatment of patients with exon 11 *KIT* mutant gastric GIST>5 cm *and*>5 mitoses per 50 hpf, or for exon 11 *KIT* mutant GIST from other sites>5 cm *or*>5 mitoses per 50 hpf. The use of imatinib in patients with GIST bearing exon 9 *KIT* mutations is controversial. Based on available data, patients with WT *KIT* and *PDGFRA* or D842V, *PDGFRA* mutant GIST should not receive adjuvant imatinib, although patients with *PDGFRA* mutation other than D842V may benefit
Metastatic disease	First line	Imatinib 400 mg daily; to consider increase to 800 mg oral daily if exon 9 *KIT* mutant. Patients with recurrent *PDGFRA* mutant or WT *KIT/PDGFR* GIST should be considered for alternative clinical studies given the low response rate with imatinib
	Second line	Sunitinib; we favor dosing at 37.5 mg oral daily without interruption
	Third line and beyond	Regorafenib; sorafenib, nilotinib, masitinib, pazopanib, or other RTK inhibitors; clinical trials; imatinib rechallenge

[a]Clinical trials are always appropriate if available

References

1. Kindblom LG, Remotti HE, Aldenborg F, Meis-Kindblom JM. Gastrointestinal pacemaker cell tumor (GIPACT): gastrointestinal stromal tumors show phenotypic characteristics of the interstitial cells of Cajal. Am J Pathol. 1998;152:1259–69.
2. DeMatteo RP, Lewis JJ, Leung D, Mudan SS, Woodruff JM, Brennan MF. Two hundred gastrointestinal stromal tumors: recurrence patterns and prognostic factors for survival. Ann Surg. 2000;231:51–8.
3. Kleinbaum EP, Lazar AJ, Tamborini E, et al. Clinical, histopathologic, molecular and therapeutic findings in a large kindred with gastrointestinal stromal tumor. Int J Cancer. 2008; 122:711–8.
4. Antonescu CR. Gastrointestinal stromal tumor (GIST) pathogenesis, familial GIST, and animal models. Semin Diagn Pathol. 2006;23:63–9.
5. Yantiss RK, Rosenberg AE, Sarran L, Besmer P, Antonescu CR. Multiple gastrointestinal stromal tumors in type I neurofibromatosis: a pathologic and molecular study. Mod Pathol. 2005;18:475–84.
6. Gold JS, van der Zwan SM, Gonen M, et al. Outcome of metastatic GIST in the era before tyrosine kinase inhibitors. Ann Surg Oncol. 2007;14:134–42.
7. Dematteo RP, Gold JS, Saran L, et al. Tumor mitotic rate, size, and location independently predict recurrence after resection of primary gastrointestinal stromal tumor (GIST). Cancer. 2008;112:608–15.
8. Rossi S, Miceli R, Messerini L, et al. Natural history of imatinib-naive GISTs: a retrospective analysis of 929 cases with long-term follow-up and development of a survival nomogram based on mitotic index and size as continuous variables. Am J Surg Pathol. 2011;35:1646–56.

9. Lagarde P, Perot G, Kauffmann A, et al. Mitotic Checkpoints and Chromosome Instability Are Strong Predictors of Clinical Outcome in Gastrointestinal Stromal Tumors. Clin Cancer Res. 2012;18(3):826–38.

10. Chi P, Chen Y, Zhang L, et al. ETV1 is a lineage survival factor that cooperates with KIT in gastrointestinal stromal tumours. Nature. 2010;467:849–53.

11. Tarn C, Rink L, Merkel E, et al. Insulin-like growth factor 1 receptor is a potential therapeutic target for gastrointestinal stromal tumors. Proc Natl Acad Sci USA. 2008;105:8387–92.

12. Janeway KA, Kim SY, Lodish M, et al. Defects in succinate dehydrogenase in gastrointestinal stromal tumors lacking KIT and PDGFRA mutations. Proc Natl Acad Sci USA. 2011; 108:314–8.

13. Pasini B, McWhinney SR, Bei T, et al. Clinical and molecular genetics of patients with the Carney-Stratakis syndrome and germline mutations of the genes coding for the succinate dehydrogenase subunits SDHB, SDHC, and SDHD. Eur J Hum Genet. 2008;16:79–88.

14. Stratakis CA, Carney JA. The triad of paragangliomas, gastric stromal tumours and pulmonary chondromas (Carney triad), and the dyad of paragangliomas and gastric stromal sarcomas (Carney-Stratakis syndrome): molecular genetics and clinical implications. J Intern Med. 2009;266:43–52.

15. West RB, Corless CL, Chen X, et al. The novel marker, DOG1, is expressed ubiquitously in gastrointestinal stromal tumors irrespective of KIT or PDGFRA mutation status. Am J Pathol. 2004;165:107–13.

16. Espinosa I, Lee CH, Kim MK, et al. A novel monoclonal antibody against DOG1 is a sensitive and specific marker for gastrointestinal stromal tumors. Am J Surg Pathol. 2008;32:210–8.

17. Dematteo RP, Ballman KV, Antonescu CR, et al. Adjuvant imatinib mesylate after resection of localised, primary gastrointestinal stromal tumour: a randomised, double-blind, placebo-controlled trial. Lancet. 2009;373:1097–104.

18. Dematteo RP, Gold JS, Saran L, et al. Tumor mitotic rate, size, and location independently predict recurrence after resection of primary gastrointestinal stromal tumor (GIST). Cancer. 2008;112:608–15.

19. Joensuu H, Eriksson M, Hatrmann J, et al. Twelve versus 36 months of adjuvant imatinib (IM) as treatment of operable GIST with a high risk of recurrence: final results of a randomized trial (SSGXVIII/AIO). ASCO Meeting Abstracts. 2011;29:LBA1.

20. Corless CL, Ballman KV, Antonescu C, et al. Relation of tumor pathologic and molecular features to outcome after surgical resection of localized primary gastrointestinal stromal tumor (GIST): results of the intergroup phase III trial ACOSOG Z9001. J Clin Oncol (Meeting Abstr). 2010;28:10006.

21. Fiore M, Palassini E, Fumagalli E, et al. Preoperative imatinib mesylate for unresectable or locally advanced primary gastrointestinal stromal tumors (GIST). Eur J Surg Oncol. 2009;35:739–45.

22. Eisenberg BL, Harris J, Blanke CD, et al. Phase II trial of neoadjuvant/adjuvant imatinib mesylate (IM) for advanced primary and metastatic/recurrent operable gastrointestinal stromal tumor (GIST): early results of RTOG 0132/ACRIN 6665. J Surg Oncol. 2009;99:42–7.

23. McAuliffe JC, Hunt KK, Lazar AJ, et al. A randomized, phase II study of preoperative plus postoperative imatinib in GIST: evidence of rapid radiographic response and temporal induction of tumor cell apoptosis. Ann Surg Oncol. 2009;16:910–9.

24. Tuveson DA, Willis NA, Jacks T, et al. STI571 inactivation of the gastrointestinal stromal tumor c-KIT oncoprotein: biological and clinical implications. Oncogene. 2001;20:5054–8.

25. Joensuu H, Roberts PJ, Sarlomo-Rikala M, et al. Effect of the tyrosine kinase inhibitor STI571 in a patient with a metastatic gastrointestinal stromal tumor. N Engl J Med. 2001;344:1052–6.

26. van Oosterom AT, Judson I, Verweij J, et al. Safety and efficacy of imatinib (STI571) in metastatic gastrointestinal stromal tumours: a phase I study. Lancet. 2001;358:1421–3.

27. Demetri GD, von Mehren M, Blanke CD, et al. Efficacy and safety of imatinib mesylate in advanced gastrointestinal stromal tumors. N Engl J Med. 2002;347:472–80.

28. Verweij J, van Oosterom A, Blay JY, et al. Imatinib mesylate (STI-571 Glivec, Gleevec) is an active agent for gastrointestinal stromal tumours, but does not yield responses in other

soft-tissue sarcomas that are unselected for a molecular target. Results from an EORTC Soft Tissue and Bone Sarcoma Group phase II study. Eur J Cancer. 2003;39:2006–11.

29. Blanke CD, Rankin C, Demetri GD, et al. Phase III randomized, intergroup trial assessing imatinib mesylate at two dose levels in patients with unresectable or metastatic gastrointestinal stromal tumors expressing the kit receptor tyrosine kinase: S0033. J Clin Oncol. 2008;26: 626–32.

30. Verweij J, Casali PG, Zalcberg J, et al. Progression-free survival in gastrointestinal stromal tumours with high-dose imatinib: randomised trial. Lancet. 2004;364:1127–34.

31. Benjamin RS, Choi H, Macapinlac HA, et al. We should desist using RECIST, at least in GIST. J Clin Oncol. 2007;25:1760–4.

32. Choi H, Charnsangavej C, Faria SC, et al. Correlation of computed tomography and positron emission tomography in patients with metastatic gastrointestinal stromal tumor treated at a single institution with imatinib mesylate: proposal of new computed tomography response criteria. J Clin Oncol. 2007;25:1753–9.

33. Blay JY, Le Cesne A, Ray-Coquard I, et al. Prospective multicentric randomized phase III study of imatinib in patients with advanced gastrointestinal stromal tumors comparing interruption versus continuation of treatment beyond 1 year: the French Sarcoma Group. J Clin Oncol. 2007;25:1107–13.

34. Demetri GD, Benjamin RS, Blanke CD, et al. NCCN Task Force report: management of patients with gastrointestinal stromal tumor (GIST)–update of the NCCN clinical practice guidelines. J Natl Compr Canc Netw. 2007;5:S1–29.

35. GSTM-AG (MetaGIST). Comparison of two doses of imatinib for the treatment of unresectable or metastatic gastrointestinal stromal tumors: a meta-analysis of 1,640 patients. J Clin Oncol. 2010;28:1247–53.

36. Zalcberg JR, Verweij J, Casali PG, et al. Outcome of patients with advanced gastro-intestinal stromal tumours crossing over to a daily imatinib dose of 800 mg after progression on 400 mg. Eur J Cancer. 2005;41:1751–7.

37. Demetri GD, van Oosterom AT, Garrett CR, et al. Efficacy and safety of sunitinib in patients with advanced gastrointestinal stromal tumour after failure of imatinib: a randomised controlled trial. Lancet. 2006;368:1329–38.

38. Blanke CD, Demetri GD, von Mehren M, et al. Long-term results from a randomized phase II trial of standard- versus higher-dose imatinib mesylate for patients with unresectable or metastatic gastrointestinal stromal tumors expressing KIT. J Clin Oncol. 2008;26:620–5.

39. Van Glabbeke MM, Owzar K, Rankin C, Simes J, Crowley J. Comparison of two doses of imatinib for the treatment of unresectable or metastatic gastrointestinal stromal tumors (GIST): a meta-analyis based on 1,640 patients. J Clin Oncol. 2007;25:Abstr 10004.

40. von Mehren M, Wang Y, Joensuu H, Blanke CD, Wehrle E, Demetri GD. Imatinib pharmacokinetics and its correlation with clinical response in patients with unresectable/metastatic gastrointestinal stromal tumor. J. Clin. Oncol. 2008;26:Abstr 4523.

41. Larson RA, Druker BJ, Guilhot F, et al. Imatinib pharmacokinetics and its correlation with response and safety in chronic-phase chronic myeloid leukemia: a subanalysis of the IRIS study. Blood. 2008;111:4022–8.

42. Forrest DL, Trainor S, Brinkman RR, et al. Cytogenetic and molecular responses to standard-dose imatinib in chronic myeloid leukemia are correlated with Sokal risk scores and duration of therapy but not trough imatinib plasma levels. Leuk Res. 2009;33:271–5.

43. Marin D, Bazeos A, Mahon F-X, et al. Adherence is the critical factor for achieving molecular responses in patients with chronic myeloid leukemia who achieve complete cytogenetic responses on imatinib. J Clin Oncol. 2010;28:2381–8.

44. DeMatteo RP, Maki RG, Singer S, Gonen M, Brennan MF, Antonescu CR. Results of tyrosine kinase inhibitor therapy followed by surgical resection for metastatic gastrointestinal stromal tumor. Ann Surg. 2007;245:347–52.

45. Gronchi A, Fiore M, Miselli F, et al. Surgery of residual disease following molecular-targeted therapy with imatinib mesylate in advanced/metastatic GIST. Ann Surg. 2007;245:341–6.

46. Raut CP, Posner M, Desai J, et al. Surgical management of advanced gastrointestinal stromal tumors after treatment with targeted systemic therapy using kinase inhibitors. J Clin Oncol. 2006;24:2325–31.
47. Rutkowski P, Nowecki Z, Nyckowski P, et al. Surgical treatment of patients with initially inoperable and/or metastatic gastrointestinal stromal tumors (GIST) during therapy with imatinib mesylate. J Surg Oncol. 2006;93:304–11.
48. Peng B, Lloyd P, Schran H. Clinical pharmacokinetics of imatinib. Clin Pharmacokinet. 2005;44:879–94.
49. Burger H, van Tol H, Brok M, et al. Chronic imatinib mesylate exposure leads to reduced intracellular drug accumulation by induction of the ABCG2 (BCRP) and ABCB1 (MDR1) drug transport pumps. Cancer Biol Ther. 2005;4:747–52.
50. Delbaldo C, Chatelut E, Re M, et al. Pharmacokinetic-pharmacodynamic relationships of imatinib and its main metabolite in patients with advanced gastrointestinal stromal tumors. Clin Cancer Res. 2006;12:6073–8.
51. Ramanathan RK, Egorin MJ, Takimoto CH, et al. Phase I and pharmacokinetic study of imatinib mesylate in patients with advanced malignancies and varying degrees of liver dysfunction: a study by the National Cancer Institute Organ Dysfunction Working Group. J Clin Oncol. 2008;26:563–9.
52. Gibbons J, Egorin MJ, Ramanathan RK, et al. Phase I and pharmacokinetic study of imatinib mesylate in patients with advanced malignancies and varying degrees of renal dysfunction: a study by the National Cancer Institute Organ Dysfunction Working Group. J Clin Oncol. 2008;26:570–6.
53. Judson I, Ma P, Peng B, et al. Imatinib pharmacokinetics in patients with gastrointestinal stromal tumour: a retrospective population pharmacokinetic study over time. EORTC Soft Tissue and Bone Sarcoma Group. Cancer Chemother Pharmacol. 2005;55:379–86.
54. Prenen H, Guetens G, De Boeck G, Highley M, van Oosterom AT, de Bruijn EA. Everolimus alters imatinib blood partition in favour of the erythrocyte. J Pharm Pharmacol. 2006;58:1063–6.
55. Deprimo SE, Huang X, Blackstein ME, et al. Circulating levels of soluble KIT serve as a biomarker for clinical outcome in gastrointestinal stromal tumor patients receiving sunitinib following imatinib failure. Clin Cancer Res. 2009;15:5869–77.
56. Norden-Zfoni A, Desai J, Manola J, et al. Blood-based biomarkers of SU11248 activity and clinical outcome in patients with metastatic imatinib-resistant gastrointestinal stromal tumor. Clin Cancer Res. 2007;13:2643–50.
57. Heinrich MC, Maki RG, Corless CL, et al. Primary and secondary kinase genotypes correlate with the biological and clinical activity of sunitinib in imatinib-resistant gastrointestinal stromal tumor. J Clin Oncol. 2008;26:5352–9.
58. George S, Blay JY, Casali PG, et al. Clinical evaluation of continuous daily dosing of sunitinib malate in patients with advanced gastrointestinal stromal tumour after imatinib failure. Eur J Cancer. 2009;45:1959–68.
59. Italiano A, Cioffi A, Coco P, et al. Patterns of care, prognosis, and survival in patients with metastatic gastrointestinal stromal tumors (GIST) refractory to first-line imatinib and second-line sunitinib. Ann Surg Oncol. 2012;19(5):1551–9.
60. Joensuu H, De Braud F, Grignagni G, et al. Vatalanib for metastatic gastrointestinal stromal tumour (GIST) resistant to imatinib: final results of a phase II study. Br J Cancer. 2011;104:1686–90.
61. Demetri GD. Differential properties of current tyrosine kinase inhibitors in gastrointestinal stromal tumors. Semin Oncol. 2011;38 Suppl 1:S10–9.
62. Le Cesne A, Blay JY, Bui BN, et al. Phase II study of oral masitinib mesilate in imatinib-naive patients with locally advanced or metastatic gastro-intestinal stromal tumour (GIST). Eur J Cancer. 2010;46:1344–51.
63. Dewaele B, Wasag B, Cools J, et al. Activity of dasatinib, a dual SRC/ABL kinase inhibitor, and IPI-504, a heat shock protein 90 inhibitor, against gastrointestinal stromal tumor-associated PDGFRAD842V mutation. Clin Cancer Res. 2008;14:5749–58.

64. Kindler HL, Campbell NP, Wroblewski K, et al. Sorafenib (SOR) in patients (pts) with imatinib (IM) and sunitinib (SU)-resistant (RES) gastrointestinal stromal tumors (GIST): Final results of a University of Chicago Phase II Consortium trial. ASCO Meeting Abstracts. 2011;29:10009.
65. Antonescu CR, Besmer P, Guo T, et al. Acquired resistance to imatinib in gastrointestinal stromal tumor occurs through secondary gene mutation. Clin Cancer Res. 2005;11:4182–90.
66. Debiec-Rychter M, Cools J, Dumez H, et al. Mechanisms of resistance to imatinib mesylate in gastrointestinal stromal tumors and activity of the PKC412 inhibitor against imatinib-resistant mutants. Gastroenterology. 2005;128:270–9.
67. Heinrich MC, Corless CL, Blanke CD, et al. Molecular correlates of imatinib resistance in gastrointestinal stromal tumors. J Clin Oncol. 2006;24:4764–74.
68. Wardelmann E, Thomas N, Merkelbach-Bruse S, et al. Acquired resistance to imatinib in gastro-intestinal stromal tumours caused by multiple KIT mutations. Lancet Oncol. 2005;6:249–51.
69. Liegl B, Kepten I, Le C, et al. Heterogeneity of kinase inhibitor resistance mechanisms in GIST. J Pathol. 2008;216:64–74.
70. Schoffski P, Reichardt P, Blay JY, et al. A phase I-II study of everolimus (RAD001) in combi-nation with imatinib in patients with imatinib-resistant gastrointestinal stromal tumors. Ann Oncol. 2010;21:1990–8.
71. Taldone T, Gozman A, Maharaj R, Chiosis G. Targeting Hsp90: small-molecule inhibitors and their clinical development. Curr Opin Pharmacol. 2008;8:370–4.
72. Wagner AJ, Morgan JA, Chugh R, et al. Inhibition of heat shock protein 90 with the novel agent IPI-504 in metastatic GIST following failure of tyrosine kinase inhibitors or other sarco-mas: Clinical results from phase I trial. J Clin Oncol. 2008;26:abstract 10503.
73. Prakash S, Sarran L, Socci N, et al. Gastrointestinal stromal tumors in children and young adults: a clinicopathologic, molecular, and genomic study of 15 cases and review of the litera-ture. J Pediatr Hematol Oncol. 2005;27:179–87.
74. Tarn C, Rink L, Merkel E, et al. Insulin-like growth factor 1 receptor is a potential therapeutic target for gastrointestinal stromal tumors. Proc Natl Acad Sci. 2008;105:8387–92.

Chapter 5
Liposarcoma

Liposarcoma is primarily a tumor that occurs (Fig. 5.1) with peak incidence between ages 50 and 70 and equal gender distribution. As described previously (see Chap. 1, Fig. 1.6), liposarcomas account for approximately 20% of all soft tissue sarcomas in adults. Anatomic distribution of liposarcoma is wide (Fig. 5.2) and is usually considered to manifest in three biological subtypes. The most common type is well-differentiated liposarcoma (sometimes called atypical lipomatous tumor [ALT]) and its high-grade variant dedifferentiated liposarcoma. The second most common is myxoid (low-grade) and round cell (high-grade) liposarcoma. The least common is (high-grade) pleomorphic liposarcoma. Each subtype has a very distinctive morphology, natural history, and genetic changes utilized in diagnosis.

Well-differentiated (WD) liposarcoma or ALT is used to describe nonmetastasizing low-grade lipomatous neoplasms that have a propensity for local recurrence. The term ALT is applied to extremity lesions, while WD liposarcoma is the preferred term for retroperitoneal and truncal lesions. It is important to realize that ALT recurs much more commonly than lipomas and is considered to have malignant potential due to the higher incidence of local recurrence. The presence of ring, giant, and marker chromosomes in the 12q15 region for both ALT and WD liposarcomas confirms that the lesions are members of the same category of tumor, hence the use of the ALT/WD liposarcoma in the World Health Organization classification. On our review of 800 patients with a histological diagnosis of liposarcoma [1], ALT rarely recurred, whereas WD liposarcoma, particularly of sclerosing type, was more likely to recur.

WD liposarcoma is locally aggressive, nonmetastasizing, and composed of mature adipocytes of variable size and focal atypia. These tumors present as deep-seated enlarging masses often of very large sizes. They have been subdivided into adipocytic or lipoma-like, sclerosing type, and inflammatory. The characteristic cytogenetic abnormality detected in most WD liposarcomas is the supranumerary ring and giant marker chromosome. *HDM2*, *CDK4*, and *HMGIC* are consistently amplified; all of these genes are located at chromosome 12q14-15 region. The high-grade counterpart of WD is dedifferentiated liposarcoma and is most common in younger patients in their third to fourth decade of life. Dedifferentiated liposarcoma

M.F. Brennan et al., *Management of Soft Tissue Sarcoma*,
DOI 10.1007/978-1-4614-5004-7_5, © Springer Science+Business Media New York 2013

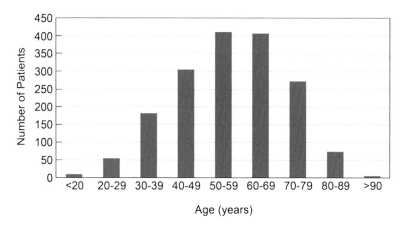

Fig. 5.1 Age distribution for adult patients with liposarcoma, all sites. MSKCC 7/1/1982–6/30/2010 n = 1,713

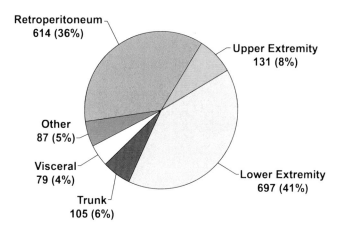

Fig. 5.2 Site distribution for adult patients with liposarcoma, all patients. MSKCC 7/1/1982–6/30/2010 n = 1,713

occurs much more frequently in the retroperitoneum compared to extremities. In the retroperitoneum, it more often presents *de novo* rather than subsequently presents in recurrences (Fig. 5.3). The kidney is often surrounded, and adherence to the capsule is seen, usually without parenchymal invasion (see "Treatment" below). The most frequent morphology of the nonlipogenic component includes myxofibrosarcoma or undifferentiated pleomorphic sarcoma (formerly termed malignant fibrous histiocytoma), although other histologies such as osteogenic sarcoma or rhabdomyosarcoma are not infrequently observed as well. Notably, these secondary histologies do not predict for a more aggressive course than the dedifferentiated liposarcoma component itself.

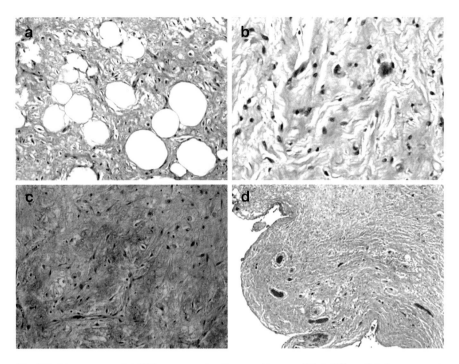

Fig. 5.3 Liposarcoma: (**a**) WD component with myxoid areas; (**b**) dedifferentiated component, nonlipogenic low grade; (**c**) dedifferentiated component high grade; (**d**) renal capsule adherence

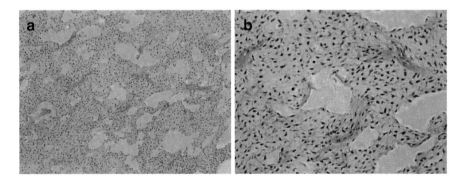

Fig. 5.4 Low-grade liposarcoma, without round cell component (**a** and **b**)

Myxoid liposarcoma (Fig. 5.4) and its high-grade counterpart round cell liposarcoma account for up to 40% of all liposarcomas. They are often large at time of presentation (Fig. 5.5). The histologic picture is composed of uniform, round or oval primitive nonlipogenic mesenchymal cells with a variable number of small signet ring lipoblasts, all in a prominent myxoid stroma. A characteristic branching vascular pattern described as "chicken wire" is commonly seen. Studies have shown

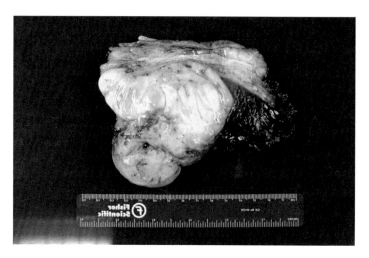

Fig. 5.5 Gross resection of low-grade myxoid liposarcoma left posterior thigh, 15.2 × 10.1 × 6.3 cm

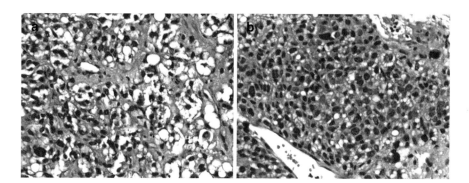

Fig. 5.6 Pleomorphic liposarcoma, needle biopsy (**a** and **b**)

that >5% of round cell defines the high-grade variant with significant risk of metastatic disease. Most commonly, the myxoid/round cell subtype occurs in the deep tissues of the extremities, usually the proximal thigh.

Pleomorphic liposarcoma (Fig. 5.6) is a highly malignant sarcoma containing variable quantities of pleomorphic lipoblasts. Mitotic activity is always high, and hemorrhage and necrosis very common, all features of a high-grade sarcoma. Pleomorphic liposarcoma accounts for fewer than 5% of all liposarcomas and is commonly present in an older age group, usually in the deep soft tissue of the extremities. Early metastasis is common, almost always to the lung. Distribution of the various histologic subtypes of liposarcoma is seen in Fig. 5.7 and by subtype and by site, Fig. 5.8.

Outcome is site dependent with lower risk of local recurrence in extremity lesions. Those tumors that did recur in our institution occurred late, often after 5 years [1]. WD liposarcoma situated in the retroperitoneum and mediastinum

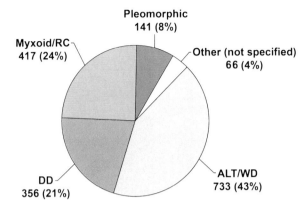

Fig. 5.7 Distribution of adult patients with liposarcoma by histology, all sites. MSKCC 7/1/1982–6/30/2010 n = 1,713. *DD* dedifferentiated, *ALT/WD* atypical lipomatous tumor/well differentiated

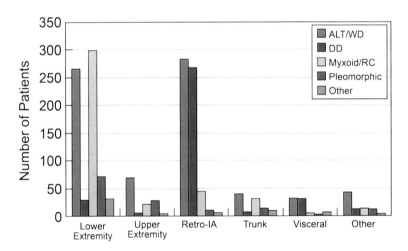

Fig. 5.8 Distribution of adult patients with liposarcoma by site and histology. MSKCC 7/1/1982–6/30/2010 n = 1,713. *DD* dedifferentiated, *ALT/WD* atypical lipomatous tumor/well differentiated, *RC* round cell, *IA* intra-abdominal

recurs consistently, often accompanied by dedifferentiation and ultimately metastasis in some. It is difficult to determine how frequent dedifferentiation occurs, but it is certainly greater than 10% and, probably in a lifetime, approaches 40%.

Imaging

Imaging is characteristic, particularly in the retroperitoneum, where well-differentiated components can be readily identified and often accompanied by subsequent dedifferentiation. On CT imaging, this portion of the tumor has fat density, typically

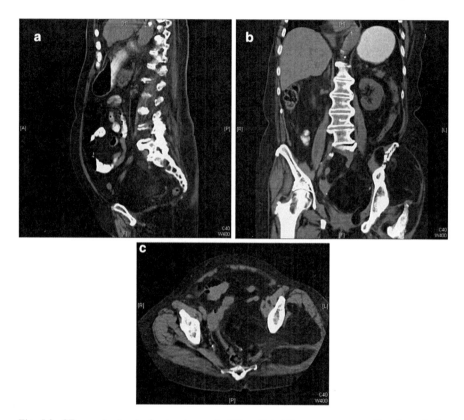

Fig. 5.9 CT scan (**a, b, c**) of extensive well-differentiated liposarcoma, extending through the pelvis into the buttock

Hounsfield units (HU). The dedifferentiated component has more variable but higher density by HU; a minimum of 0 HU for defining the dedifferentiated component may be useful in characterizing these tumors, but this concept has not been examined prospectively. Once a recurrence has occurred, the lesions are often multifocal and unlikely to be cured by further operative procedures. In the retroperitoneum, lesions are large, often with a well-differentiated component that can be present for years (Figs. 5.9 and 5.10). The majority usually develops a dedifferentiated component, and it is this higher-grade component that increases the risk of progression with displacement, but not invasion of intra-abdominal organs (Fig. 5.11). The largest of these tumors can reach large size and extend into the buttock and thigh (Figs. 5.12 and 5.13). Pleomorphic liposarcoma has a relatively high risk of metastasis to multiple sites including lung, soft tissue, bone, and liver (Fig. 5.14). Myxoid/round cell liposarcoma has an unusual predilection for unusual sites of soft tissue metastasis (Fig. 5.15) and subsequent death, making surveillance for metastases a challenge, as noted below in the section on radiation therapy.

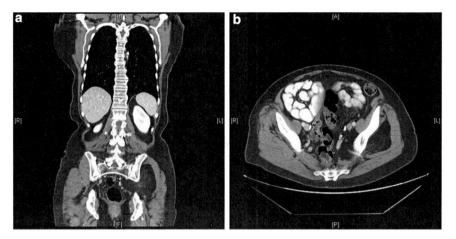

Fig. 5.10 Well-differentiated liposarcoma of pelvis and buttock with encasement of L5 nerve root and superior gluteal vessels (**a, b**)

Diagnosis

The genetics of each type of liposarcoma makes them as distinct from one another as breast adenocarcinoma is from renal cell carcinoma, and their biology and the results of treatment vary substantially. WD and dedifferentiated liposarcomas have characteristic amplifications of chromosome 12q, giant chromosomes, ring chromosomes, and marker chromosomes, in particular loci around genes encoding *CDK4* and *HDM2* (the human version of *MDM2*). Myxoid-round cell liposarcomas usually contain t(12;16) with *FUS-DDIT3* (genes formerly termed *TLS* and *CHOP*, respectively) and occasionally t(12;22) *EWSR1-DDIT3* (see Chap. 1, Table 1.1). Both are distinct from pleomorphic liposarcoma, which has genetic characteristics more in common with undifferentiated pleomorphic sarcoma (UPS, formerly termed malignant fibrous histiocytoma [MFH]) than the other forms of liposarcoma.

Treatment

The dominant treatment of all liposarcoma subtypes remains surgical resection. The extent of surgical resection is dependent both on the site of the lesion and the underlying histopathology. As with all sarcomas, complete gross resection is essential. The extent of the resection beyond complete gross resection will vary by site and by type. ALT often presents late as a large lesion and has a somewhat tenuous membrane or pseudocapsule at the time of initial dissection, and simple but large excision is adequate. High-grade sarcomas require a more extensive resection with a 2 cm margin of normal tissue but limited by adjacent neurovascular structures.

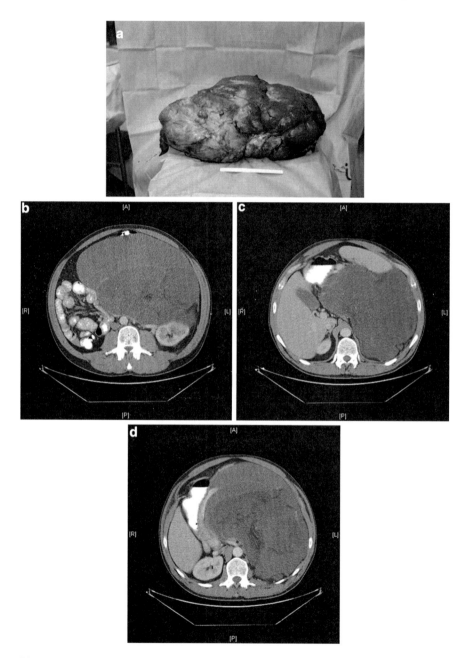

Fig. 5.11 Gross specimen (**a**) and CT of well-differentiated liposarcoma with dedifferentiated elements, showing displacement of (**b**) kidney, (**c**) spleen, and (**d**) pancreas

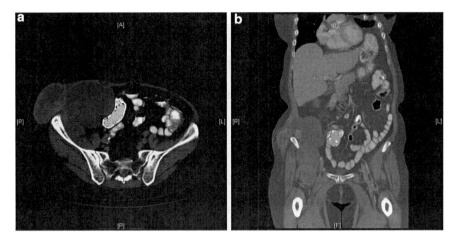

Fig. 5.12 CT of dedifferentiated liposarcoma with retroperitoneal transpelvic extension into thigh (**a** and **b**)

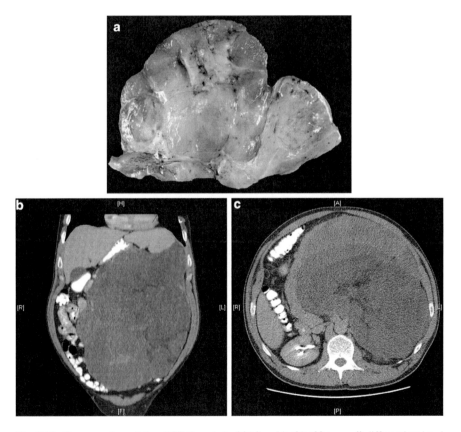

Fig. 5.13 Gross specimen (**a**) and CT (**b** and **c**) of 31 lbs, 44×31×23 cm well-differentiated and dedifferentiated liposarcoma

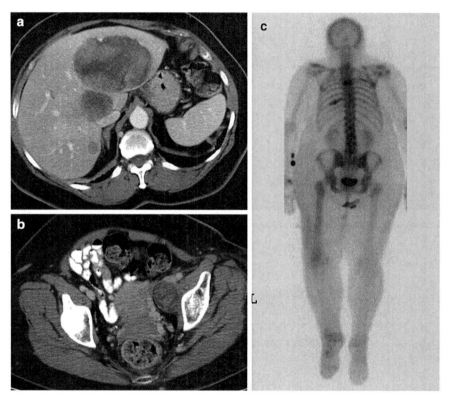

Fig. 5.14 Axial CT (**a** and **b**) and PET scan (**c**) of metastatic pleomorphic liposarcoma to liver, retroperitoneum, and bone

The focus on the extremity is continued preservation of function as local recurrence has only limited, if any, effect on long-term survival.

The object at the first operation in the retroperitoneum is complete gross resection. We have not shown a benefit to more extended resections to involve adjacent but uninvolved organs [2]. It is important to appreciate that the kidney is rarely involved by parenchymal invasion and capsular adherence can be treated by capsular excision (Fig. 5.3). Recurrence is common and multifocal recurrence very common. On the majority of occasions when there is no identifiable high-grade or dedifferentiated recurrence, low-grade recurrence can be followed symptomatically. Aggressive use of chemotherapy or radiation in this situation is not justified.

Where the patient is symptomatic, reoperation can be advised with some evidence that even an incomplete resection can palliate symptoms and be associated with prolonged survival [3]. In the extremity, bone invasion is very uncommon, but periosteal adherence is possible and requires periosteal stripping. The latter is associated with increased risk of fracture if adjuvant radiation is employed [4]. In the retroperitoneum, recurrent lesions, in contradistinction to primary lesions, can often invade or involve previously dissected tissue especially viscera and mesentery. This can often present in solvable local problems with great morbidity (Fig. 5.16).

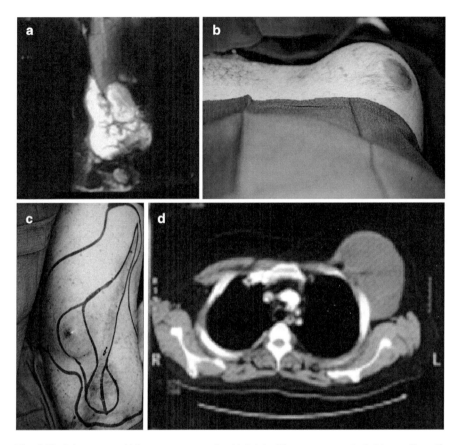

Fig. 5.15 Primary myxoid liposarcoma posterior thigh (a) with metastases to the left breast (b, c, d)

Radiation Therapy

Radiation therapy for a variety of clinical situations with liposarcoma remains a matter of controversy. As a generalization, local radiation therapy can limit local recurrence particularly in extremity lesions. Attempts at performing randomized trials for selective populations in other sites have failed. In the main, radiation therapy is most commonly used preoperatively for retroperitoneal and intra-abdominal lesions and very selectively for low-grade extremity lesions. Conversely, as low-grade retroperitoneal WD liposarcoma can exist for many years without symptoms or progression, overvigorous utilization of radiation therapy in these patients is not justified and is accompanied by significant morbidity. In a manuscript examining the benefit of radiation to patients with positive surgical margins, it does seem clear that if a patient received preoperative radiation therapy, then additional postoperative radiation therapy is not of benefit even in the presence of positive microscopic margins [5]. It has been suggested that myxoid liposarcoma is more radiosensitive than other liposarcomas or other soft tissue sarcomas [6]. This suggests that radiation

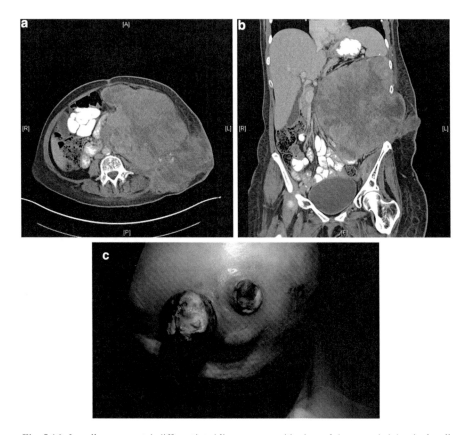

Fig. 5.16 Locally recurrent dedifferentiated liposarcoma with visceral, bony, and abdominal wall invasion

therapy can be utilized when metastatic disease from myxoid liposarcoma is identified. As noted above, myxoid liposarcoma is one of the sarcomas that commonly recur in nonpulmonary sites in comparison to other soft tissue sarcomas of the extremity, such as soft tissue, spine, and bony pelvis [7], and radiation therapy can be effective in palliation of disease in this and other sites (Fig. 5.15). It is also notable that such bony metastases of myxoid liposarcoma are often not observed with CT scan, PET, or bone scan, but only visible by MRI [7, 8].

Many groups have utilized radiation therapy more aggressively than we do, but the data to support such an approach is limited and the potential complications significant.

Systemic Therapy: General Considerations

It is particularly important to recall the three major forms of liposarcoma when deciding upon systemic therapy for patients with metastatic disease [9–20]. The recurrence patterns of these tumors differ substantially, with retroperitoneal WD and dedifferentiated liposarcoma recurring much more commonly in the abdomen than metastasizing. Sites for the unusual dedifferentiated-well-differentiated liposarcoma that does metastasize include other fatty sites of the body or bone as frequently as lung. Myxoid-round cell liposarcoma particularly metastasizes to other fatty sites of the body (e.g., mediastinum, bone marrow of the spine/pelvis) [7, 8], making assessment of response as challenging as identifying the key metastatic sites of disease in the first place.

Adjuvant Therapy

Given the 0% response rate for WD and very low response rate for dedifferentiated liposarcoma to doxorubicin-ifosfamide [21], it is clear that adjuvant chemotherapy is not indicated for this diagnosis. Given the resemblance of pleomorphic liposarcoma to UPS (see Chap. 7) and sensitivity to doxorubicin-ifosfamide, use of adjuvant therapy for this diagnosis should be discussed on a case-by-case basis for those patients with high-risk disease. The Royal Marsden paper [21] and two studies including patients receiving adjuvant or neoadjuvant therapy for myxoid liposarcoma [22, 23] indicate the relative sensitivity to chemotherapy of myxoid-round cell liposarcoma. However, data regarding adjuvant chemotherapy are conflicting when considering extremity sarcomas, with many negative and few positive studies of patients with an array of histologies [24]. The Pervaiz 2008 meta-analysis suggests a clinically meaningful effect of chemotherapy on overall survival [25].

If there is an "adult" sarcoma histology in which chemotherapy may be helpful (along with synovial sarcoma), it is myxoid/round cell liposarcoma, and for young patients with higher-risk disease, we will offer systemic adjuvant or neoadjuvant chemotherapy for tumors over 5 cm in size. This recommendation may be an over-reading or underreading of the literature, and treating physicians are encouraged to review the primary data.

Treatment of Metastatic Disease

Subsets of liposarcoma and their response to chemotherapy in the recurrent or metastatic setting were not well defined before the publication from the Royal Marsden group of the results of chemotherapy for patients with metastatic liposarcoma, grouped by liposarcoma subtype [21]. This has been the most instructive paper in highlighting the differences in doxorubicin-ifosfamide therapy for each of the diagnoses. In this study of 88 patients receiving chemotherapy for recurrent or metastatic liposarcoma, Jones et al. found patients with myxoid liposarcoma had a significantly higher response rate compared to all other liposarcoma patients, 48% (95%CI; 28–69) and 18% (95%CI; 8–31). Fourteen percent of patients had received adjuvant therapy, typically with doxorubicin-ifosfamide. Despite the higher response rate for the lower-grade tumor, there was a longer time to progression for the high-grade version of the tumor (round cell liposarcoma) in comparison to myxoid lipos-arcoma, 16 months versus 4 months (with wide and overlapping confidence intervals), indicating at least some activity of chemotherapy in both myxoid and round cell liposarcomas. Notably, the response rate (largely using RECIST [Response Evaluation Criteria In Solid Tumors]) for patients with WD liposarcoma was 0. No data were provided on the specific utility of trabectedin, known to be active in myxoid-round cell liposarcoma [26].

Other studies examining patients with primary and metastatic liposarcoma demonstrate [23] or deduce [22] that myxoid-round cell liposarcoma is relatively sensitive to doxorubicin- or ifosfamide-based chemotherapy.

Patients with myxoid and round cell liposarcoma demonstrate significant sensitivity to the minor groove-binding agent trabectedin (ET743), approved for clinical use in Europe, although not approved in the United States as of 2011 [26]. Although real and reproducible activity was seen in a number of phase II studies with trabectedin in myxoid-round cell liposarcoma, the randomized phase II study of patients with all forms of leiomyosarcoma and liposarcoma treated with trabectedin as a 24-hour infusion versus 1-hour infusion showed RECIST 1.0 response rates of 6% and 2%, respectively [27]. Of note, trabectedin was active in both schedules, though median progression-free survival was only modestly different, at 3.7 months for the 24-hour arm q 3 weeks versus 2.3 months for the 3-hours weekly infusion arm ($p < 0.02$ after multivariate adjustment) [27] (Fig. 5.17). Although the data on time to progression as a function of sarcoma subtype were not published, in the authors' experience, the responses to trabectedin were in patients with myxoid/round cell liposarcoma and largely only stable disease for patients with leiomyosarcoma or well-differentiated or dedifferentiated liposarcoma.

While the paper by Jones et al. noted activity of doxorubicin-ifosfamide in pleomorphic liposarcoma [21], there are only anecdotal data that pleomorphic liposarcoma can respond to gemcitabine-docetaxel, with two of three patients on a randomized study responding to gemcitabine-based therapy [28], suggesting a unique sensitivity of this form of liposarcoma, which we have seen in patients treated off study. Similarly, gemcitabine-docetaxel has occasionally been associated with minor responses of the dedifferentiated form of liposarcoma, although we have not observed responses of WD liposarcoma to any form of systemic therapy to date.

Similarly, responses of any of these forms of liposarcoma to kinase-directed agents have been largely fruitless to date [29–32], indicating the need to focus more on the activity seen with trabectedin in these sarcomas as well as the role by which these largely aneuploid tumors (save myxoid-round cell liposarcoma) maintain their aneuploidy without undergoing apoptosis (Tables 5.1, 5.2, and 5.3).

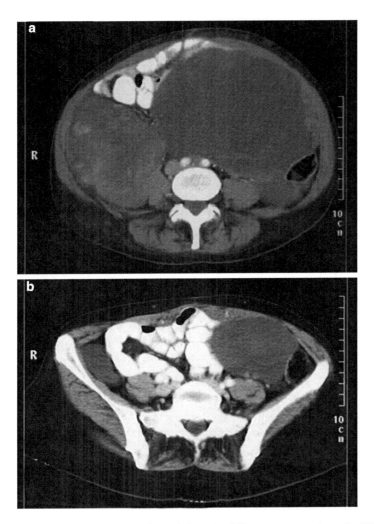

Fig. 5.17 Axial CT scan of response of myxoid/round cell liposarcoma to trabectedin (ET743)–
(**a**) at diagnosis (**b**) after 7 months of treatment

Outcomes

Mortality rates for liposarcoma vary widely depending on the underlying histopathology and have been reported to vary from 1% to 90%, firmly establishing the
importance of histological subtyping. Recurrence is common and, depending on site
and histopathology, has equal wide range. In addition to the histological subtype,
histological grade remains a dominant factor in outcome, often reflecting the extent
of differentiation or dedifferentiation. We have recently described a subtype-specific
nomogram for patients with primary liposarcoma [33], which allows better

Table 5.1 Recommendations for systemic therapy for patients with well-differentiated/dedifferentiated liposarcoma[a]

Clinical scenario		Comments
Adjuvant chemotherapy		Not employed
Metastatic/recurrent disease[a]	First line	Anthracycline[a] or anthracycline-ifosfamide
	Second line	Gemcitabine alone or in combination with docetaxel or vinorelbine
		Trabectedin (in Europe)
	Third line	Clinical trial; supportive care

[a]Only the dedifferentiated component may respond; clinical trials are always an appropriate option

Table 5.2 Recommendations for systemic therapy for patients with myxoid-round cell liposarcoma

Clinical scenario		Comments
Adjuvant chemotherapy		Anthracycline-ifosfamide for 4–6 cycles in patients with high-risk myxoid-round cell liposarcoma
Metastatic disease	First line	Anthracycline or anthracycline-ifosfamide
	Second line	Ifosfamide if not used in first line; gemcitabine-docetaxel appears inactive
		Trabectedin in Europe (myxoid-round cell and possibly well-differentiated/dedifferentiated liposarcomas only)
	Third line	Clinical trial; supportive care

Table 5.3 Recommendations for systemic therapy for patients with pleomorphic liposarcoma*

Clinical scenario		Comments
Adjuvant chemotherapy		Remains controversial, to be discussed on a case-by-case basis
Metastatic disease	First line	Anthracycline ± ifosfamide[a] or gemcitabine alone or in combination with docetaxel or vinorelbine
	Second line	Agent(s) not used in first line
	Third line	Clinical trial; supportive care

[a]PEGylated liposomal doxorubicin (Doxil®/Caelyx®) if poor performance status or elderly
*Clinical trials are always appropriate if available

characterization of outcome. The clear delineation between the subtypes is seen (Fig. 5.18), and a nomogram has been established based on over 800 patients presenting with primary liposarcoma to our institution. The breakdown by histological subtype was 46% WD, 18% dedifferentiated, 18% myxoid, 10% round cell, and 8% pleomorphic.

Outcome is also dependent on site (Fig. 5.19) and the ability to obtain a complete gross resection. Once a complete gross resection has been achieved, a negative microscopic margin contributes a small but limited benefit. In the retroperitoneum, microscopic margin has not been identified as an important issue for recurrence or survival.

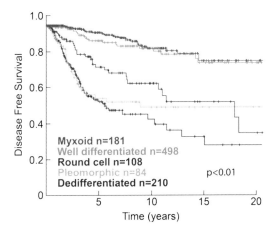

Fig. 5.18 Disease-specific survival of adult patients with primary liposarcoma by histology. MSKCC 7/1/1982–6/30/2010 n = 1,081

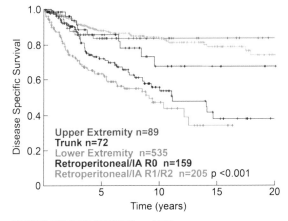

Fig. 5.19 Disease-specific survival of adult patients with primary liposarcoma by site. MSKCC 7/1/1982–6/30/2010 n = 1,060

MSKCC 7/1/1982-6/30/2010 n=1060
**RO and R1 for all sites except Retro-IA which is R0 vs R1/R2

Outcome Following Metastasis

While there can be patients with responses to trabectedin for three or more years, responses to systemic therapy are not durable for the majority of patients. As an upper boundary, a European summary of 51 patients treated with trabectedin noted their myxoid/round cell liposarcoma population had a median progression-free survival of 14 months [34], while the Jones paper from Royal Marsden noted better survival for patients with lower-grade liposarcomas, despite a lower response rate [21]. Inhibitors of CDK4 and HDM2 are now being studied as new potential approaches for patients with recurrent WD/DD liposarcoma [35, 36]. WD/DD liposarcoma remains a frustrating disease for patients, surgeons, radiation oncologists, and medical oncologists alike.

References

1. Kooby DA, Antonescu CR, Brennan MF, et al. Atypical lipomatous tumor/well-differentiated liposarcoma of the extremity and trunk wall: importance of histological subtype with treatment recommendations. Ann Surg Oncol. 2004;11(1):78–84.
2. Russo P, Brady MS, Conlon K, et al. Adult urological sarcoma. J Urol. 1992;147(4):1032–6. discussion 1036–7.
3. Shibata D, Lewis JJ, Leung DH, et al. Is there a role for incomplete resection in the management of retroperitoneal liposarcomas? J Am Coll Surg. 2001;193(4):373–9.
4. Alektiar KM, Hu K, Anderson L, et al. High-dose-rate intraoperative radiation therapy (HDR-IORT) for retroperitoneal sarcomas. Int J Radiat Oncol Biol Phys. 2000;47(1):157–63.
5. Al Yami A, Griffin AM, Ferguson PC, et al. Positive surgical margins in soft tissue sarcoma treated with preoperative radiation: is a postoperative boost necessary? Int J Radiat Oncol Biol Phys. 2010;77(4):1191–7.
6. Chung PW, Deheshi BM, Ferguson PC, et al. Radiosensitivity translates into excellent local control in extremity myxoid liposarcoma: a comparison with other soft tissue sarcomas. Cancer. 2009;115(14):3254–61.
7. Schwab JH, Boland PJ, Antonescu C, et al. Spinal metastases from myxoid liposarcoma warrant screening with magnetic resonance imaging. Cancer. 2007;110(8):1815–22.
8. Schwab JH, Boland P, Guo T, et al. Skeletal metastases in myxoid liposarcoma: an unusual pattern of distant spread. Ann Surg Oncol. 2007;14(4):1507–14.
9. Verweij J, Baker LH. Future treatment of soft tissue sarcomas will be driven by histological subtype and molecular aberrations. Eur J Cancer. 2010;46(5):863–8.
10. Romeo S, Dei Tos AP. Soft tissue tumors associated with EWSR1 translocation. Virchows Arch. 2010;456(2):219–34.
11. Rieker RJ, Weitz J, Lehner B, et al. Genomic profiling reveals subsets of dedifferentiated liposarcoma to follow separate molecular pathways. Virchows Arch. 2010;456(3):277–85.
12. Guillou L, Aurias A. Soft tissue sarcomas with complex genomic profiles. Virchows Arch. 2010;456(2):201–17.
13. Pires de Camargo V, Van de Rijn M, Maestro R, et al. Other targetable sarcomas. Semin Oncol. 2009;36(4):358–71.
14. Goransson M, Andersson MK, Forni C, et al. The myxoid liposarcoma FUS-DDIT3 fusion oncoprotein deregulates NF-kappaB target genes by interaction with NFKBIZ. Oncogene. 2009;28(2):270–8.
15. Italiano A, Bianchini L, Keslair F, et al. HMGA2 is the partner of MDM2 in well-differentiated and dedifferentiated liposarcomas whereas CDK4 belongs to a distinct inconsistent amplicon. Int J Cancer. 2008;122(10):2233–41.
16. Italiano A, Cardot N, Dupre F, et al. Gains and complex rearrangements of the 12q13-15 chromosomal region in ordinary lipomas: the "missing link" between lipomas and liposarcomas? Int J Cancer. 2007;121(2):308–15.
17. Antonescu CR. The role of genetic testing in soft tissue sarcoma. Histopathology. 2006;48(1):13–21.
18. Dei Tos AP. Liposarcoma: new entities and evolving concepts. Ann Diagn Pathol. 2000;4(4):252–66.
19. Mertens F, Fletcher CD, Dal Cin P, et al. Cytogenetic analysis of 46 pleomorphic soft tissue sarcomas and correlation with morphologic and clinical features: a report of the CHAMP Study Group. Chromosomes and MorPhology. Genes Chromosomes Cancer. 1998;22(1):16–25.
20. Turc-Carel C, Limon J, Dal Cin P, et al. Cytogenetic studies of adipose tissue tumors. II. Recurrent reciprocal translocation t(12;16)(q13;p11) in myxoid liposarcomas. Cancer Genet Cytogenet. 1986;23(4):291–9.
21. Jones RL, Fisher C, Al-Muderis O, et al. Differential sensitivity of liposarcoma subtypes to chemotherapy. Eur J Cancer. 2005;41(18):2853–60.

22. Eilber FC, Eilber FR, Eckardt J, et al. The impact of chemotherapy on the survival of patients with high-grade primary extremity liposarcoma. Ann Surg. 2004;240(4):686–95.
23. Patel SR, Burgess MA, Plager C, et al. Myxoid liposarcoma. Experience with chemotherapy. Cancer. 1994;74(4):1265–9.
24. Pisters PW, O'Sullivan B, Maki RG. Evidence-based recommendations for local therapy for soft tissue sarcomas. J Clin Oncol. 2007;25(8):1003–8.
25. Pervaiz N, Colterjohn N, Farrokhyar F, et al. A systematic meta-analysis of randomized controlled trials of adjuvant chemotherapy for localized resectable soft-tissue sarcoma. Cancer. 2008;113(3):573–81.
26. Grosso F, Sanfilippo R, Virdis E, et al. Trabectedin in myxoid liposarcomas (MLS): a long-term analysis of a single-institution series. Ann Oncol. 2009;20(8):1439–44.
27. Demetri GD, Chawla SP, von Mehren M, et al. Efficacy and safety of trabectedin in patients with advanced or metastatic liposarcoma or leiomyosarcoma after failure of prior anthracyclines and ifosfamide: results of a randomized phase II study of two different schedules. J Clin Oncol. 2009;27(25):4188–96.
28. Maki RG, Wathen JK, Patel SR, et al. Randomized phase II study of gemcitabine and docetaxel compared with gemcitabine alone in patients with metastatic soft tissue sarcomas: results of sarcoma alliance for research through collaboration study 002 [corrected]. J Clin Oncol. 2007;25(19):2755–63.
29. Chawla SP, Tolcher AW, Sankhala KK, et al. Updated interim results of a phase 2 study of the mTOR inhibitor AP23573 in patients with advanced sarcomas of soft tissue or bone. In: Connective Tissue Oncology Society 15th Annual Meeting, Vol. 15. Boca Raton; 2005. Abstract 447.
30. Chugh R, Wathen JK, Maki RG, et al. Phase II multicenter trial of imatinib in 10 histologic subtypes of sarcoma using a bayesian hierarchical statistical model. J Clin Oncol. 2009;27(19):3148–53.
31. Maki RG, D'Adamo DR, Keohan ML, et al. Phase II study of sorafenib in patients with metastatic or recurrent sarcomas. J Clin Oncol. 2009;27(19):3133–40.
32. Sleijfer S, Ray-Coquard I, Papai Z, et al. Pazopanib, a multikinase angiogenesis inhibitor, in patients with relapsed or refractory advanced soft tissue sarcoma: a phase II study from the European organisation for research and treatment of cancer-soft tissue and bone sarcoma group (EORTC study 62043). J Clin Oncol. 2009;27(19):3126–32.
33. Dalal KM, Kattan MW, Antonescu CR, et al. Subtype specific prognostic nomogram for patients with primary liposarcoma of the retroperitoneum, extremity, or trunk. Ann Surg. 2006;244(3):381–91.
34. Grosso F, Jones RL, Demetri GD, et al. Efficacy of trabectedin (ecteinascidin-743) in advanced pretreated myxoid liposarcomas: a retrospective study. Lancet Oncol. 2007;8(7):595–602.
35. Muller CR, Paulsen EB, Noordhuis P, et al. Potential for treatment of liposarcomas with the MDM2 antagonist Nutlin-3A. Int J Cancer. 2007;121(1):199–205.
36. Singer S, Socci ND, Ambrosini G, et al. Gene expression profiling of liposarcoma identifies distinct biological types/subtypes and potential therapeutic targets in well-differentiated and dedifferentiated liposarcoma. Cancer Res. 2007;67(14):6626–36.

Chapter 6
Leiomyosarcoma

Leiomyosarcoma (LMS) is one of the most common forms of soft-tissue sarcoma, with approximately 2,500 cases per year in the United States in 2010. The age distribution of adult leiomyosarcoma is seen in Fig. 6.1.

Leiomyosarcoma occurs in multiple different sites in the body (Fig. 6.2). Approximately half are located in the retroperitoneum or intra-abdominal sites, most commonly in the uterus. Leiomyosarcoma can arise in major vessels including the inferior vena cava (Figs. 6.3, 6.4, and 6.5). It is important to recognize that leiomyosarcomas are excellent examples of the difference in biology of the tumor based on anatomic site. For example, cutaneous leiomyosarcomas are lesions with a much better prognosis, appearing as small cutaneous nodules and classified as low grade regardless of histological appearance.

Leiomyosarcomas are easier to characterize based on the relatively consistent presence of markers such as desmin and smooth muscle actin easily noted using standard immunohistochemistry (Fig. 6.6), and thus there may be greater concordance between pathologists in the diagnosis of leiomyosarcoma than other forms of soft-tissue sarcoma. However, there is heterogeneity appreciated even in this group of sarcomas. Leiomyosarcomas may contain epithelioid or myxoid changes, with unclear relevance for outcome but posing diagnostic challenges to pathologists. Similar to GIST with different mutation patterns in *KIT* and different outcomes depending on the primary tumor site (gastric, small bowel, other), it is also evident that there are important biological differences in leiomyosarcomas depending on their site of origin.

Imaging

In the extremity, MRI is usually preferred although CT provides similar information. In the retroperitoneum, CT and MRI provide differing information but the MRI, on occasion, showing better vascular delineation. Unfortunately, in incompletely

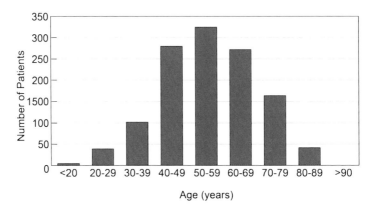

Fig. 6.1 Distribution by age of adult patients with leiomyosarcoma, all sites. MSKCC 7/1/1982–6/30/2010 n = 1,229

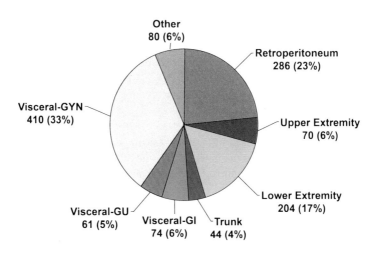

Fig. 6.2 Distribution by site of adult patients with leiomyosarcoma. MSKCC 7/1/1982–6/30/2010 n = 1,229 *GYN* gynecologic, *GU* genitourinary, *GI* gastrointestinal

resected lesions, local-regional progression is common (Fig. 6.7). Metastases are readily identified on CT, with the liver as a common site for visceral primaries (Fig. 6.8) and lung the most common metastatic sites for uterine and extremity primaries.

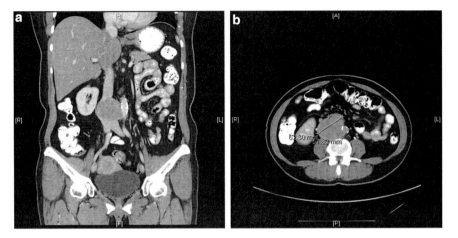

Fig. 6.3   CT scan (**a** & **b**) of high-grade leiomyosarcoma of inferior vena cava

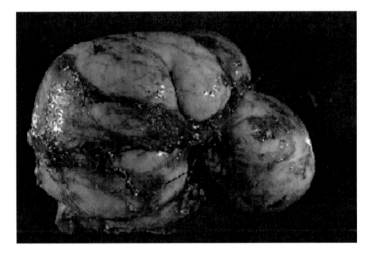

Fig. 6.4   Gross specimen of leiomyosarcoma of inferior vena cava

Diagnosis, Molecular Pathology

Leiomyosarcomas must be differentiated from leiomyomas, cellular schwannomas, as well as other sarcomas such as GIST, depending on the anatomic location. The differentiation between leiomyoma and leiomyosarcoma is particularly difficult in the uterus, where even benign lesions may have a high mitotic rate. As a result, for

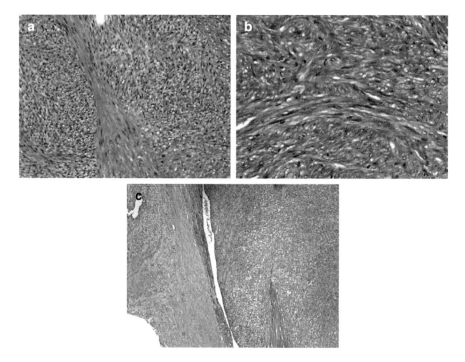

Fig. 6.5 Microscopic features (**a**, **b**, **c**) of leiomyosarcoma, with IVC wall invasion

borderline uterine lesions, the term smooth muscle tumor of uncertain mitotic potential (STUMP) is used [1]. It has been suggested that high levels of CA125 can help to distinguish the uterine leiomyosarcoma from uterine leiomyoma, but this remains to be confirmed [2]. Historically, many of the gastrointestinal leiomyosarcomas have proven to be GIST based on immunoreactivity to *KIT*.

A similar designation is given to another rare low-grade lesion termed Epstein-Barr virus-associated smooth muscle tumor (EBV-SMT), found in patients on chronic immunosuppressive therapy or with HIV disease. EBV-SMT usually presents in unusual anatomical locations and can be multifocal, which mimics metastases, and is characterized by very slow but persistent growth. Similarly perivascular epithelial cell tumors (PEComas) must be differentiated from leiomyosarcomas, the former expressing both markers of smooth muscle and melanocytes [3]. Leiomyosarcomas are typically composed of eosinophilic spindle cells arranged in intersecting fascicles at 90° angles and associated with variable amounts of necrosis, mitotic activity, and atypia, depending on the grade of the lesion (Fig. 6.9).

By immunohistochemistry, leiomyosarcomas are positive for desmin, smooth muscle actin, muscle specific actin, and caldesmon, and rarely other markers such as cytokeratins or EMA in the epithelioid subtype. Leiomyosarcomas have an

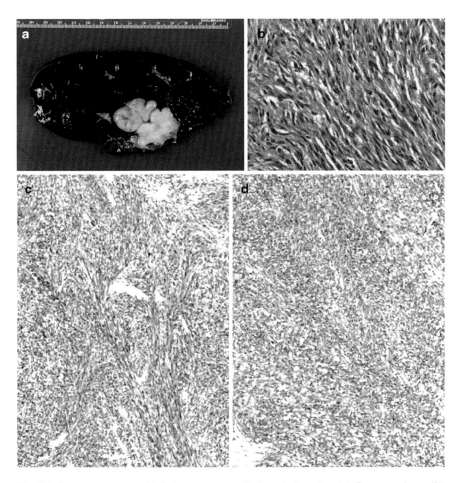

Fig. 6.6 Leiomyosarcoma of inferior vena cava with hepatic invasion, (a) Gross specimen, (b) microscopic features, immunohistochemistry for (c) desmin and (d) smooth muscle actin (SMA)

aneuploid karyotype [4–6]. More than half of leiomyosarcomas examined show karyotypes with profound structural aberrations, e.g., numerical changes and deletions of chromosomes 1, 13, 14, 16, 18, and 22, but the frequency of any specific aberration is <20%.

Treatment

As with other sarcomas, the primary treatment is surgical with complete resection necessary for prolonged survival. Lesions of unusual sites such as the inferior vena cava can require some technically challenging resections and reconstruction [7].

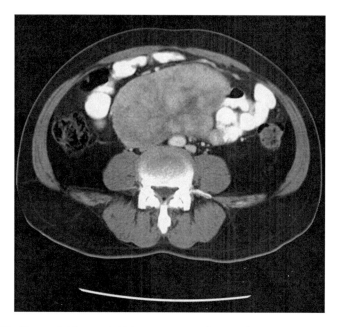

Fig. 6.7 CT of incompletely resected leiomyosarcoma of retroperitoneum

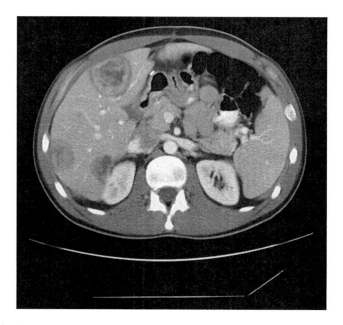

Fig. 6.8 CT of metastatic leiomyosarcoma to liver

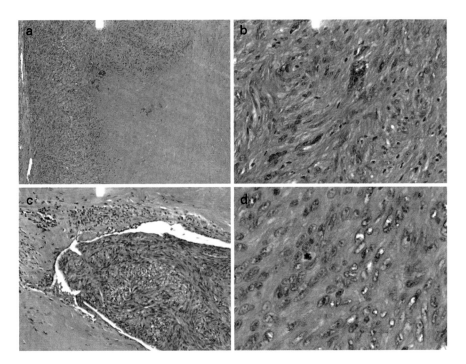

Fig. 6.9 Histologic features of high-grade leiomyosarcoma (**a, b, c, d**)

It has long been suggested that the replacement of the vena cava is required, but we have found that that is not necessary, and the majority of patients, as long as they have adequate venous drainage from at least one kidney, can safely have the vena cava tied distal to the inflow of the hepatic veins without major long-term sequelae. As the inferior vena cava is commonly occluded at the time of presentation, collaterals have developed such that caval replacement is not necessary. However, the extensive collaterals can complicate the procedure, as all such vessels not involved by tumor should be preserved. Diligent attention in the immediate postoperative period to the prevention of peripheral edema is such that significant edema is prevented and resolved, usually followed by clinical improvement and resolution of swelling of the lower extremities within 6–8 weeks of the procedure. Exercise tolerance appears limited in some patients following inferior vena cava (IVC) ligation, perhaps owing to the vasodilation and venous pooling that occurs with exercise. Situations where the vena cava can be simply patched are preferable to its ligation if possible. A simple alternative using peritoneum to patch the vena cava [8] has been supplanted by other alternatives such as bovine pericardium.

Radiation Therapy

As with other soft-tissue sarcomas, adjuvant radiation is generally employed for tumors over 5 cm in size or those with difficult anatomic constraints such as those of the head and neck. External beam radiation, either in the adjuvant or neoadjuvant setting, is appropriate for high-grade leiomyosarcomas over 5 cm in size [9, 10] or brachytherapy for high-grade soft-tissue sarcomas over 5 cm in size [11]. There remains controversy regarding the use of radiation therapy in the adjuvant setting for uterine sarcomas, though published data indicate no clear benefit in terms of progression free or overall survival, though local recurrences were reduced [12, 13]. In a large tumor registry analysis, overall survival was not affected by adjuvant radiation, though lower local-regional recurrence risk was associated with adjuvant radiation therapy [14]. In our practice, adjuvant radiation is employed for uterine sarcomas only for overt involvement of pelvic wall structures.

Systemic Therapy

Adjuvant Chemotherapy

Adjuvant chemotherapy with doxorubicin or with gemcitabine-docetaxel has been examined prospectively in patients with uterine leiomyosarcomas. The Gynecologic Oncology Group conducted the first prospective randomized trial comparing adjuvant chemotherapy to no further therapy in patients with stage I or II uterine sarcoma, the majority of which were leiomyosarcomas. No significant improvement was noted in progression-free interval or overall survival with chemotherapy [15].

In a pilot study of patients with any stage primary uterine leiomyosarcoma rendered free of disease, promising results were seen in terms of progression free and overall survival with four cycles of gemcitabine-docetaxel chemotherapy [16]. The relative success of this study, at least in comparison to historical controls, has led to a further phase II evaluation of the sequential use of four cycles of gemcitabine-docetaxel then four cycles of doxorubicin therapy in the adjuvant setting after resection of primary, nonmetastatic uterine leiomyosarcoma [17]. A total of 47 women with disease limited to the uterus were enrolled. With median follow-up of 27.4 months, 78% of women were progression-free at 2 years, and median progression-free survival was 39.3 months [17].

These data may lead to a randomized studies examining this question further in leiomyosarcomas of the uterus and other sites alike. The authors have learned that a number of oncologists use adjuvant doxorubicin-gemcitabine-docetaxel, despite lack of proof of any survival benefit. The 2011 standard of care as noted by the first author of the study is surgery alone without adjuvant chemotherapy [18].

Treatment of Recurrence

With single site recurrence, surgical resection can be anticipated and is potentially curative. As leiomyosarcomas are the commonest histology resected in the lung, pulmonary resections should be considered where possible. Otherwise, systemic therapy may be employed with palliative intent.

Metastatic Disease

Analysis of a variety of randomized studies dissecting out the response rate for leiomyosarcomas versus other subtypes of sarcomas is useful to delineate the differential response of leiomyosarcoma versus others such as liposarcoma, synovial sarcoma, or undifferentiated pleomorphic sarcoma (formerly MFH, malignant fibrous histiocytoma) [19]. It should be noted that subset analyses cannot substitute for primary trials of chemotherapy but still can be useful in generating hypotheses.

In considering leiomyosarcomas as a whole, doxorubicin is clearly active, but ifosfamide appears to add relatively little to the response rate, based on both primary data and retrospective analysis clinical trials [20, 21]. Some of the data are difficult to parse since there is obvious contamination of the leiomyosarcoma group with what would today be termed GIST, which represents the majority of the sarcomas of the gastrointestinal tract. Dacarbazine (DTIC) and the related oral compound temozolomide have at least minor activity against leiomyosarcoma but little to no activity against other sarcoma subtypes [22, 23]. Doxorubicin-DTIC combinations are also active against leiomyosarcoma [19, 24], but there is not obvious synergy of the combination in comparison to the single agents.

In studies of uterine sarcomas specifically (largely leiomyosarcomas), the Gynecologic Oncology Group compared doxorubicin alone to doxorubicin and dacarbazine in a randomized trial. Response rates and overall survival did not differ between the two arms; the response rate to doxorubicin of 28 women with leiomyosarcoma was 25% [25]. There is at least a weak association of estrogen or tamoxifen exposure to uterine leiomyosarcoma development [26–29]. However, estrogen receptor- or progesterone receptor-positive leiomyosarcomas only rarely respond to hormonal therapy such as aromatase inhibitors [30]. For an asymptomatic patient with low-volume metastatic disease, it may provide a less toxic option for care than standard cytotoxic chemotherapy.

The above studies raise the idea that leiomyosarcomas from different anatomical primary sites could respond differently to chemotherapy. The difference in response rates for different sites of leiomyosarcoma is highlighted in the trials from cooperative groups [20, 21, 31]. Although only 20–25% of uterine leiomyosarcomas responded to chemotherapy, uterine leiomyosarcoma was approximately twice as responsive to chemotherapy compared to leiomyosarcomas arising from the GI tract (mostly GISTs). These data are at odds with the cumulative EORTC meta-analysis of therapy for metastatic sarcomas; [32] however, in this EORTC analysis, leiomyosarcomas were not stratified with respect to site; poorly responding GIST were likely grouped together with better responding leiomyosarcomas of other sites.

The distinction of histology, anatomic site, and chemotherapy responsiveness extends to the gemcitabine-docetaxel combination. While there is activity of gemcitabine-docetaxel in leiomyosarcoma from a variety of anatomic sites, phase II data support the contention that uterine primaries respond better than those from other sites [33–38]. Randomized and nonrandomized data also support the idea that combination therapy is superior to single agent gemcitabine [34, 35, 38–41] and that activity of gemcitabine-docetaxel is similar in first or second line for metastatic disease [34, 35]. Conversely, there is at least one randomized study exclusively of patients with leiomyosarcoma that indicates the equivalence of gemcitabine and gemcitabine-docetaxel [42]. It is also notable that the gemcitabine-docetaxel combination may have even greater activity against other sarcomas, including UPS, pleomorphic liposarcoma, and pleomorphic rhabdomyosarcoma than leiomyosarcoma (all of which are sarcomas with aneuploid karyotypes) [38]. Other options for gemcitabine combinations for soft-tissue sarcoma include those using vinorelbine [43] or dacarbazine [44]. The data regarding dacarbazine are notable for the observation of an overall survival advantage for the combination [44], as was seen for the gemcitabine-docetaxel combination [38].

There are also data supportive of the activity of the DNA minor groove binding agent ET-743 (trabectedin) in patients with recurrent or metastatic leiomyosarcoma, although the response rate for leiomyosarcoma appears significantly below that of patients with myxoid-round cell liposarcoma [45–48]. With data from one randomized phase II study and support from other clinical trials, trabectedin was approved in Europe for use against metastatic sarcomas, while the drug was not approved using similar data in the United States. As of 2011, trabectedin is only available in the United States at limited sites on an expanded access program.

While there has been little activity of kinase-directed agents in clinical trials involving sarcoma patients, the addition of antiangiogenic and other agents has not been adequately addressed. Bevacizumab has been added to doxorubicin and to gemcitabine-docetaxel in phase II studies. In the former study, only 2/17 patients with leiomyosarcoma had a response to doxorubicin with bevacizumab, lower than expected given the single agent activity of doxorubicin in leiomyosarcoma. Of equal or greater concern was the finding of six patients with grade 2–4 cardiac toxicity (usually reversible) on study [49]. It would appear difficult to move forward with this combination of agents given these data.

Conversely, a beneficial effect of bevacizumab with gemcitabine-docetaxel has not been ruled out. In a phase I-II study of the three agents given together, the RECIST response rate was 44% (11/25). However, bowel perforation, pneumothorax, wound dehiscence, and hemorrhage were all seen on study. A phase III study underway by the Gynecologic Oncology Group will hopefully be able to determine if this observed toxicity is balanced by improved outcomes [50].

Table 6.1 Recommendations for systemic therapy for patients with leiomyosarcoma[a]

Clinical scenario		Comments
Adjuvant chemotherapy		No data specifically support its use as of 2013; some physicians will use the 2008 Pervaiz meta-analysis to justify adjuvant chemotherapy, however.
Metastatic disease	First line	Anthracycline[b] or gemcitabine alone or in combination[c]
	Second line	Agent not used in first line
	Third line	Dacarbazine or temozolomide; trabectedin in Europe; pazopanib
	Fourth line	Ifosfamide (in fit patient); clinical trial; supportive care

[a]Clinical trials are always appropriate if available. Hormonal therapy, e.g., an aromatase inhibitor, is an option in uterine and retroperitoneal leiomyosarcomas, which are more commonly ER + or PR +
[b]PEGylated liposomal doxorubicin (Doxil®/Caelyx®) if poor KPS or elderly
[c]Weekly gemcitabine-docetaxel has activity. There are no data comparing weekly low-dose therapy to a gemcitabine d1/d8, docetaxel d8 schedule. Gemcitabine in combination with either vinorelbine or dacarbazine may also have some degree of synergy

Clearly we collectively must determine which molecular features of leiomyosarcoma are related to chemotherapy responsiveness. Whether subsets of leiomyosarcoma defined by immunohistochemistry [46] or by analysis of mRNA gene expression arrays, miRNA arrays, comparative genomic hybridization (CGH), or other more sophisticated techniques can predict for chemotherapy responsiveness or overall outcome remains a topic for future research.

In summary, leiomyosarcomas, although relatively uniform at first glance histologically, vary in their biological profile as well as responsiveness to chemotherapy based on anatomic site. Doxorubicin, DTIC, gemcitabine-docetaxel, and trabectedin all have activity in metastatic disease, although there is no proven role of any chemotherapy in the adjuvant setting as of 2011. Further progress in defining subsets responsive to therapy and determination of the mechanism by which leiomyosarcoma aneuploidy is maintained should help lead to new ideas for therapy (Table 6.1).

Outcome

For extremity leiomyosarcoma, actuarial disease-specific survival is approximately 70%. Survival based on size for primary extremity lesions, i.e., ≤5 cm, 5–10 cm, and >10 cm, is shown in Fig. 6.10. Considering all primary sizes for retroperitoneal leiomyosarcomas together, the outcomes are poor and consistent with their typically large size at presentation (Fig. 6.11).

Fig. 6.10 Disease-specific
survival for adult patients
with primary extremity
leiomyosarcoma, by size.
MSKCC 7/1/1982–6/30/2010
n = 213

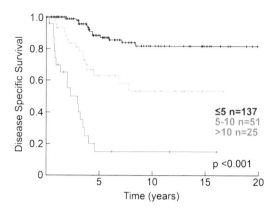

Fig. 6.11 Disease-specific
survival for adult patients
with retroperitoneal
leiomyosarcoma. MSKCC
7/1/1982–6/30/2010 n = 146

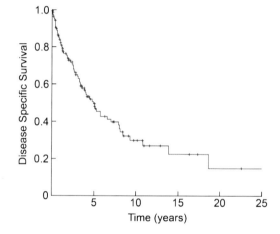

References

1. Miettinen M, Fetsch JF. Evaluation of biological potential of smooth muscle tumours. Histopathology. 2006;48:97–105.
2. Juang CM, Yen MS, Horng HC, Twu NF, Yu HC, Hsu WL. Potential role of preoperative serum CA125 for the differential diagnosis between uterine leiomyoma and uterine leiomyosarcoma. Eur J Gynaecol Oncol. 2006;27:370–4.
3. Folpe AL, Mentzel T, Lehr HA, Fisher C, Balzer BL, Weiss SW. Perivascular epithelioid cell neoplasms of soft tissue and gynecologic origin: a clinicopathologic study of 26 cases and review of the literature. Am J Surg Pathol. 2005;29:1558–75.
4. Guillou L, Aurias A. Soft tissue sarcomas with complex genomic profiles. Virchows Arch. 2010;456(2):201–17.
5. Meza-Zepeda LA, Kresse SH, Barragan-Polania AH, et al. Array comparative genomic hybridization reveals distinct DNA copy number differences between gastrointestinal stromal tumors and leiomyosarcomas. Cancer Res. 2006;66:8984–93.

6. Sandberg AA. Updates on the cytogenetics and molecular genetics of bone and soft tissue tumors: leiomyosarcoma. Cancer Genet Cytogenet. 2005;161:1–19.
7. Hollenbeck ST, Grobmyer SR, Kent KC, Brennan MF. Surgical treatment and outcomes of patients with primary inferior vena cava leiomyosarcoma. J Am Coll Surg. 2003;197:575–9.
8. Suzman MS, Smith AJ, Brennan MF. Fascio-peritoneal patch repair of the IVC: a workhorse in search of work? J Am Coll Surg. 2000;191:218–20.
9. Davis AM, O'Sullivan B, Turcotte R, et al. Late radiation morbidity following randomization to preoperative versus postoperative radiotherapy in extremity soft tissue sarcoma. Radiother Oncol. 2005;75:48–53.
10. O'Sullivan B, Davis AM, Turcotte R, et al. Preoperative versus postoperative radiotherapy in soft-tissue sarcoma of the limbs: a randomised trial. Lancet. 2002;359:2235–41.
11. Pisters PW, Harrison LB, Leung DH, Woodruff JM, Casper ES, Brennan MF. Long-term results of a prospective randomized trial of adjuvant brachytherapy in soft tissue sarcoma. J Clin Oncol. 1996;14:859–68.
12. Reed NS, Mangioni C, Malmstrom H, et al. Phase III randomised study to evaluate the role of adjuvant pelvic radiotherapy in the treatment of uterine sarcomas stages I and II: an European Organisation for Research and Treatment of Cancer Gynaecological Cancer Group Study (protocol 55874). Eur J Cancer. 2008;44:808–18.
13. Wright JD, Seshan VE, Shah M, et al. The role of radiation in improving survival for early-stage carcinosarcoma and leiomyosarcoma. Am J Obstet Gynecol. 2008;199(536):531–8.
14. Sampath S, Schultheiss TE, Ryu JK, Wong JY. The role of adjuvant radiation in uterine sarcomas. Int J Radiat Oncol Biol Phys. 2010;76(3):728–34.
15. Omura GA, Blessing JA, Major F, et al. A randomized clinical trial of adjuvant adriamycin in uterine sarcomas: a Gynecologic Oncology Group Study. J Clin Oncol. 1985;3:1240–5.
16. Hensley ML, Ishill N, Soslow R, et al. Adjuvant gemcitabine plus docetaxel for completely resected stages I-IV high-grade uterine leiomyosarcoma: Results of a prospective study. Gynecol Oncol. 2009;112:563–7.
17. Hensley ML, Wathen K, Maki RG, et al. Adjuvant treatment of high-risk primary uterine leiomyosarcoma with gemcitabine/docetaxel, followed by doxorubicin: results of phase II multicenter trial SARC005. J Clin Oncol. 2010;28:abstr 10021.
18. Hensley ML. Role of chemotherapy and biomolecular therapy in the treatment of uterine sarcomas. Best Pract Res Clin Obstet Gynaecol. 2011;25:773–82.
19. Borden EC, Amato DA, Rosenbaum C, et al. Randomized comparison of three adriamycin regimens for metastatic soft tissue sarcomas. J Clin Oncol. 1987;5:840–50.
20. Edmonson JH, Ryan LM, Blum RH, et al. Randomized comparison of doxorubicin alone versus ifosfamide plus doxorubicin or mitomycin, doxorubicin, and cisplatin against advanced soft tissue sarcomas. J Clin Oncol. 1993;11:1269–75.
21. Sleijfer S, Ouali M, van Glabbeke M, et al. Prognostic and predictive factors for outcome to first-line ifosfamide-containing chemotherapy for adult patients with advanced soft tissue sarcomas: an exploratory, retrospective analysis on large series from the European Organization for Research and Treatment of Cancer-Soft Tissue and Bone Sarcoma Group (EORTC-STBSG). Eur J Cancer. 2010;46:72–83.
22. Gottlieb JA, Benjamin RS, Baker LH, et al. Role of DTIC (NSC-45388) in the chemotherapy of sarcomas. Cancer Treat Rep. 1976;60:199–203.
23. Talbot SM, Keohan ML, Hesdorffer M, et al. A phase II trial of temozolomide in patients with unresectable or metastatic soft tissue sarcoma. Cancer. 2003;98:1942–6.
24. Zalupski M, Metch B, Balcerzak S, et al. Phase III comparison of doxorubicin and dacarbazine given by bolus versus infusion in patients with soft-tissue sarcomas: a Southwest Oncology Group study. J Natl Cancer Inst. 1991;83:926–32.
25. Omura GA, Major FJ, Blessing JA, et al. A randomized study of adriamycin with and without dimethyl triazenoimidazole carboxamide in advanced uterine sarcomas. Cancer. 1983;52:626–32.
26. Botsis D, Koliopoulos C, Kondi-Pafitis A, Creatsas G. Myxoid leiomyosarcoma of the uterus in a patient receiving tamoxifen therapy: a case report. Int J Gynecol Pathol. 2006;25:173–5.

27. Yildirim Y, Inal MM, Sanci M, et al. Development of uterine sarcoma after tamoxifen treatment for breast cancer: report of four cases. Int J Gynecol Cancer. 2005;15:1239–42.
28. Sabatini R, Di Fazio F, Loizzi P. Uterine leiomyosarcoma in a postmenopausal woman treated with tamoxifen: case report. Eur J Gynaecol Oncol. 1999;20:327–8.
29. McCluggage WG, Varma M, Weir P, Bharucha H. Uterine leiomyosarcoma in patient receiving tamoxifen therapy. Acta Obstet Gynecol Scand. 1996;75:593–5.
30. O'Cearbhaill R, Zhou Q, Iasonos A, et al. Treatment of advanced uterine leiomyosarcoma with aromatase inhibitors. Gynecol Oncol. 2010;116(3):424–9.
31. Antman K, Crowley J, Balcerzak SP, et al. An intergroup phase III randomized study of doxorubicin and dacarbazine with or without ifosfamide and mesna in advanced soft tissue and bone sarcomas. J Clin Oncol. 1993;11:1276–85.
32. Van Glabbeke M, Verweij J, Judson I, Nielsen OS. Progression-free rate as the principal endpoint for phase II trials in soft-tissue sarcomas. Eur J Cancer. 2002;38:543–9.
33. Bay JO, Ray-Coquard I, Fayette J, et al. Docetaxel and gemcitabine combination in 133 advanced soft-tissue sarcomas: a retrospective analysis. Int J Cancer. 2006;119:706–11.
34. Hensley ML, Blessing JA, Degeest K, Abulafia O, Rose PG, Homesley HD. Fixed-dose rate gemcitabine plus docetaxel as second-line therapy for metastatic uterine leiomyosarcoma: a Gynecologic Oncology Group phase II study. Gynecol Oncol. 2008;109:323–8.
35. Hensley ML, Blessing JA, Mannel R, Rose PG. Fixed-dose rate gemcitabine plus docetaxel as first-line therapy for metastatic uterine leiomyosarcoma: a Gynecologic Oncology Group phase II trial. Gynecol Oncol. 2008;109:329–34.
36. Hensley ML, Maki R, Venkatraman E, et al. Gemcitabine and docetaxel in patients with unresectable leiomyosarcoma: results of a phase II trial. J Clin Oncol. 2002;20:2824–31.
37. Leu KM, Ostruszka LJ, Shewach D, et al. Laboratory and clinical evidence of synergistic cytotoxicity of sequential treatment with gemcitabine followed by docetaxel in the treatment of sarcoma. J Clin Oncol. 2004;22:1706–12.
38. Maki RG, Wathen JK, Patel SR, et al. Randomized phase II study of gemcitabine and docetaxel compared with gemcitabine alone in patients with metastatic soft tissue sarcomas: results of sarcoma alliance for research through collaboration study 002 [corrected]. J Clin Oncol. 2007;25:2755–63.
39. Look KY, Sandler A, Blessing JA, Lucci 3rd JA, Rose PG. Phase II trial of gemcitabine as second-line chemotherapy of uterine leiomyosarcoma: a Gynecologic Oncology Group (GOG) Study. Gynecol Oncol. 2004;92:644–7.
40. Okuno S, Edmonson J, Mahoney M, Buckner JC, Frytak S, Galanis E. Phase II trial of gemcitabine in advanced sarcomas. Cancer. 2002;94:3225–9.
41. Okuno S, Ryan LM, Edmonson JH, Priebat DA, Blum RH. Phase II trial of gemcitabine in patients with advanced sarcomas (E1797): a trial of the Eastern Cooperative Oncology Group. Cancer. 2003;97:1969–73.
42. Duffaud F, Bui BN, Penel N, et al. A FNCLCC French Sarcoma Group–GETO multicenter randomized phase II study of gemcitabine versus gemcitabine and docetaxel in patients with metastatic or relapsed leiomyosarcoma. J Clin Oncol. 2008;26:Abstr 10511.
43. Dileo P, Morgan JA, Zahrieh D, et al. Gemcitabine and vinorelbine combination chemotherapy for patients with advanced soft tissue sarcomas: results of a phase II trial. Cancer. 2007;109:1863–9.
44. Garcia-Del-Muro X, Lopez-Pousa A, Maurel J, et al. Randomized phase II study comparing gemcitabine plus dacarbazine versus dacarbazine alone in patients with previously treated soft tissue sarcoma: a Spanish Group for Research on Sarcomas study. J Clin Oncol. 2011; 29:2528–33.
45. Amant F, Coosemans A, Renard V, Everaert E, Vergote I. Clinical outcome of ET-743 (Trabectedin; Yondelis) in high-grade uterine sarcomas: report on five patients and a review of the literature. Int J Gynecol Cancer. 2009;19:245–8.
46. Demetri GD, Chawla SP, von Mehren M, et al. Efficacy and safety of trabectedin in patients with advanced or metastatic liposarcoma or leiomyosarcoma after failure of prior anthracyclines and ifosfamide: results of a randomized phase II study of two different schedules. J Clin Oncol. 2009;27:4188–96.

47. Tewari D, Saffari B, Cowan C, Wallick AC, Koontz MZ, Monk BJ. Activity of trabectedin (ET-743, Yondelis) in metastatic uterine leiomyosarcoma. Gynecol Oncol. 2006;102:421–4.
48. Grosso F, Jones RL, Demetri GD, et al. Efficacy of trabectedin (ecteinascidin-743) in advanced pretreated myxoid liposarcomas: a retrospective study. Lancet Oncol. 2007;8:595–602.
49. D'Adamo DR, Anderson SE, Albritton K, et al. Phase II study of doxorubicin and bevacizumab for patients with metastatic soft-tissue sarcomas. J Clin Oncol. 2005;23:7135–42.
50. Verschraegen CF, Arias-Pulido H, Lee SJ, et al. Phase IB study of the combination of docetaxel, gemcitabine, and bevacizumab in patients with advanced or recurrent soft tissue sarcoma: the Axtell regimen. Ann Oncol. 2012;23(3):785–90.

Chapter 7
Undifferentiated Pleomorphic Sarcoma (UPS; Malignant Fibrous Histiocytoma: MFH) and Myxofibrosarcoma

The most common term for a generic high-grade sarcoma has evolved over the years from fibrosarcoma to malignant fibrous histiocytoma (MFH) and now to high-grade undifferentiated pleomorphic sarcoma (UPS). The new nomenclature is utilized to differentiate this tumor from tumors that are truly histiocytic, i.e., histiocytic sarcoma, recognizing that the microscopic morphology of such tumors was not specific for sarcomas. Specific varieties of what was called MFH in the past have proved to be unique entities. For example, myxofibrosarcoma is now a clearly defined sarcoma subtype that was formerly termed myxoid MFH. Myxofibrosarcoma occurs more frequently in the subcutaneous tissue and has infiltrating pattern (Fig. 7.1). Angiomatoid MFH is reclassified as angiomatoid fibrous histiocytoma, having mostly a benign clinical course and occurring in children and young adults. The situation is further complicated since the term MFH is still employed in the bone (and treated most commonly as osteogenic sarcoma in children).

The age distribution for adult myxofibrosarcoma is shown in Fig. 7.2. The summary of the various sites now identified as having myxofibrosarcoma is seen in Fig. 7.3.

Imaging

There are no characteristics that discern UPS/myxofibrosarcoma from other sarcomas radiologically (Fig. 7.4). The lungs are the most common site of metastasis and should be monitored by x-ray or CT.

Diagnosis/Molecular Pathology

The cells in UPS appear to be fibroblastic or myofibroblastic but by definition should not show differentiation toward a more specific line of differentiation. The differential diagnosis will depend on the anatomic site of the body in which the tumor is

M.F. Brennan et al., *Management of Soft Tissue Sarcoma*,
DOI 10.1007/978-1-4614-5004-7_7, © Springer Science+Business Media New York 2013

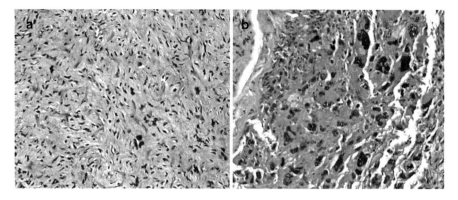

Fig. 7.1 (**a**) Myxofibrosarcoma: spindle and pleomorphic cells embedded in a predominantly myxoid stroma and associated with a rich vascular network. (**b**) High-grade pleomorphic-type UPS (undifferentiated pleomorphic sarcoma) bizarre, multinucleated cells, with hyperchromasia and anaplasia

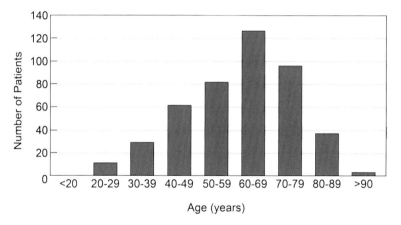

Fig. 7.2 Distribution by age for adult patients with myxofibrosarcoma, all sites. MSKCC 7/1/1982–6/30/2010 n = 445

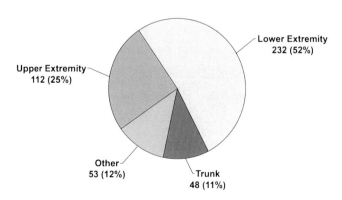

Fig. 7.3 Distribution by site for adult patients with myxofibrosarcoma. MSKCC 7/1/1982–6/30/2010 n = 445

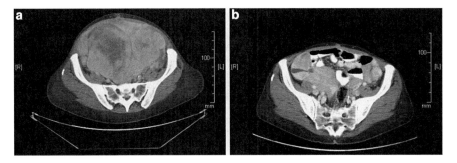

Fig. 7.4 CT of malignant fibrous histiocytoma/undifferentiated pleomorphic sarcoma of abdomen (**a**) and response to treatment at 4 months (**b**)

identified. For example, in the retroperitoneum, most (if not all) lesions with pleomorphic morphology represent dedifferentiated liposarcoma. Cytogenetically, UPS are aneuploid tumors without recurrent or characteristic genetic abnormalities. Conversely, angiomatoid fibrous histiocytoma is characterized by a t(2;22) resulting in *EWSR1-CREB1* in most cases and rarely by a t(12;22) or t(12;16) secondary to *EWSR1-ATF1* or *FUS-ATF1* [1–4]. Finding such a translocation rules out the diagnosis of UPS. Myxofibrosarcomas have a characteristic light microscopic pattern but like UPS have no specific characteristic genetic abnormality. Interestingly, a spectrum of tumors ranging from embryonal rhabdomyosarcoma and UPS has been defined in an elegant series of mouse model experiments, suggesting the primitive nature of UPS may be from their derivation from muscular satellite cells in which tumor suppressor *Rb1* is lost [5].

Not mentioned in this section are the rarer diagnoses that also appear to be related to fibroblastic or myofibroblastic cells, such as low-grade fibromyxoid sarcoma (Evans tumor), sclerosing epithelioid fibrosarcoma, dermatofibrosarcoma protuberans, or even rarer inflammatory myofibroblastic tumor or acral myxoinflammatory fibroblastic sarcoma (see Chap. 12). These diagnoses have only become evident with the careful application of immunohistochemical and molecular techniques for a group of sarcomas that are otherwise relatively rare and difficult to subclassify.

Natural History

A major concern with myxofibrosarcoma, even when compared to UPS, is local recurrence. The margins of myxofibrosarcoma are often difficult to appreciate and difficult to manage.

Patterns of failure are both local and distant. Local recurrence is related to the diffuse growth pattern and the infiltrative nature. The lung is the most common site for distant metastasis, but satellite lesions are often seen in the area of the primary lesion particularly in low-grade myxofibrosarcoma of the extremity. Grade is a factor in outcome and low-grade lesions having a reasonably good prognosis but high-grade lesions having a very significant rate of both local and distant metastasis.

Treatment

Primary treatment is surgical. The ability to gain negative margins in these lesions is often most challenging. Only rarely is skin involved and so skin grafts should be uncommon.

Radiation Therapy

We do not have specific data as to the utilization of radiation therapy, but the assumption is that it provides, based on randomized trials, an improvement in local control without impacting on survival.

Metastatic Disease

There are three lines of therapy to consider for UPS/MFH as of 2013: anthracyclines, ifosfamide, and gemcitabine-docetaxel (or gemcitabine alone or in combination with vinorelbine).

In our experience, UPS can respond to doxorubicin or ifosfamide, but very rarely to dacarbazine. Thanks to a careful analysis of patients treated prospectively in EORTC studies, it appears both ifosfamide and doxorubicin are useful systemic agents for metastatic sarcoma [6]. As a by-product of a randomized study of gemcitabine-docetaxel vs. gemcitabine for patients with recurrent/metastatic soft-tissue sarcomas [7], we learned that UPS/MFH is sensitive to gemcitabine-docetaxel and to gemcitabine to a lesser degree, with sensitivity perhaps even greater than that of leiomyosarcoma (Fig. 7.4). Formal studies of gemcitabine-docetaxel vs. doxorubicin-ifosfamide in soft-tissue sarcomas are underway and will hopefully provide supportive data from this clinical trial.

While clinical trials have been performed generally examining gemcitabine on day 1 and day 8, and docetaxel at a large dose on day 8, with the randomized study noted above, as many as 50% of patients had to stop therapy for toxicity within 6 months of treatment [7]. Gemcitabine and docetaxel can both be given on a low-dose weekly schedule, with gemcitabine 600–900 mg/m² day 1 and day 8, docetaxel 20–35 mg/m² day 1, day 8, with or without growth factors, q 21 days, a variation of a three week out of four-treatment schedule used for treatment of other cancers [8, 9]. Whether this schedule is as effective as the high-dose docetaxel regimen is to be seen but provides another treatment option for patients who are more frail or with poor performance status to tolerate the admitted toxic day 8 docetaxel at 100 (or even 75) mg/m^2.

Gemcitabine with either vinorelbine or dacarbazine are other options for combination therapy [10, 11]. Eribulin has at least some activity in recurrent/metastatic soft-tissue sarcomas but is not well examined in UPS specifically [12].

Kinase-directed therapy such as imatinib, sorafenib, pazopanib, and sunitinib does not appear to have significant activity in UPS/MFH, though there are relatively sparse data specifically testing sunitinib against UPS/MFH [13–16]. A response in a patient with UPS/MFH was seen in a phase II clinical trial of imatinib, but this appears to be the exception rather than the rule; similarly such agents have been largely inactive in leiomyosarcomas as well, another aneuploid sarcoma subtype. Pazopanib may have at least minor activity in UPS/MFH [16]. We postulate that agents that inhibit the tumor cell cycle or have activity against epigenetic factors within the aneuploid tumor cell may prove a more useful approach than kinase inhibitors, as may combinations of with chemotherapeutic agents.

Adjuvant Chemotherapy

Given the sensitivity of some patients with UPS/MFH to doxorubicin/ifosfamide in the metastatic setting, consideration can be given to the use of these agents in the adjuvant setting. While most of these individual studies are negative [17, 18], a few of these studies are positive for overall survival benefit [19, 20], and the most recent meta-analysis of adjuvant therapy studies, which unfortunately excludes a large but negative study from EORTC [18], indicates benefit of adjuvant therapy for patients who receive doxorubicin-ifosfamide-based therapy [21]. Given the relatively high risk of larger tumors (e.g., those over 10 cm), consideration can be given to adjuvant chemotherapy with the understanding of the conflicting data, knowing that a high percentage of such patients will require the use of chemotherapy at some point in their course of treatment (Table 7.1).

Table 7.1 Recommendations for systemic therapy for patients with UPS[a]

Clinical scenario	Comments	
Adjuvant chemotherapy		Remains controversial and should be discussed on a case-by-case basis
Metastatic disease	First line	Anthracycline ± ifosfamide[b] or gemcitabine alone or in combination (docetaxel, vinorelbine, or possibly dacarbazine)
	Second line	Agent(s) not used in first line; pazopanib
	Third line	Agents not used in first or second line; clinical trial; dacarbazine in patient without trial options

[a]Clinical trials are always appropriate if available
[b]PEGylated liposomal doxorubicin (Doxil®/Caelyx®) if poor KPS or elderly

Fig. 7.5 Local disease-free survival for adult patients with primary malignant fibrous histiocytoma/ undifferentiated pleomorphic sarcoma, all sites. MSKCC 7/1/1982–6/30/2010 n = 772

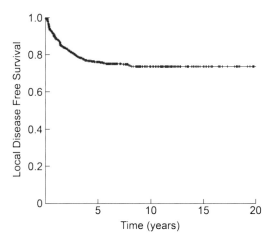

Fig. 7.6 Disease-specific survival for adult patients with primary malignant fibrous histiocytoma/ undifferentiated pleomorphic sarcoma, all sites. MSKCC 7/1/1982–6/30/2010 n = 772

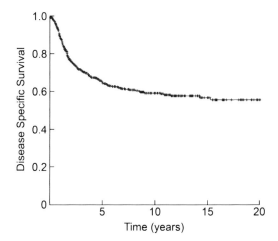

Outcome

Local disease-free survival (Fig. 7.5) for patients with UPS is approximately 75% at 10 years with a local recurrence uncommon. Patients have a substantial risk of metastatic disease, with disease-specific survival of approximately 60% (Fig. 7.6) at 10 years and late metastatic recurrence possible but most uncommon. In contrast, myxofibrosarcoma has a higher local relapse rate of at least 40% at 10 years (Fig. 7.7), while the metastatic risk is similar between the true myxofibrosarcoma group and patients who have UPS. There are perhaps more patients with late relapses and death from myxofibrosarcoma compared to UPS (Fig. 7.8).

Fig. 7.7 Local recurrence-free survival for adult patients with primary myxofibrosarcoma, all sites. MSKCC 7/1/1982–6/30/2010 n = 361

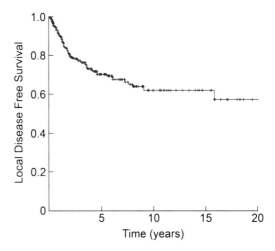

Fig. 7.8 Disease-specific survival for adult patients with primary myxofibrosarcoma, all sites. MSKCC 7/1/1982–6/30/2010 n = 361

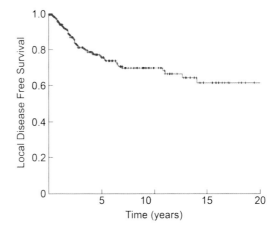

References

1. Antonescu CR, Dal Cin P, Nafa K, et al. EWSR1-CREB1 is the predominant gene fusion in angiomatoid fibrous histiocytoma. Genes Chromosomes Cancer. 2007;46(12):1051–60.
2. Hallor KH, Mertens F, Jin Y, et al. Fusion of the EWSR1 and ATF1 genes without expression of the MITF-M transcript in angiomatoid fibrous histiocytoma. Genes Chromosomes Cancer. 2005;44(1):97–102.
3. Romeo S, Dei Tos AP. Soft tissue tumors associated with EWSR1 translocation. Virchows Arch. 2010;456(2):219–34.
4. Tanas MR, Rubin BP, Montgomery EA, et al. Utility of FISH in the diagnosis of angiomatoid fibrous histiocytoma: a series of 18 cases. Mod Pathol. 2010;23(1):93–7.
5. Rubin BP, Nishijo K, Chen HI, et al. Evidence for an unanticipated relationship between undifferentiated pleomorphic sarcoma and embryonal rhabdomyosarcoma. Cancer Cell. 2011;19(2): 177–91.
6. Sleijfer S, Ouali M, van Glabbeke M, et al. Prognostic and predictive factors for outcome to first-line ifosfamide-containing chemotherapy for adult patients with advanced soft tissue

sarcomas: an exploratory, retrospective analysis on large series from the European organization for research and treatment of cancer-soft tissue and bone sarcoma group (EORTC-STBSG). Eur J Cancer. 2010;46(1):72–83.

7. Maki RG, Wathen JK, Patel SR, et al. Randomized phase II study of gemcitabine and docetaxel compared with gemcitabine alone in patients with metastatic soft tissue sarcomas: results of sarcoma alliance for research through collaboration study 002 [corrected]. J Clin Oncol. 2007;25(19):2755–63.

8. Hainsworth JD, Carrell D, Drengler RL, et al. Weekly combination chemotherapy with docetaxel and gemcitabine as first-line treatment for elderly patients and patients with poor performance status who have extensive-stage small cell lung carcinoma: a Minnie Pearl Cancer Research Network phase II trial. Cancer. 2004;100(11):2437–41.

9. O'Shaughnessy JA, Pluenneke R, Sternberg J, et al. Phase II trial of weekly docetaxel/gemcitabine as first-line chemotherapy in patients with locally recurrent or metastatic breast cancer. Clin Breast Cancer. 2006;6(6):505–10.

10. Dileo P, Morgan JA, Zahrieh D, et al. Gemcitabine and vinorelbine combination chemotherapy for patients with advanced soft tissue sarcomas: results of a phase II trial. Cancer. 2007;109(9):1863–9.

11. Garcia-Del-Muro X, Lopez-Pousa A, Maurel J, et al. Randomized phase II study comparing gemcitabine plus dacarbazine versus dacarbazine alone in patients with previously treated soft tissue sarcoma: a Spanish Group for Research on Sarcomas study. J Clin Oncol. 2011;29(18):2528–33.

12. Schoffski P, Ray-Coquard IL, Cioffi A, et al. Activity of eribulin mesylate in patients with soft-tissue sarcoma: a phase 2 study in four independent histological subtypes. Lancet Oncol. 2011;12(11):1045–52.

13. Chugh R, Wathen JK, Maki RG, et al. Phase II multicenter trial of imatinib in 10 histologic subtypes of sarcoma using a bayesian hierarchical statistical model. J Clin Oncol. 2009;27(19):3148–53.

14. D'Adamo DR, Keohan M, Schuetze S, et al. Clinical results of a phase II study of sorafenib in patients (pts) with non-GIST sarcomas (CTEP study #7060). J Clin Oncol. 2007; 25(18S): Abstr 10001.

15. George S, Merriam P, Maki RG, et al. Multicenter phase II trial of sunitinib in the treatment of nongastrointestinal stromal tumor sarcomas. J Clin Oncol. 2009;27(19):3154–60.

16. Sleijfer S, Ray-Coquard I, Papai Z, et al. Pazopanib, a multikinase angiogenesis inhibitor, in patients with relapsed or refractory advanced soft tissue sarcoma: a phase II study from the European organisation for research and treatment of cancer-soft tissue and bone sarcoma group (EORTC study 62043). J Clin Oncol. 2009;27(19):3126–32.

17. Gortzak E, Azzarelli A, Buesa J, et al. A randomised phase II study on neo-adjuvant chemotherapy for 'high-risk' adult soft-tissue sarcoma. Eur J Cancer. 2001;37(9):1096–103.

18. Woll PJ, Van Glabbeke M, Hohenberger P, et al. Adjuvant chemotherapy with doxorubicin and ifosfamide in resected soft tissue sarcoma: interim analysis of a randomised phase III trial. J Clin Oncol. 2007; 25(18S): Abstr 10008.

19. Frustaci S, Gherlinzoni F, De Paoli A, et al. Adjuvant chemotherapy for adult soft tissue sarcomas of the extremities and girdles: results of the Italian randomized cooperative trial. J Clin Oncol. 2001;19(5):1238–47.

20. Frustaci S, De Paoli A, Bidoli E, et al. Ifosfamide in the adjuvant therapy of soft tissue sarcomas. Oncology. 2003;65 Suppl 2:80–4.

21. Pervaiz N, Colterjohn N, Farrokhyar F, et al. A systematic meta-analysis of randomized controlled trials of adjuvant chemotherapy for localized resectable soft-tissue sarcoma. Cancer. 2008;113(3):573–81.

Chapter 8
Synovial Sarcoma

Synovial sarcomas present typically as a mass lesion usually on the extremities. Historically thought to be associated with peripheral joints, it is clear that there is no association of this sarcoma with synovium *per se*. Clinical presentation is that of younger age groups than other sarcomas, predominantly a disease of adolescent and young adulthood. As our data set includes patients over age 16, we underemphasize the presence in adolescents (Fig. 8.1). Site distribution for this adult cohort is shown in Fig. 8.2.

Imaging

As with other sarcomas, CT and MRI are the bases of imaging (Fig. 8.3). Synovial sarcomas may occur in the mediastinum, pleura, or lung as a primary site, but do not have particular radiological features to discern them from other sarcomas, other than occasional calcifications. Imaging more frequently demonstrates bone invasion (Fig. 8.4) in comparison to other sarcoma subtypes.

Diagnosis, Molecular Pathology

While being of uncertain histogenesis, mouse models indicate the satellite cells of skeletal muscle as a possible cell of origin for synovial sarcoma [1]. Monophasic and biphasic variants of synovial sarcoma are well recognized; 2/3 of synovial sarcomas are monophasic (Figs. 8.5 and 8.6). Monophasic synovial sarcoma cells are arranged in intersecting fascicles and show a monotonous cytomorphology. They often have a hemangiopericytoma-like vascular pattern and not infrequently contain intralesional calcification. The biphasic variant looks similar in its spindled areas, interrupted by evidence of glandular differentiation, lined with low cuboidal to columnar epithelioid cells. There is a rarer poorly differentiated variant that has

M.F. Brennan et al., *Management of Soft Tissue Sarcoma*,
DOI 10.1007/978-1-4614-5004-7_8, © Springer Science+Business Media New York 2013

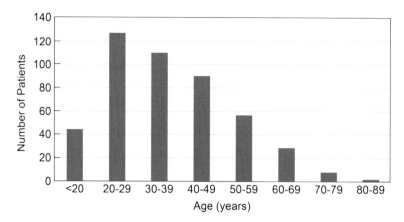

Fig. 8.1 Distribution by age of adult patients with synovial sarcoma, all sites. MSKCC 7/1/1982–6/30/2010 n = 467

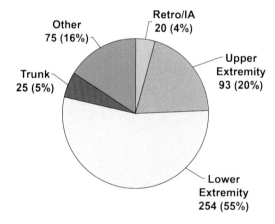

Fig. 8.2 Distribution by site of adult patients with synovial sarcoma. MSKCC 7/1/1982–6/30/2010 n = 467 Retro/IA = retroperitoneal/intra abdominal

evidence of a more aggressive small round cell component and rhabdoid features and could be mistaken for Ewing sarcoma or rhabdomyosarcoma [2]. EMA and cytokeratins can stain both the glandular and spindle components of tumors.

The characteristic translocation of synovial sarcoma is t(X;18)(p11.2;q11.2) [3], with *SS18* on chromosome 18 (formerly termed *SYT*) fused to *SSX1*, *SSX2*, or rarely *SSX4* [4, 5]. A tumor with such a translocation by FISH, RT-PCR, or cytogenetics confirms the diagnosis of synovial sarcoma, helping with the differential diagnosis [6]. Most biphasic tumors contain *SS18-SSX1*, while monophasic tumors have a roughly equal chance of containing *SS18-SSX1* or *SS18-SSX2*. *SS18-SSX2* synovial sarcomas

Fig. 8.3 MRI of extensive thigh synovial sarcoma

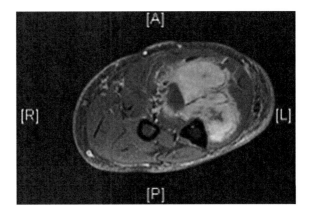

Fig. 8.4 T2 fat-saturated MRI image of a synovial sarcoma of the thigh demonstrating invasion of the femur

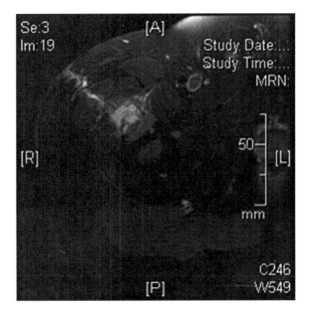

are nearly all monophasic [7]. The variation between *SSX1* and *SSX2* expression in synovial sarcoma impacts differentiation seen in synovial sarcomas, through expression of genes *Snail* or *Slug*, both of which can suppress E-cadherin expression [8, 9]. E-cadherin mutations are also a common finding in synovial sarcoma [10].

As a consequence of the *SS18-SSX* fusion gene, the diagnosis of synovial sarcoma has now been seen in what historically would be considered unusual sites

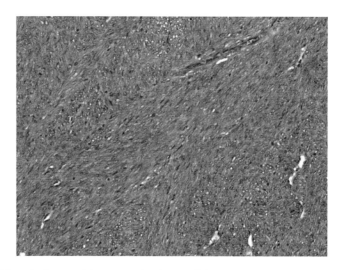

Fig. 8.5 Monophasic synovial sarcoma showing a cellular but monotonous proliferation of spindle cells arranged in long, intersecting fascicles. Typically no nuclear pleomorphism or necrosis is noted (HE, × 200)

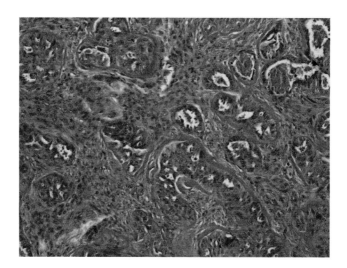

Fig. 8.6 Biphasic synovial sarcoma showing well-defined glandular spaces, in the background of a spindle cell component and thick, refractile collagenous stroma (HE, 200×)

such as the prostate, retroperitoneum, and diaphragm. They are an excellent example for the use of molecular diagnosis to characterize tumors that were thought to occur in a particular age group or in a particular site and realize that they can occur at any age and in any site.

Treatment

Treatment is primarily surgical, with the use of radiation in selected patients (usually primary size >5 cm) as an adjuvant to minimize the risk of local recurrence. Adjuvant chemotherapy (see below) has been suggested as valuable and more valuable than in other sarcomatous tumor types, particularly in regimens including ifosfamide [11].

Radiation Therapy

The general principles already outlined apply to synovial sarcoma. While brachyther-apy can be considered, external beam radiation is most commonly used. Preoperative external beam radiation is associated with a smaller field, lower dose, but higher risk of wound complications; postoperative radiation employs larger fields, higher dose, and higher risk of long-term complications such as radiation site fibrosis. While we typically employ radiation for synovial sarcoma >5 cm in greatest dimen-sion, for areas where local control is difficult, such as the head and neck, radiation can be considered for smaller lesions, bearing in mind the risks of short- and long-term toxicities vs. the risk of local failure. The use of concurrent chemotherapy and radiation remains investigational.

Chemotherapy

There remains debate as to the benefit of chemotherapy in the adjuvant setting for patients with soft-tissue sarcoma. While a new meta-analysis of prior adjuvant che-motherapy clinical trials demonstrated an overall survival advantage with the use of adjuvant chemotherapy [11], this study did not examine individual data of patients in performing the meta-analysis, unlike a similar effort published in 1997 [12]. These data are in conflict with the largest single study of adjuvant therapy from the EORTC, which showed no benefit in overall survival in patients who received chemotherapy [13]. An analysis of patients from University of California at Los Angeles and MSKCC indicated that those patients who received chemotherapy fared better than the MSKCC nomogram would have predicted, a nomogram including patients who most had not received chemotherapy in the adjuvant setting [14] (Figs. 8.7 and 8.8).

Given the relative chemotherapy sensitivity of synovial sarcoma, this is one sce-nario (along with myxoid-round cell liposarcoma and sarcomas more common in a pediatric population) in which we generally administer chemotherapy in the adju-vant setting for higher-risk tumors, i.e., those over 5 cm in greatest dimension. We will generally employ 5–6 cycles of AIM, i.e., doxorubicin 75 mg/m^2 and ifosf-amide 9 g/m^2 in split doses over 3 days (doxorubicin IV push, ifosfamide over 3 h,

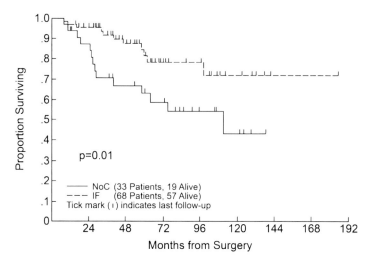

Fig. 8.7 Primary extremity synovial sarcoma – disease-specific survival by ifosfamide (IF) treatment (Used with permission from Eilber et al. [14])

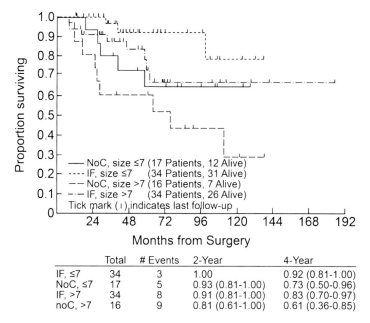

	Total	# Events	2-Year	4-Year
IF, ≤7	34	3	1.00	0.92 (0.81-1.00)
NoC, ≤7	17	5	0.93 (0.81-1.00)	0.73 (0.50-0.96)
IF, >7	34	8	0.91 (0.81-1.00)	0.83 (0.70-0.97)
noC, >7	16	9	0.81 (0.61-1.00)	0.61 (0.36-0.85)

Fig. 8.8 Primary extremity synovial sarcoma – disease-specific survival by size and ifosfamide (IF) treatment (Used with permission from Eilber et al. [14])

with mesna). A schedule used at MD Anderson Cancer Center employs doxorubicin 75 mg/m² and ifosfamide 10 g/m² per cycle. Neutrophil growth factors (i.e., filgrastim or pegfilgrastim) are necessary to aid recovery from the neutropenia and mucositis common with this regimen.

Treatment of Recurrence

Local Recurrence

An attempt at surgical resection of locally recurrent disease is appropriate for patients. Local recurrence may be the result of either technical issues (close / positive margins in the primary) or aggressive biology of the tumor. In many cases, this will mean greater morbidity or sacrifice of critical structures such as nerves, veins, arteries, or bone, some of which cannot be spared without loss of the extremity. In synovial sarcomas of the hand, a ray amputation may still be limb preserving, but in synovial sarcomas recurrent in the foot, a transmetatarsal or below the knee amputation may be the only options for tumor control. Re-irradiation is typically not feasible in someone who has already received a lifetime dose to a particular anatomic site. However, we have shown that in some patients having received prior irradiation, additional irradiation by the brachytherapy technique is possible with minimal morbidity [15, 16].

Local recurrence is a poor prognostic sign, often premonitory for overt metastatic disease. In patients with local recurrence, it is wise to reimage the patient to confirm lack of metastatic disease before proceeding with surgery. If metastatic disease is found, the degree of metastatic involvement and local control issues are weighed to develop the best treatment plan for a patient.

Systemic Treatment

Limb perfusion with tumor necrosis factor (TNF) and chemotherapy has been successfully employed in patients with locally recurrent sarcomas when amputation is the only local control option [17–19]. Limb perfusion is EMA-approved in Europe and available at specialized centers, but the lack of the availability of TNF in the United States has limited limb perfusion in the United States to chemotherapy only. The use of TNF with chemotherapy adds both tumor anti-vascular effects and also apparently allows for greater intratumoral uptake of chemotherapy [17]. Systemic therapy for a purely local recurrence of tumor is typically ineffective save for the occasional patient in whom there will be stabilization of disease. Synovial sarcoma may represent one of the few histologies in which there can be frank shrinking of tumor with chemotherapy in the locally recurrent setting.

For metastatic disease, ifosfamide and anthracyclines are the most active agents and can be used singly or in combination depending on prior exposure and need to palliate symptoms. In contrast to MFH/UPS and leiomyosarcoma, gemcitabine-docetaxel has nearly no activity, at least in adults. Trabectedin (ET743) [20] is active in at least a minority of patients and can be employed when available; eribulin may also have minor activity [21]. We have had modest success with the occasional patient with cisplatin-etoposide (Fig. 8.9), or even oral etoposide alone, 50 mg oral daily, 7 days on, 7 days off, for patients with poor performance status. Phase II and phase III data indicate activity of pazopanib in synovial sarcoma, which was not observed with sorafenib or sunitinib in other phase II studies, thus

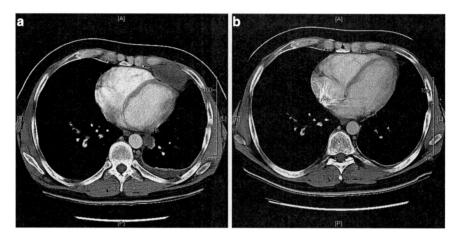

Fig. 8.9 Response of metastatic synovial sarcoma to ifosfamide chemotherapy

Table 8.1 Recommendations for systemic therapy for patients with synovial sarcoma[a]

Clinical scenario	Comments	
Adjuvant chemotherapy		Doxorubicin/ifosfamide (AIM) x 5–6 cycles for high-risk tumors
Metastatic disease	First line	Ifosfamide ± doxorubicin (if not employed before). Some investigators use a higher dose of ifosfamide than previously employed
	Second line	Doxorubicin if not employed previously; pegylated liposomal doxorubicin can be used in a poor prognosis patient.[b] Trabectedin (if available)
	Third line +	Pazopanib; clinical trial, e.g. histone deacetylase (HDAC) inhibitor; etoposide as a single agent or possibly in combinations; gemcitabine-docetaxel appears largely inactive

[a]Clinical trials are always appropriate if available. Gemcitabine and combinations appear inactive
[b]Pegylated liposomal doxorubicin (Doxil®/Caelyx®) if poor KPS or elderly

making it perhaps the most viable option for an oral multitargeted tyrosine kinase inhibitor for systemic therapy [22].

As of 2012, patients who are HLA-A0201+ may enroll in a trial at the US National Cancer Institute of autologous NY-ESO-1-directed T cells derived from patients. Patients have demonstrated signs of radiological and clinical benefit from this approach [23]. The process of training and expanding the CD8+ T cells from a patient sample is 3–6 months. Other immunotherapeutic studies focused on the NY-ESO-1 may be worth considering as well, given the near universal expression of NY-ESO-1 in synovial sarcomas (Table 8.1).

Newer approaches for systemic therapy are needed, and one approach that will require systematic examination is that of (histone) deacetylase inhibitors or other DNA modifying agents, given the strong preclinical rationale developed over the last several years by the laboratory of Nielsen et al. [24–26].

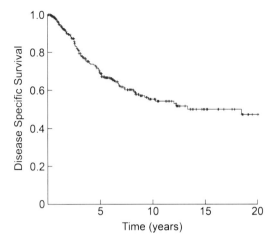

Fig. 8.10 Disease-specific survival of adult patients with synovial sarcoma, all sites. MSKCC 7/1/1982–6/30/2010 n = 297

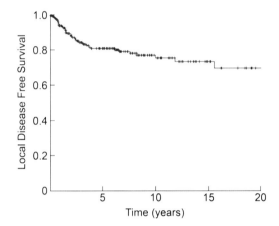

Fig. 8.11 Local recurrence-free survival of adult patients with synovial sarcoma, all sites. MSKCC 7/1/1982–6/30/2010 n = 297

Outcome

SS18-SSX gene fusion type has been suggested to have some significance in predicting outcome. In a description of the experience from our institution [27], it was found that patients with *SSX2* gene fusions fare worse than those with *SSX1* fusion, but these data were contradicted by other data showing no significant difference in outcome based on fusion type [28]. Our earlier analyses [29] looking at 112 patients suggested that the majority presented with a relatively small lesion involving the lower extremity. Less than 10% of those patients have had a local recurrence, but up to 30% have developed metastatic disease. As this was an analysis of extremity-only patients, the lung was the commonest site. In that article, we first identified the importance of bone invasion in these lesions, with bone invasion being relatively uncommon in other types of sarcoma.

Disease-specific survival and local recurrence for adults with synovial sarcoma are shown in Figs. 8.10 and 8.11.

References

1. Haldar M, Hancock JD, Coffin CM, et al. A conditional mouse model of synovial sarcoma: insights into a myogenic origin. Cancer Cell. 2007;11(4):375–88.
2. van de Rijn M, Barr FG, Xiong QB, et al. Poorly differentiated synovial sarcoma: an analysis of clinical, pathologic, and molecular genetic features. Am J Surg Pathol. 1999;23(1):106–12.
3. Turc-Carel C, Dal Cin P, Limon J, et al. Involvement of chromosome X in primary cytogenetic change in human neoplasia: nonrandom translocation in synovial sarcoma. Proc Natl Acad Sci USA. 1987;84(7):1981–5.
4. Lasota J, Jasinski M, Debiec-Rychter M, et al. Detection of the SYT-SSX fusion transcripts in formaldehyde-fixed, paraffin-embedded tissue: a reverse transcription polymerase chain reaction amplification assay useful in the diagnosis of synovial sarcoma. Mod Pathol. 1998;11(7): 626–33.
5. Skytting B, Nilsson G, Brodin B, et al. A novel fusion gene, SYT-SSX4, in synovial sarcoma. J Natl Cancer Inst. 1999;91(11):974–5.
6. Coindre JM, Pelmus M, Hostein I, et al. Should molecular testing be required for diagnosing synovial sarcoma? A prospective study of 204 cases. Cancer. 2003;98(12):2700–7.
7. Kawai A, Woodruff J, Healey JH, et al. SYT-SSX gene fusion as a determinant of morphology and prognosis in synovial sarcoma. N Engl J Med. 1998;338(3):153–60.
8. Saito T, Nagai M, Ladanyi M. SYT-SSX1 and SYT-SSX2 interfere with repression of E-cadherin by snail and slug: a potential mechanism for aberrant mesenchymal to epithelial transition in human synovial sarcoma. Cancer Res. 2006;66(14):6919–27.
9. Saito T, Oda Y, Kawaguchi K, et al. E-cadherin mutation and Snail overexpression as alternative mechanisms of E-cadherin inactivation in synovial sarcoma. Oncogene. 2004;23(53):8629–38.
10. Saito T, Oda Y, Sugimachi K, et al. E-cadherin gene mutations frequently occur in synovial sarcoma as a determinant of histological features. Am J Pathol. 2001;159(6):2117–24.
11. Pervaiz N, Colterjohn N, Farrokhyar F, et al. A systematic meta-analysis of randomized controlled trials of adjuvant chemotherapy for localized resectable soft-tissue sarcoma. Cancer. 2008;113(3):573–81.
12. Sarcoma Meta-Analysis Collaboration. Adjuvant chemotherapy for localised resectable soft-tissue sarcoma of adults: meta-analysis of individual data. Lancet. 1997;350(9092):1647–54.
13. Woll PJ, van Glabbeke M, Hohenberger P, et al. Adjuvant chemotherapy (CT) with doxorubicin and ifosfamide in resected soft tissue sarcoma (STS): interim analysis of a randomised phase III trial. J Clin Oncol (Meet Abstr). 2007;25 Suppl 18:10008.
14. Eilber FC, Brennan MF, Eilber FR, et al. Chemotherapy is associated with improved survival in adult patients with primary extremity synovial sarcoma. Ann Surg. 2007;246(1):105–13.
15. Shiu MH, Hilaris BS, Harrison LB, et al. Brachytherapy and function-saving resection of soft tissue sarcoma arising in the limb. Int J Radiat Oncol Biol Phys. 1991;21(6):1485–92.
16. Nori D, Schupak K, Shiu MH, et al. Role of brachytherapy in recurrent extremity sarcoma in patients treated with prior surgery and irradiation. Int J Radiat Oncol Biol Phys. 1991;20(6): 1229–33.
17. Eggermont AM, de Wilt JH, ten Hagen TL. Current uses of isolated limb perfusion in the clinic and a model system for new strategies. Lancet Oncol. 2003;4(7):429–37.
18. Eggermont AM, Schraffordt Koops H, Lienard D, et al. Isolated limb perfusion with high-dose tumor necrosis factor-alpha in combination with interferon-gamma and melphalan for nonresectable extremity soft tissue sarcomas: a multicenter trial. J Clin Oncol. 1996;14(10):2653–65.
19. Grunhagen DJ, de Wilt JH, Graveland WJ, et al. The palliative value of tumor necrosis factor alpha-based isolated limb perfusion in patients with metastatic sarcoma and melanoma. Cancer. 2006;106(1):156–62.
20. Fayette J, Coquard IR, Alberti L, et al. ET-743: a novel agent with activity in soft tissue sarcomas. Oncologist. 2005;10(10):827–32.
21. Schoffski P, Ray-Coquard IL, Cioffi A, et al. Activity of eribulin mesylate in patients with soft-tissue sarcoma: a phase 2 study in four independent histological subtypes. Lancet Oncol. 2011;12(11):1045–52.

22. Sleijfer S, Ray-Coquard I, Papai Z, et al. Pazopanib, a multikinase angiogenesis inhibitor, in patients with relapsed or refractory advanced soft tissue sarcoma: a phase II study from the European organisation for research and treatment of cancer-soft tissue and bone sarcoma group (EORTC study 62043). J Clin Oncol. 2009;27(19):3126–32.
23. Robbins PF, Morgan RA, Feldman SA, et al. Tumor regression in patients with metastatic synovial cell sarcoma and melanoma using genetically engineered lymphocytes reactive with NY-ESO-1. J Clin Oncol. 2011;29(7):917–24.
24. Lubieniecka JM, de Bruijn DR, Su L, et al. Histone deacetylase inhibitors reverse SS18-SSX-mediated polycomb silencing of the tumor suppressor early growth response 1 in synovial sarcoma. Cancer Res. 2008;68(11):4303–10.
25. Nguyen A, Su L, Campbell B, et al. Synergism of heat shock protein 90 and histone deacetylase inhibitors in synovial sarcoma. Sarcoma. 2009;2009:794901.
26. Su L, Sampaio AV, Jones KB, et al. Deconstruction of the SS18-SSX fusion oncoprotein complex: insights into disease etiology and therapeutics. Cancer Cell. 2012;21(3):333–47.
27. Ladanyi M. Correlates of SYT-SSX fusion type in synovial sarcoma: getting more complex but also more interesting? J Clin Oncol. 2005;23(15):3638–9.
28. Guillou L, Benhattar L, Bonichon F, et al. Histologic grade, but not SYT-SSX fusion type, is an important prognostic factor in patients with synovial sarcoma: a multicenter, retrospective analysis. J Clin Oncol. 2004;22(20):4040–50.
29. Lewis JJ, Antonescu CR, Leung DH, et al. Synovial sarcoma: a multivariate analysis of prognostic factors in 112 patients with primary localized tumors of the extremity. J Clin Oncol. 2000;18(10):2087–94.

Chapter 9
Malignant Peripheral Nerve Sheath Tumor (MPNST) and Triton Tumor

Malignant peripheral nerve sheath tumors (MPNSTs) are tumors that arise from cellular components of a normal nerve, i.e., Schwann cells and perineurial cells. They are relatively uncommon and very aggressive soft-tissue tumors seen in two settings, sporadic and associated with neurofibromatosis (NF) type 1. Despite the two clinical scenarios, the biological background, loss of *NF1* expression by deletion or mutation, is believed to be similar. Older, abandoned terms for MPNST include neurofibrosarcoma, malignant schwannoma, and neurogenic sarcoma.

Presentation

MPNST arises as a mass lesion that is often painful. Approximately one-third will be associated with NF type 1. Age distribution (Fig. 9.1) and site distribution (Fig. 9.2) for adult patients at MSKCC are shown. A different series had a median age of 33 with a male predominance and a median size of 9.5 cm [1].

In NF type 1 (NF1), it is most common to observe MPNST to arise in plexiform neurofibromas that undergo malignant transformation, typically in the sciatic nerve, lumbosacral, or brachial plexus (Fig. 9.3). Remarkably, 10% or fewer of patients with NF1 (also termed von Recklinghausen disease) will develop an MPNST. Conversely, other tumors are more common in NF1 patients, including benign dermal neurofibromas which are nearly universal, and plexiform neurofibromas, which occur in as many as half of NF1 patients, and optic gliomas (as many as 10–15%) [2].

Imaging

Imaging as for other primary high-grade sarcomas is predominantly MRI and CT, with one not being preferred over the other (Figs. 9.4 and 9.5). For tumors involving the brachial or lumbosacral plexus, MRI may have an advantage in outlining extent of tumor. The use of PET scan to discern plexiform neurofibroma from MPNST is

M.F. Brennan et al., *Management of Soft Tissue Sarcoma*,
DOI 10.1007/978-1-4614-5004-7_9, © Springer Science+Business Media New York 2013

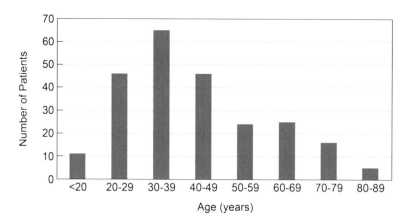

Fig. 9.1 Age distribution of adult patients with malignant peripheral nerve sheath tumor. MSKCC 7/1/82–6/30/2010 n = 238

Fig. 9.2 Anatomic primary site distribution of adult patients with malignant peripheral nerve sheath tumor. MSKCC 7/1/82–6/30/2010 n = 238. Retro/IA = retroperitoneal/intraabdominal

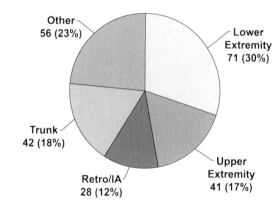

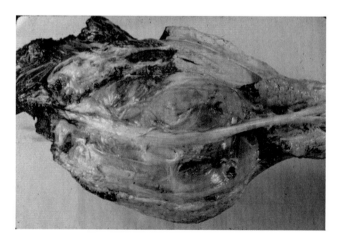

Fig. 9.3 Gross pathology image of a sciatic nerve malignant peripheral nerve sheath tumor, highlighting the nerve entering and exiting the tumor

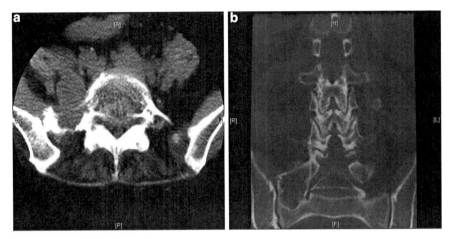

Fig. 9.4 Noncontrast axial (**a**) and coronal (**b**) CT images of a malignant peripheral nerve sheath tumor of a *right*-sided lumbar nerve root developing after sacral irradiation

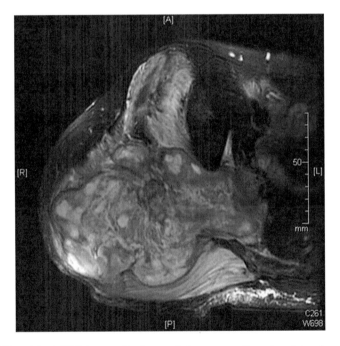

Fig. 9.5 T2-weighted MRI image of a large sciatic nerve malignant peripheral nerve sheath tumor

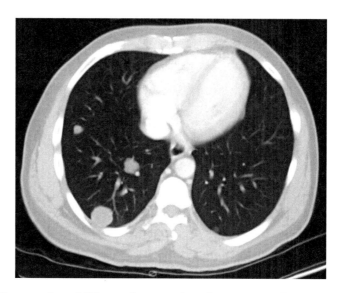

Fig. 9.6 Contrast-enhanced CT scan of a metastatic malignant peripheral nerve sheath tumor to lung

investigational [3], but rarely helpful in the presence of neurofibromas, in our experience. Unfortunately, metastatic disease is all too common (Fig. 9.6) and appears to be more common than with many other forms of soft-tissue sarcoma.

Diagnosis/Pathology

MPNSTs have a characteristic microscopic pattern of a high-grade spindle cell lesion arranged in intersecting fascicles and geographic areas of necrosis (Figs. 9.7 and 9.8). It can be difficult to discern MPNST from poorly differentiated monophasic synovial sarcoma or melanoma, especially in the head and neck area, and care must be taken with this differential diagnosis [4, 5]. A significant number of reported MPNST may represent spindle cell melanoma.

Triton tumor is a name given to MPNST with rhabdomyosarcomatous divergent differentiation [6]. Masson gave this tumor its name in 1932 after observing that it appeared microscopically similar to the supernumerary limbs in Tritons (salamanders of the genus *Triturus*) grown by implantation of the cut end of the sciatic nerve into the soft tissues of the back. Triton tumors are also highly aggressive [6] and are managed similarly with other MPNST.

A variety of gene expression profiling and other molecular and genetic analyses have been performed, comparing MPNSTs to other sarcomas [7, 8], to Schwann cells [9], and to plexiform neurofibromas [10–13]. These data confirm somewhat

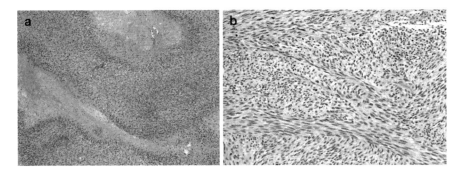

Fig. 9.7 Microscopic image anatomy of high grade malignant peripheral nerve sheath tumor (H&E). (**a**) Low power showing typical large areas of geographic necrosis, 100×. (**b**) Higher power showing intersecting fascicles composed of monotonous spindle cells with hyperchromatic nuclei and high mitotic activity, 200×

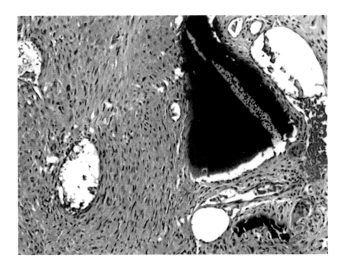

Fig. 9.8 Radiation-induced high grade malignant peripheral nerve sheath tumor with bone invasion, H&E, 100×

older studies regarding expression of *EGFR* in MPNST [14] as well as *PDGFR-alpha, -beta,* and *KIT* [15–17] and highlight important genes/pathways activated in MPNST, including neural crest stem cell markers (*TWIST1* and *SOX9*), apoptosis (survivin/*BIRC5, TP73*), ras-raf signaling (*RASF2, HMMR*), and the Hedgehog pathway (*DHH, Ptch2*). Amplification and deletions are seen in a variety of genes beyond *NF1* as well, such as *p16INK4A, TP73, MET,* and *NEDL1,* and *HGF* consistent with the co-opting of critical growth pathways in MPNST beyond NF1-ras-raf signaling [18–21].

Neurofibromatosis Type 1 and Outcome

In neurofibromatosis type 1, the underlying gene abnormality is deletion or loss of *NF1* on chromosome 17, causing loss of a functional protein (neurofibromin) that is normally a suppressor of p21-ras. The *NF2* gene, on chromosome 22, is more commonly associated with benign central nervous system tumors.

The preponderance of data from several review studies indicates that MPNSTs arise earlier in patients with NF1 and fare worse than people who have an MPNST arise spontaneously [22–29]. However, when MPNSTs from NF type 1 patients and those arising sporadically were compared in a large surgical series corrected for other known prognostic factors such as size and site, these differences disappeared (Fig. 9.9) [30].

A recent analysis of 120 cases from the Mayo Clinic [25] suggests that the prevalence of MPNST in neurofibromatosis was ~5% and the tumors occurred at an earlier age (Fig. 9.10) and outcome was worse (Fig. 9.11); however, most MPNSTs associated with neurofibromatosis are large and high grade, with known poor prognostic factors.

Treatment

The primary treatment is surgical, and as they typically arise from major nerve plexuses, potential morbidity is high. Primary disease presents multiple problems in terms of local control. For tumors arising from large nerves, the loss of function is obvious. With MPNST arising from plexiform neurofibromas, it is often difficult to discern which portion of the large nerve plexus is affected by tumor and which area is not. As benign neurofibromata can be PET avid, ^{18}F-FDG-PET is rarely helpful. There is obviously greater morbidity associated with loss of multiple nerve roots, which must be balanced with the understanding of the poor prognosis of such patients even with optimal surgery. It is not unusual to see tumor recurrences that skip portions of normal nerve, frustrating attempts at local control. On occasions, the lesions are so large and involve such major nerves that amputation is necessary. In our earlier series, almost one-third came to amputation either primarily or because of otherwise unresectable recurrence.

Radiation Therapy

The clinical situation is made more difficult by either early development of metastatic disease for most patients with larger (>5 cm) tumors or the development of multiple primary tumors simultaneously in some patients. As with other large primary sarcomas, radiation therapy is standard of care in the adjuvant setting, but the local-regional relapse rate is still significant [31].

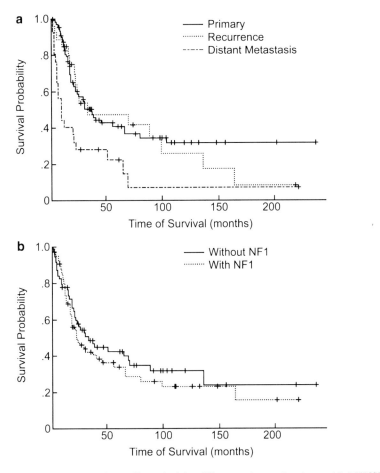

Fig. 9.9 Kaplan-Meier curves of overall survival for different cohorts of patients with MPNST. (**a**) Patients with metastatic disease (*dotted line*) fare worse than those with localized primary disease (*dark solid line*, p=0.0025). There was no difference in disease-specific survival for patients with primary vs. recurrent disease (*light solid line*, p=0.92). (**b**) There is no statistical difference in overall survival comparing patients with NF1-associated MPNST (*light solid line*) vs. those with sporadic MPNST (*dark solid line*) (Used with permission from: Zou et al. [30])

Chemotherapy

Our general practice is to not offer adjuvant chemotherapy for patients with primary MPNST, given the relative lack of activity of chemotherapy in the metastatic setting. Adjuvant chemotherapy is administered by some physicians in consideration of the high risk of metastatic disease. In our experience, the RECIST response rate for doxorubicin-ifosfamide is under 10% using doxorubicin at 75 mg/m^2 per cycle and ifosfamide at 9 g/m^2/cycle.

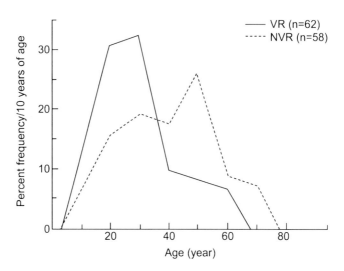

Fig. 9.10 MPNST in patients with NF1 (*solid line*) develops earlier than those with sporadic MPNST (*dotted line*) (Used with permission from Ducatman et al. [25]) *VR* - von Recklinghausen *NVR* - non-von Recklinghausen

Fig. 9.11 Data from an independent series from Fig. 9.10 indicating inferior overall survival for patients with NF1 associated MPNST (*solid line*) compared to patients with sporadic MPNST (*dotted line*) (From Ducatman et al. [25]) *VR* - von Recklinghausen *NVR* - non-von Recklinghausen

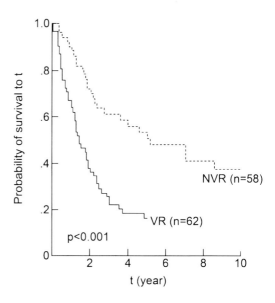

For metastatic disease, similar poor options exist for therapy. There is a low response rate in our experience with both doxorubicin-ifosfamide and gemcitabine combinations for patients with MPNST, with perhaps the greatest response rate for a single agent from ifosfamide. Cisplatin may have minor activity, and given the overexpression of *TOP2A* in MPNST [32], one might expect etoposide or doxorubicin to have greater activity in MPNST than other sarcomas, but it is not clear if

Table 9.1 Recommendations for systemic therapy for patients with malignant peripheral nerve sheath tumor

Clinical scenario		Comments
Adjuvant chemotherapy		Difficult to recommend outside the setting of a clinical trial given the poor response rate in the metastatic setting
Metastatic disease	First line	(Doxorubicin)-ifosfamide
	Second line	Clinical trial; sorafenib (or other B-raf inhibitor) difficult to recommend routinely Pazopanib. Erlotinib is inactive in one phase II study. We have not observed dramatic results with gemcitabine-based therapy in a small number of patients treated. Combinations of agents including TOR inhibitors have been suggested from preclinical models

such relative overexpression represents a marker for sensitivity or resistance to topoisomerase II inhibitors.

Among targeted agents, although EGFR is expressed in MPNST, erlotinib was inactive in one multicenter phase II [33]. Similarly, by virtue of elimination of NF1 expression in MPNST and activation of ras-raf pathways, sorafenib was of interest for metastatic disease, but only minor responses (and no RECIST responses) were observed in a phase II study of sorafenib in MPNST patients [34]. The minor responses in the latter study indicate that a better raf inhibitor could be associated with greater activity and also calls for examination of combinations of other agents, e.g., those agents that block mTOR [35]. Identification of other treatment strategies seems paramount [36, 37]. Since <10% of patients with neurofibromatosis type 1 develop MPNST, it stands to reason that mutation or deletion of *NF1* is associated with the preneoplastic lesion, i.e., a neurofibroma, but that other genetic changes (e.g., alterations in *Rb* or *TP53*) are necessary to yield an MPNST, making targeting such tumors potentially much more difficult. (Table 9.1)

Outcome

As with other high-grade sarcomas, margin positivity predicts an unfavorable local recurrence rate but does not appear to be causative for death from disease as amputation is not associated with improved survival [1]. Local recurrence-free survival and disease-specific survival curves for patients with MPNST are shown in Figs. 9.12 and 9.13. A recent review from the Mayo Clinic of 175 patients found a local recurrence rate of 22% and 5- and 10-year disease-specific survival of 60% and 45%, respectively, with known poor prognostic factors of grade and large size [38].

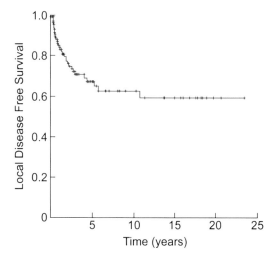

Fig. 9.12 Local recurrence-free survival for adult patients with primary MPNST. MSKCC 7/1/82–6/30/2010 n = 141

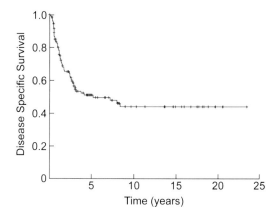

Fig. 9.13 Disease-specific survival for adult patients with primary MPNST. MSKCC 7/1/82–6/30/2010 n = 141

References

1. Vauthey JN, Woodruff JM, Brennan MF. Extremity malignant peripheral nerve sheath tumors (neurogenic sarcomas): a 10-year experience. Ann Surg Oncol. 1995;2(2):126–31.
2. Widemann BC. Current status of sporadic and neurofibromatosis type 1-associated malignant peripheral nerve sheath tumors. Curr Oncol Rep. 2009;11(4):322–8.
3. Basu S, Nair N. Potential clinical role of FDG-PET in detecting sarcomatous transformation in von Recklinghausen's disease: a case study and review of the literature. J Neurooncol. 2006;80(1):91–5.
4. Leong AS, Wannakrairot P. A retrospective analysis of immunohistochemical staining in identification of poorly differentiated round cell and spindle cell tumors–results, reagents and costs. Pathology. 1992;24(4):254–60.

5. Lodding P, Kindblom LG, Angervall L. Metastases of malignant melanoma simulating soft tissue sarcoma A clinico-pathological, light- and electron microscopic and immunohistochemical study of 21 cases. Virchows Arch A Pathol Anat Histopathol. 1990;417(5):377–88.

6. Woodruff JM, Chernik NL, Smith MC, et al. Peripheral nerve tumors with rhabdomyosarcomatous differentiation (malignant "Triton" tumors). Cancer. 1973;32(2):426–39.

7. Nielsen TO, West RB, Linn SC, et al. Molecular characterisation of soft tissue tumours: a gene expression study. Lancet. 2002;359(9314):1301–7.

8. Segal NH, Pavlidis P, Antonescu CR, et al. Classification and subtype prediction of adult soft tissue sarcoma by functional genomics. Am J Pathol. 2003;163(2):691–700.

9. Miller SJ, Rangwala F, Williams J, et al. Large-scale molecular comparison of human schwann cells to malignant peripheral nerve sheath tumor cell lines and tissues. Cancer Res. 2006; 66(5):2584–91.

10. Holtkamp N, Mautner VF, Friedrich RE, et al. Differentially expressed genes in neurofibromatosis 1-associated neurofibromas and malignant peripheral nerve sheath tumors. Acta Neuropathol. 2004;107(2):159–68.

11. Holtkamp N, Reuss DE, Atallah I, et al. Subclassification of nerve sheath tumors by gene expression profiling. Brain Pathol. 2004;14(3):258–64.

12. Levy P, Bieche I, Leroy K, et al. Molecular profiles of neurofibromatosis type 1-associated plexiform neurofibromas: identification of a gene expression signature of poor prognosis. Clin Cancer Res. 2004;10(11):3763–71.

13. Levy P, Vidaud D, Leroy K, et al. Molecular profiling of malignant peripheral nerve sheath tumors associated with neurofibromatosis type 1, based on large-scale real-time RT-PCR. Mol Cancer. 2004;3:20.

14. Watson MA, Perry A, Tihan T, et al. Gene expression profiling reveals unique molecular subtypes of Neurofibromatosis Type I-associated and sporadic malignant peripheral nerve sheath tumors. Brain Pathol. 2004;14(3):297–303.

15. Badache A, De Vries GH. Neurofibrosarcoma-derived Schwann cells overexpress platelet-derived growth factor (PDGF) receptors and are induced to proliferate by PDGF BB. J Cell Physiol. 1998;177(2):334–42.

16. Badache A, Muja N, De Vries GH. Expression of Kit in neurofibromin-deficient human Schwann cells: role in Schwann cell hyperplasia associated with type 1 neurofibromatosis. Oncogene. 1998;17(6):795–800.

17. Dang I, Nelson JK, DeVries GH. c-Kit receptor expression in normal human Schwann cells and Schwann cell lines derived from neurofibromatosis type 1 tumors. J Neurosci Res. 2005;82(4):465–71.

18. Mantripragada KK, Diaz de Stahl T, Patridge C, et al. Genome-wide high-resolution analysis of DNA copy number alterations in NF1-associated malignant peripheral nerve sheath tumors using 32K BAC array. Genes Chromosomes Cancer. 2009;48(10):897–907.

19. Mantripragada KK, Spurlock G, Kluwe L, et al. High-resolution DNA copy number profiling of malignant peripheral nerve sheath tumors using targeted microarray-based comparative genomic hybridization. Clin Cancer Res. 2008;14(4):1015–24.

20. Upadhyaya M, Han S, Consoli C, et al. Characterization of the somatic mutational spectrum of the neurofibromatosis type 1 (NF1) gene in neurofibromatosis patients with benign and malignant tumors. Hum Mutat. 2004;23(2):134–46.

21. Upadhyaya M, Kluwe L, Spurlock G, et al. Germline and somatic NF1 gene mutation spectrum in NF1-associated malignant peripheral nerve sheath tumors (MPNSTs). Hum Mutat. 2008;29(1):74–82.

22. Carli M, Ferrari A, Mattke A, et al. Pediatric malignant peripheral nerve sheath tumor: the Italian and German soft tissue sarcoma cooperative group. J Clin Oncol. 2005;23(33): 8422–30.

23. Cashen DV, Parisien RC, Raskin K, et al. Survival data for patients with malignant schwannoma. Clin Orthop Relat Res. 2004;426:69–73.

24. deCou JM, Rao BN, Parham DM, et al. Malignant peripheral nerve sheath tumors: the St. Jude children's research hospital experience. Ann Surg Oncol. 1995;2(6):524–9.
25. Ducatman BS, Scheithauer BW, Piepgras DG, et al. Malignant peripheral nerve sheath tumors. A clinicopathologic study of 120 cases. Cancer. 1986;57(10):2006–21.
26. Evans DG, Baser ME, McGaughran J, et al. Malignant peripheral nerve sheath tumours in neurofibromatosis 1. J Med Genet. 2002;39(5):311–4.
27. Hruban RH, Shiu MH, Senie RT, et al. Malignant peripheral nerve sheath tumors of the buttock and lower extremity. A study of 43 cases. Cancer. 1990;66(6):1253–65.
28. Sordillo PP, Helson L, Hajdu SI, et al. Malignant schwannoma–clinical characteristics, survival, and response to therapy. Cancer. 1981;47(10):2503–9.
29. Wong WW, Hirose T, Scheithauer BW, et al. Malignant peripheral nerve sheath tumor: analysis of treatment outcome. Int J Radiat Oncol Biol Phys. 1998;42(2):351–60.
30. Zou C, Smith KD, Liu J, et al. Clinical, pathological, and molecular variables predictive of malignant peripheral nerve sheath tumor outcome. Ann Surg. 2009;249(6):1014–22.
31. Gupta G, Mammis A, Maniker A. Malignant peripheral nerve sheath tumors. Neurosurg Clin N Am. 2008;19(4):533–43.
32. Skotheim RI, Kallioniemi A, Bjerkhagen B, et al. Topoisomerase-II alpha is upregulated in malignant peripheral nerve sheath tumors and associated with clinical outcome. J Clin Oncol. 2003;21(24):4586–91.
33. Albritton KH, Rankin C, Coffin CM, et al. Phase II study of erlotinib in metastatic or unresectable malignant peripheral nerve sheath tumors (MPNST). ASCO Meet Abstr. 2006;24 Suppl 18:9518.
34. Maki RG, D'Adamo DR, Keohan ML, et al. Phase II study of sorafenib in patients with metastatic or recurrent sarcomas. J Clin Oncol. 2009;27(19):3133–40.
35. Johansson G, Mahller YY, Collins MH, et al. Effective in vivo targeting of the mammalian target of rapamycin pathway in malignant peripheral nerve sheath tumors. Mol Cancer Ther. 2008;7(5):1237–45.
36. Yang J, Ylipaa A, Sun Y, et al. Genomic and molecular characterization of malignant peripheral nerve sheath tumor identifies the IGF1R pathway as a primary target for treatment. Clin Cancer Res. 2011;17(24):7563–73.
37. Zou CY, Smith KD, Zhu QS, et al. Dual targeting of AKT and mammalian target of rapamycin: a potential therapeutic approach for malignant peripheral nerve sheath tumor. Mol Cancer Ther. 2009;8(5):1157–68.
38. Stucky CC, Johnson KN, Gray RJ, et al. Malignant peripheral nerve sheath tumors (MPNST): the mayo clinic experience. Ann Surg Oncol. 2012;19(3):878–85.

Chapter 10
Desmoid Tumor/Deep-Seated Fibromatosis (Desmoid-Type Fibromatosis)

Desmoids are enigmatic clonal malignancies of myofibroblastic cells that do not have the ability to metastasize, but cause morbidity and occasionally mortality by locally aggressive growth. They are sometimes termed deep fibromatoses, to distinguish them from superficial fibromatoses such as Dupuytren contracture, trigger finger, or Peyronie disease.

Desmoids can occur at any anatomic site (Fig. 10.1), and the age at presentation is variable (Fig. 10.2). A clinical classification of desmoids distinguishes three scenarios. In the first, a desmoid arises in the abdominal wall in the setting of pregnancy. This form of desmoid tumor may be hormonally driven and frequently dissipates postpartum. The second common clinical scenario is that of spontaneous development of a desmoid in the extremity or trunk (Fig. 10.3). These tumors are most frequently associated with mutation in the beta-catenin gene (*CTNNB1*). There are some patients with antecedent trauma that, unlike sarcomas, may be related to the development of the tumor. The final common scenario is the development of a mesenteric desmoid, frequently in the setting of familial adenomatous polyposis (FAP), with its characteristic loss of expression of the adenomatous polyposis coli (*APC*) gene. FAP-associated desmoids are more commonly diffuse and can be associated with bowel perforation or bowel obstruction. A proportion of desmoids that have no *CTNNB1* mutation instead demonstrate loss of *APC* as an apparent mechanism of development.

At least 10% of all patients with familial adenomatous polyposis (FAP) develop mesenteric desmoids [1], although desmoids in such patients occasionally arise at other sites. The lesions that develop in the vicinity of the proximal mesenteric arterial and venous drainage increase the risk of severe morbidity from either overaggressive treatment or from progression of disease, creating a fundamentally difficult situation with respect to management.

In the patient with FAP, the desmoid tumor is assuming a more prominent role in the death of the patient following the prevention of metastatic colon cancer by prophylactic colectomy and is now the most common cause of death for patients with FAP who have colectomy [1].

M.F. Brennan et al., *Management of Soft Tissue Sarcoma*,
DOI 10.1007/978-1-4614-5004-7_10, © Springer Science+Business Media New York 2013

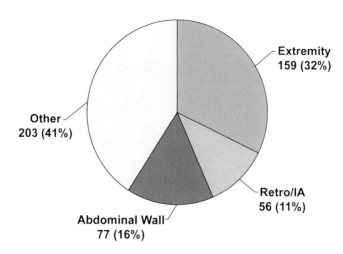

Fig. 10.1 Primary site distribution of adult patients with desmoid tumor/deep fibromatosis. MSKCC 7/1/1982–6/30/2010. n = 495 Retro/IA = retroperitoneal/intra-abdominal

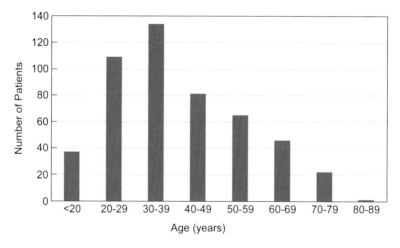

Fig. 10.2 Age distribution of adult patients with desmoid tumor/deep fibromatosis. MSKCC 7/1/1982–6/30/2010 n = 495

FAP may not be the only diagnosis associated with development of desmoid tumors. There appears to be a nonrandom association between development of GIST (gastrointestinal stromal tumor) and desmoid tumors [2]. The degree of this association will probably best be determined by examination of large national databases such as that of SEER or other national registries.

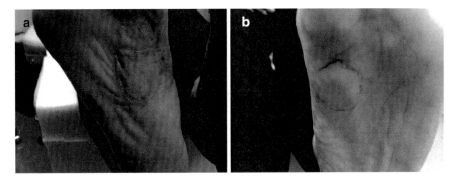

Fig. 10.3 Images of a patient with bilateral plantar desmoid tumor who also had Dupuytren contracture of both hands (**a** and **b**)

Clinical Presentation

The clinical presentation is usually that of a localized, firm to hard mass often in the proximal extremity or in the abdominal wall. The diagnosis is suspected when a lesion is in a classic position, e.g., the abdominal wall of a parturient female or in the retroperitoneum of a patient with a familial polyposis [3, 4].

Imaging

Both CT and MRI are utilized in diagnostic imaging (Fig. 10.4). The T2 signal on MRI imaging may serve as a surrogate for the relative cellularity of the lesion, with T2 bright lesions being more cellular and T2 dark lesions representing more collagenous and acellular areas of a tumor [5, 6]. We have observed two radiographic patterns of desmoids, either nodular, with rounded surfaces, or diffuse, with tentacles of tumor extending into surrounding tissues. The latter pattern is most commonly encountered in the mesenteric variety of desmoids.

Diagnosis: Molecular

Desmoids are myofibroblastic proliferations that can be sometimes difficult to discern from scar tissue, nodular fasciitis, and other diagnoses (Fig. 10.5). As expected, desmoids associated with FAP demonstrate inactivation of adenomatous polyposis coli (*APC*) gene by mutation or deletion. Sporadic desmoids frequently contain beta-catenin (*CTNNB1*) mutations, typically in codons 41 or 45 of exon 3 [7]. Both APC and beta-catenin are elements of the Wnt signaling pathway. Alterations in APC and CTNNB1 lead to stabilization of nuclear beta-catenin and subsequent binding to members of the T cell factor/lymphoid enhancer factor (TCF/LEF) family

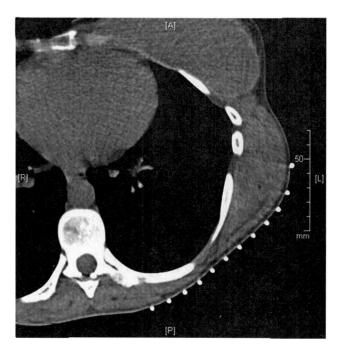

Fig. 10.4 Noncontrast CT image (with CT markers) of a patient with a left subscapular desmoid tumor

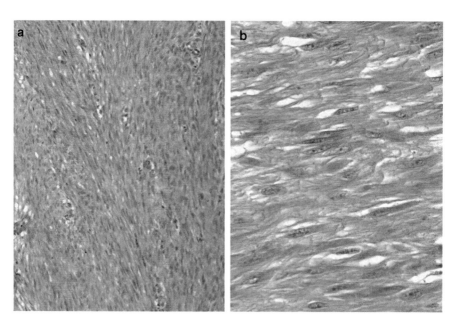

Fig. 10.5 Light microscopy of desmoid tumor (deep seated fibromatosis), H&E staining. (**a**) Low-power image demonstrating uniform spindle cells arranged in long intersecting fascicles (100×); (**b**) higher-power image demonstrating bland spindle cells with open chromatin and small nucleoli, separated by abundant collagenous stroma. The cells typically lack hyperchromasia or cytologic pleomorphism that would suggest a spindle cell soft tissue sarcoma

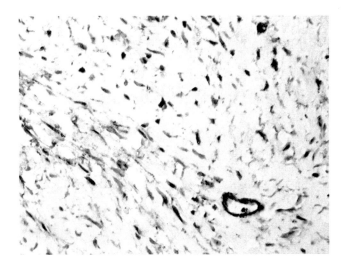

Fig. 10.6 Immunohistochemical staining demonstrating nuclear beta-catenin in a desmoid tumor of the abdomen (200×)

of transcription factors. The site of *APC* mutation in patients with FAP dictates the risk of developing desmoid tumors [8, 9].

Domont [10] reported that 85% of desmoid tumors contain a *CTNNB1* mutation, predominantly in codons 41 or 45 of exon 3, which can be used as a diagnostic tool. In addition, there may be prognostic information based on the type of mutation in *CTNNB1* observed. In particular, the exon 3 S45F mutation appears to be associated with increased recurrence rate, while wild-type *CTNNB1* or mutations in codon 41 may indicate a desmoid less likely to recur [7, 11].

Nuclear beta-catenin positivity by immunohistochemistry appears to be a useful ancillary tool, where it is difficult to differentiate between recurrent desmoid and simple scar tissue (Fig. 10.6) [12, 13]. Other lesions in the differential diagnosis include nodular fasciitis, fibrosarcomas, GIST (gastrointestinal stromal tumor), leiomyosarcoma, and other sarcomas, depending on the anatomic location. Other tumors that can contain *CTNNB1* mutations include pilomatrix carcinomas of skin, hepatoblastoma, and solid pseudopapillary tumor of pancreas, among others, so it is unlikely to make errors in diagnosis on this basis. Desmoids express ER (estrogen receptor)-beta, which is distinct from the form found in breast cancer (ER-alpha), but perhaps the reason some desmoids are sensitive to estrogen blockade or deprivation [14].

Natural History

The enigmatic behavior of the desmoid tumor has been well recognized and is part of the reason that management varies from one institution to another [4, 15, 16]. The natural behavior is of an infiltrative and persistent lesion without metastatic potential.

Some lesions show only sluggish change and few symptoms, while others can grow with a relentless course. Some are easily removed by wide excision, while others appear in difficult areas such as the axilla or near the root of mesentery, where anatomic limitations make primary management difficult [3, 4, 17, 18]. Only limited numbers of desmoids are ultimately unresectable or unresectable without amputation, and desmoids may respond to either radiation therapy or systemic therapy, be it hormonal agents, cytotoxic chemotherapy, or kinase-specific agents such as sorafenib, sunitinib, or imatinib [19–21]. Any response to treatment must be weighed against the finding of occasional patients with spontaneous improvement in their desmoids. The differences in anatomic location, association with FAP, growth rate, and potential utility of multiple modalities for this diagnosis make comparison of different series of patients complicated.

Treatment

The primary treatment of the desmoid tumor is surgical resection. However, this treatment decision must be finely balanced between the aggressiveness of the lesion and the aggressiveness of the surgical process [3, 18, 22–24]. It has been suggested that small bowel autograft or allograft are options for the patient with desmoids or as a consequence of aggressive resection that has resulted in loss of small intestine and dependence upon intravenous nutrition [25]. Emphasis, however, remains on complete gross resection in the setting of minimal morbidity; both the quoted series and our own experience with people who have sought out bowel transplantation for desmoids of the mesentery have suggested a high short-term mortality rate and longer-term morbidity rate from the procedure.

Given the variable nature of progression in these tumors, some suggestion has been to follow a wait-and-see policy. For more indolent lesions, serial observation by exam and imaging may be useful, but this finding should be predicated on information from the patient examination and imaging studies [23]. It is important to emphasize that a conservative approach to surgery in patients with desmoids is always an option and should certainly be considered when the side effects of the treatment are significant.

Treatment of Recurrence

Treatment of recurrence has become increasingly conservative. We have moved from extraordinary aggression to trying to select only those patients with recurrence who are symptomatic or who have high probability of becoming symptomatic. The real challenge, however, is the person who has marked progression with small bowel loss with potential demise. The challenge remains to identify those patients who are going to progress versus those patients who have an indolent course. Desmoids with wild-type *CTNNB1* or exon 3 codon 41 mutations may fare better than those with the S45F mutation, but this favorable group represents only a minority of desmoids.

Systemic Therapy

Despite many case reports of the use of nonsteroidal anti-inflammatory agents in desmoid tumors, we have not observed significant activity of such agents in patients with desmoid tumors. The utility of antiestrogen therapy is well recognized and often a good first line of therapy in relatively asymptomatic patients with growing tumors [26, 27]. The first series reporting the activity of systemic chemotherapy came from MD Anderson in 1993, in which the activity of doxorubicin with dacarbazine was readily demonstrated [20]. We have employed this chapter and others as templates for potentially active agents, deconstructing combinations into individual agents, given the increased toxicity of combination therapy, and the lack of recognized synergy of any particular combination. Other series have reported on the activity of vinblastine and methotrexate, vinorelbine and methotrexate, or hydroxyurea [28–31].

We reported our experience with systemic therapy for desmoids (68 patients, 157 lines of therapy) in 2009 [19]. The most active agents in our analysis included anthracyclines and antiestrogens. The activity of anthracyclines was further confirmed in a retrospective analysis in France [32]. Progression-free survival rates of ~70% at 3–5 years were commonly observed, and there were few relapses in patients after a patient had a response. In another review [33], the group at MD Anderson examined the use of systemic therapy for nonresectable lesions. Of the 29 patients who received systemic therapy, there was one complete response, 11 partial responses, and two with stable disease. Like our own and other series, these data are difficult to evaluate with the variable nature of the disease; as seen in other series, only one patient died due to uncontrolled progression of the desmoid, again emphasizing the importance of balancing the morbidity of any treatment against the subsequent morbidity of the disease and the risk for demise. Responses to any one of a number of interventions are possible (Fig. 10.7).

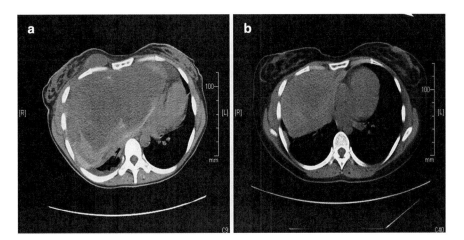

Fig. 10.7 Noncontrast CT images of a 35-year-old female patient with aggressive chest wall desmoid with cardiovascular collapse who responded to sorafenib. (**a**) Pretreatment and (**b**) 28 months after starting sorafenib

Table 10.1 Recommendations for therapy for patients with desmoid tumor/deep fibromatosis[a]

Primary disease	Observation in selected patients; surgical extirpation. Systemic therapy as noted below can be considered in patients with locally advanced disease in whom morbidity would be great
Adjuvant therapy after primary disease resection	Radiation to be considered in patients with overt positive margins
Recurrence	Observation, surgery, or systemic therapy
Multifocal, recurrent, or unresectable disease (or unresectable without amputation): first line	Antiestrogens (tamoxifen, toremifene, anastrozole, letrozole, GnRH agonist)
Recurrent intra-abdominal desmoids refractory to other therapy	Pegylated liposomal doxorubicin (Doxil/Caelyx), doxorubicin, doxorubicin-dacarbazine first line; other active agents include methotrexate, vinorelbine, vinblastine, hydroxyurea
Extremity desmoids refractory to other therapy	Sorafenib, sunitinib, pazopanib or possibly other tyrosine kinase inhibitors; systemic agents as immediately above

[a]Note: Clinical trials of novel agents are recommended when available

Several series report on the activity of imatinib in desmoid tumors. While responses are durable in some patients, the Response Evaluation Criteria in Solid Tumor (RECIST) response rate is only 6–15% [34–37]. In our own patients, imatinib was inferior to both anthracycline-based and antiestrogens [19]. A recent report [34] describes a series of patients who were not curable by surgical resection or in whom surgery would lead to an inappropriate functional impairment were treated with imatinib 300 mg twice daily with response outcome at 2 and 4 months being measured. Fifty-one patients were studied, and 4-month progression-free survival of 94–88% was identified. One-year progression-free survival was 66%. It would appear that proven benefit of imatinib in this often slow-growing and spontaneously stable tumor is of little value. An objective RECIST response rate of 6% (3 of 51) was identified.

The activity of second-generation small-molecule tyrosine kinase inhibitors was first suggested by Skubitz et al. [38], who noted a patient who failed imatinib but responded to sunitinib [38]. We observed clinical improvement in an index patient on sorafenib and have used it in an off-label setting. In a retrospective analysis of treated patients, the RECIST response rate appears to be significantly greater than imatinib (~30%), but this is a retrospective analysis of patients in an off-trial setting, and the durability of response is unknown [39]. A proportion of patients we treated with sorafenib showed progression of tumor within weeks or months of stopping sorafenib, while others have continued without further disease progression. Patients with extremity tumor appear to fare better than those with desmoids in other sites, and those with FAP appear to benefit least from such an approach. The relationship of *CTNNB1 or APC* mutations to response to sorafenib is unknown as well. Also interesting are anecdotes of desmoid patients with responses to gamma-secretase inhibitors, which are at least somewhat logical given that gamma-secretase expression is at least in part controlled by beta-catenin signaling, but such agents require prospective evaluation. Pazopanib and other tyrosine kinase inhibitors may also demonstrate benefit against desmoids, but this hypothesis requires prospective evaluation (Table 10.1).

Treatment by Observation

There is an increasing tendency to follow some patients with observation only. In a series of 142 patients who were treated with observation (n = 83) or assorted medical therapy (n = 59), 47% were treated with vinblastine/methotrexate chemotherapy, 34% had hormonal treatment, and 19% of the observation group were younger, more likely female, and asymptomatic [23]. There was no difference in progression-free survival (Fig. 10.8). Figure 10.9 is an example of a patient with 15-year follow-up of a desmoid of the pelvis and hip initially recommended to have a hemipelvectomy, having been followed with observation alone.

Radiation Therapy

Historically, radiation therapy is widely used in the management of desmoids for any persistent disease and in particular for any patient with positive margins. However, it is now clear that at least two-thirds of patients who have positive margins do not recur and the uniform utilization of radiation therapy is not indicated, paying particular attention to younger patients [4, 40, 41]. Radiation therapy can be utilized for control in the symptomatic patient with an unresectable lesion.

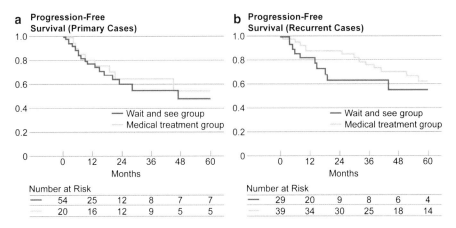

Fig. 10.8 Progression-free survival for patients with (**a**) primary and (**b**) recurrent desmoid tumors who underwent observation only (*dark lines*) or medical therapy (*light-colored lines*). Patients may undergo a period of surveillance and only a proportion of them will show tumor growth over 2–3-year median follow-up (Used with permission from Fiore et al. [23])

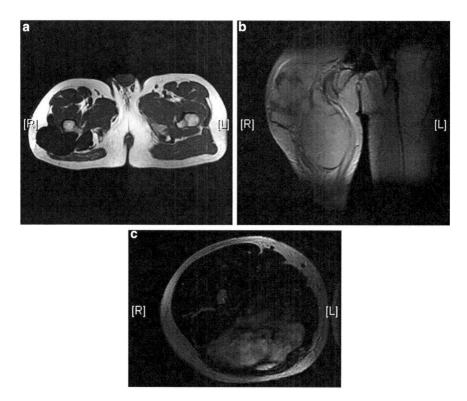

Fig. 10.9 MRI images of a desmoid tumor of the pelvis and thigh in a patient who had received a recommendation for hemipelvectomy at presentation. No change in the tumor was observed in 15 years of follow-up

Patterns of Failure

As described above, the desmoid is a locally infiltrative lesion. The pattern of failure is highly dependent on the presence of the initial lesion. Multifocal lesions have been described [22] and are difficult to understand on a biological basis outside of a field effect on a precursor cell that duplicates and becomes part of each affected area of the limb. Multifocal desmoids are most commonly seen in young women, in the distal extremity both proximal and distal, and multifocal recurrence is common. With age, these appear to progress much more in an indolent fashion suggesting a hormonal association, although this supposition is unproved. Antiestrogens do not appear any more active against multifocal desmoids, also questioning the relationship of multifocal desmoids to estrogen signaling.

Outcome

The local disease-free survival of patients presenting with a primary lesion is shown in Fig. 10.10 with 40% recurrence. Site-dependent local recurrence-free survival is in Fig. 10.11, and disease-specific survival is in Fig. 10.12.

The relationship of recurrence by microscopic margin is a subject of great debate (Table 10.2), and it is difficult to evaluate series where reoperation is performed. It is also hard to evaluate those patients receiving radiation therapy. Both modalities have been used selectively making outcome analysis difficult. Once a patient has a recurrence, however, further recurrences can be anticipated. Perhaps the greater question is why patients with positive margins do not recur, rather than why those

Fig. 10.10 Local disease-free survival for adult patients with primary desmoid tumor/deep fibromatosis. MSKCC 7/1/1982–6/30/2010 n = 361

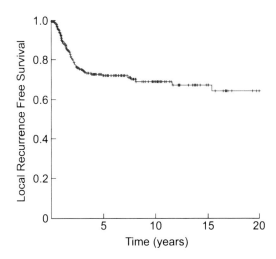

Fig. 10.11 Local disease-free survival by primary site for adult patients with desmoid tumor/deep fibromatosis, including patients with primary disease and local recurrence. MSKCC 7/1/1982–6/30/2010 n = 477

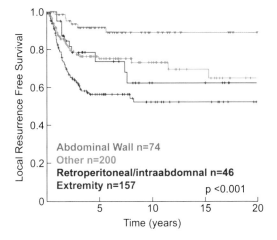

Fig. 10.12 Disease-specific survival by primary site for adult patients with desmoid tumor/deep fibromatosis, including patients with primary disease and local recurrence. MSKCC 7/1/1982–6/30/2010 n=477

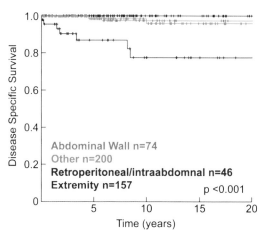

with positive margins do recur. Local recurrence occurs in approximately 25%, and it is important to understand that the natural history is very long. The results of local recurrence by site and by margin status are included in Figs. 10.13 and 10.14.

One analysis [33] examined two groups of 189 patients treated in two time intervals, 1995–2005 and 1965–1994. The progressive trend to use more systemic therapy identified and suggested an improved local recurrence rate in the latter group. These data are difficult to validate in the absence of a randomized trial. The chapter authors' recommendation was that patients resected with positive margins receive radiation therapy and that those patients who have lesions with significant operative risk of morbidity should receive preoperative radiation therapy. This is not an approach that we have taken, given that in patients with positive margins, only 30% recur at any time in their course [4]. We argue that it is hard to justify the uniform use of radiation therapy which at best limits local recurrence from 30% to 15% (Fig. 10.15a, b).

A new analysis of outcomes after initial resection of primary desmoids derived from European series provides insight into clinical risk stratification [42]. In a multivariate analysis, age, tumor size, and tumor site were independent risk factors. Scoring each of the unfavorable prognostic factors (age over 37 at time of presentation [crude hazard ratio 1.97], size>7 cm [crude HR 1.64], and extra-abdominal primary [vs. abdominal wall as lowest risk group, HR 2.55]) yielded three groups with distinguishable risk of local recurrence (0 and 1 risk factors, 2 risk factors, and 3). In the multivariate analysis, intra-abdominal location was worse than abdominal wall, but there was only a trend to inferiority for this anatomic site in multivariate analysis (HR 1.95, $p=0.084$). These findings will become of even greater value once molecular data regarding beta-catenin mutations are linked to the clinical data.

Our most recent analysis [43], where we analyzed 495 patients (382 primary, 113 recurrent) all treated in a single institution, suggested an overall local recurrence rate of 30% at 10 years. Greater than 90% of those who recurred did so within 5 years. Less than 2% died, all after R2 resection.

Table 10.2 Larger series (n >100) examining local recurrence of extremity and trunk desmoids

Author	Year	Number of patients	Primary desmoid (n)	Recurrent desmoid (n)	Median follow-up (months)	5-year PFS (%) with R0 margins	5-year PFS (%) with R1 margins	p-value
Posner [16]	1989	128	78	53	88	85	50	0.002
Merchant [4]	1998	105	105	–	49	70	78	0.51
Ballo [44]	1999	189	85	104	112	75	50	0.003
Gronchi [45]	2003	203	128	–	130	82	79	0.5
			–	75	153	65	47	0.16
Stoeckle [46]	2008	106	69	37	123	n.d.	n.d.	–
Fiore [23]	2009	142	74	68	33	n.d.	n.d.	–
Salas [42]	2011	426	426	–	52	64	62	n.s.

n number of patients, n.d. not done, n.s. not significant, PFS progression-free survival

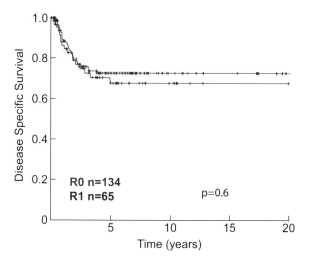

Fig. 10.13 Local disease-free survival by primary site for adult patients with desmoid tumor/deep fibromatosis of the extremity and trunk, classified by margin status, R0 versus R1. MSKCC 7/1/1982–6/30/2010 n = 199

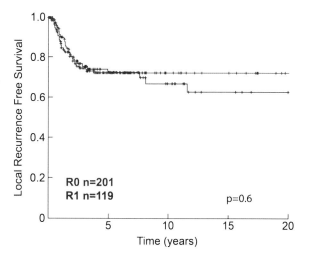

Fig. 10.14 Local disease-free survival by primary site for adult patients with desmoid tumor/deep fibromatosis of all sites, classified by margin status, R0 versus R1. MSKCC 7/1/1982–6/30/2010 n = 320

The important factors predicting recurrence were location, where extremity was more likely to recur than chest wall, more likely than intra-abdominal, more likely than other, and more likely than abdominal wall. Age less than 25 and less than 65 were more likely to recur. Size >10 cm was an important factor in increased recurrence. Positive microscopic margin (R1) was not a predictor of increased recurrence, and we could not show a benefit to radiation treatment. In fact, with a diminishing use of radiation (7% after 1996, 30% before 1997), there was no impact on local recurrence. This has allowed the generation of a predictive nomogram.

Fig. 10.15 Local disease-free survival by primary site for adult patients with desmoid tumor/deep fibromatosis of the extremity with (**a**) R0 n = 82 or (**b**) R1 resection n = 57, classified by use of external beam radiation. MSKCC 7/1/19182–6/30/2010 *EBRT* external beam radiation therapy

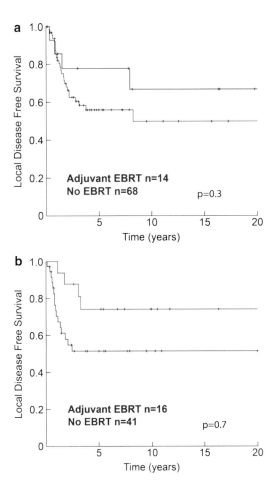

References

1. Half E, Bercovich D, Rozen P. Familial adenomatous polyposis. Orphanet J Rare Dis. 2009;4:22.
2. Dumont AG, Rink L, Godwin AK, et al. A nonrandom association of gastrointestinal stromal tumor (GIST) and desmoid tumor (deep fibromatosis): case series of 28 patients. Ann Oncol. 2012;23:1335–40.
3. Smith AJ, Lewis JJ, Merchant NB, et al. Surgical management of intra-abdominal desmoid tumours. Br J Surg. 2000;87(5):608–13.
4. Merchant NB, Lewis JJ, Woodruff JM, et al. Extremity and trunk desmoid tumors: a multifactorial analysis of outcome. Cancer. 1999;86(10):2045–52.
5. Sundaram M, Duffrin H, McGuire MH, et al. Synchronous multicentric desmoid tumors (aggressive fibromatosis) of the extremities. Skeletal Radiol. 1988;17(1):16–9.
6. Sundaram M, McGuire MH, Herbold DR. Magnetic resonance imaging of soft tissue masses: an evaluation of fifty-three histologically proven tumors. Magn Reson Imaging. 1988;6(3): 237–48.

7. Lazar AJ, Tuvin D, Hajibashi S, et al. Specific mutations in the beta-catenin gene (CTNNB1) correlate with local recurrence in sporadic desmoid tumors. Am J Pathol. 2008;173(5): 1518–27.
8. Davies DR, Armstrong JG, Thakker N, et al. Severe Gardner syndrome in families with mutations restricted to a specific region of the APC gene. Am J Hum Genet. 1995;57(5):1151–8.
9. Caspari R, Olschwang S, Friedl W, et al. Familial adenomatous polyposis: desmoid tumours and lack of ophthalmic lesions (CHRPE) associated with APC mutations beyond codon 1444. Hum Mol Genet. 1995;4(3):337–40.
10. Domont J, Benard J, Lacroix L, et al. Detection of β-catenin mutations in primary extra-abdominal fibromatosis (EAF): an ancillary diagnostic tool. J Clin Oncol (Meet Abstr). 2008; 26 Suppl 15:10518.
11. Lazar AJ, Hajibashi S, Lev D. Desmoid tumor: from surgical extirpation to molecular dissection. Curr Opin Oncol. 2009;21(4):352–9.
12. Alman BA, Li C, Pajerski ME, et al. Increased beta-catenin protein and somatic APC mutations in sporadic aggressive fibromatoses (desmoid tumors). Am J Pathol. 1997;151(2):329–34.
13. Carlson JW, Fletcher CD. Immunohistochemistry for beta-catenin in the differential diagnosis of spindle cell lesions: analysis of a series and review of the literature. Histopathology. 2007; 51(4):509–14.
14. Deyrup AT, Tretiakova M, Montag AG. Estrogen receptor-beta expression in extraabdominal fibromatoses: an analysis of 40 cases. Cancer. 2006;106(1):208–13.
15. Rock MG, Pritchard DJ, Reiman HM, et al. Extra-abdominal desmoid tumors. J Bone Joint Surg Am. 1984;66(9):1369–74.
16. Posner MC, Shiu MH, Newsome JL, et al. The desmoid tumor. Not a benign disease. Arch Surg. 1989;124(2):191–6.
17. Gaposchkin CG, Bilsky MH, Ginsberg R, et al. Function-sparing surgery for desmoid tumors and other low-grade fibrosarcomas involving the brachial plexus. Neurosurgery. 1998;42(6): 1297–301. discussion 1301–1293.
18. Lewis JJ, Boland PJ, Leung DH, et al. The enigma of desmoid tumors. Ann Surg. 1999;229(6):866–72. discussion 872–863.
19. Pires de Camargo V, Keohan ML, D'Adamo DR, et al. Clinical outcomes of systemic therapy for patients with deep fibromatosis (desmoid tumor). Cancer. 2010;116(9):2258–65.
20. Patel SR, Evans HL, Benjamin RS. Combination chemotherapy in adult desmoid tumors. Cancer. 1993;72(11):3244–7.
21. Patel SR, Benjamin RS. Desmoid tumors respond to chemotherapy: defying the dogma in oncology. J Clin Oncol. 2006;24(1):11–2.
22. Fong Y, Rosen PP, Brennan MF. Multifocal desmoids. Surgery. 1993;114(5):902–6.
23. Fiore M, Rimareix F, Mariani L, et al. Desmoid-type fibromatosis: a front-line conservative approach to select patients for surgical treatment. Ann Surg Oncol. 2009;16(9):2587–93.
24. Bonvalot S, Eldweny H, Haddad V, et al. Extra-abdominal primary fibromatosis: aggressive management could be avoided in a subgroup of patients. Eur J Surg Oncol. 2008;34(4):462–8.
25. Tryphonopoulos P, Weppler D, Levi DM, et al. Transplantation for the treatment of intra-abdominal fibromatosis. Transplant Proc. 2005;37(2):1379–80.
26. Bus PJ, Verspaget HW, van Krieken JH, et al. Treatment of mesenteric desmoid tumours with the anti-oestrogenic agent toremifene: case histories and an overview of the literature. Eur J Gastroenterol Hepatol. 1999;11(10):1179–83.
27. Kinzbrunner B, Ritter S, Domingo J, et al. Remission of rapidly growing desmoid tumors after tamoxifen therapy. Cancer. 1983;52(12):2201–4.
28. Meazza C, Bisogno G, Gronchi A, et al. Aggressive fibromatosis in children and adolescents: the Italian experience. Cancer. 2010;116(1):233–40.
29. Bertagnolli MM, Morgan JA, Fletcher CD, et al. Multimodality treatment of mesenteric desmoid tumours. Eur J Cancer. 2008;44(16):2404–10.
30. Weiss AJ, Horowitz S, Lackman RD. Therapy of desmoid tumors and fibromatosis using vinorelbine. Am J Clin Oncol. 1999;22(2):193–5.

31. Meazza C, Casanova M, Trecate G, et al. Objective response to hydroxyurea in a patient with heavily pre-treated aggressive fibromatosis. Pediatr Blood Cancer. 2010;55(3):587–8.
32. Garbay D, Le Cesne A, Penel N, et al. Chemotherapy in patients with desmoid tumors: a study from the French Sarcoma Group (FSG). Ann Oncol. 2012;23(1):182–6.
33. Lev D, Kotilingam D, Wei C, et al. Optimizing treatment of desmoid tumors. J clin oncol: official J Am Soc Clin Oncol. 2007;25(13):1785–91.
34. Chugh R, Wathen JK, Patel SR, et al. Efficacy of imatinib in aggressive fibromatosis: results of a phase II multicenter Sarcoma Alliance for Research through Collaboration (SARC) trial. Clin Cancer Res. 2010;16(19):4884–91.
35. Penel N, Le Cesne A, Bui BN, et al. Imatinib for progressive and recurrent aggressive fibromatosis (desmoid tumors): an FNCLCC/French Sarcoma Group phase II trial with a long-term follow-up. Ann Oncol. 2011;22:452–7.
36. de Camargo VP, Keohan ML, D'Adamo DR, et al. Clinical outcomes of systemic therapy for patients with deep fibromatosis (desmoid tumor). Cancer. 2010;116(9):2258–65.
37. Heinrich MC, Joensuu H, Demetri GD, et al. Phase II, open-label study evaluating the activity of imatinib in treating life-threatening malignancies known to be associated with imatinib-sensitive tyrosine kinases. Clin Cancer Res. 2008;14(9):2717–25.
38. Skubitz KM, Manivel JC, Clohisy DR, et al. Response of imatinib-resistant extra-abdominal aggressive fibromatosis to sunitinib: case report and review of the literature on response to tyrosine kinase inhibitors. Cancer Chemother Pharmacol. 2009;64(3):635–40.
39. Gounder M, Lefkowitz RA, Keohan ML, et al. Activity of sorafenib against desmoid tumor/ deep fibromatoses. Clin Cancer Res. 2011;17:4082–90.
40. Hosalkar HS, Fox EJ, Delaney T, et al. Desmoid tumors and current status of management. Orthop Clin North Am. 2006;37(1):53–63.
41. Seinfeld J, Kleinschmidt-Demasters BK, Tayal S, et al. Desmoid-type fibromatoses involving the brachial plexus: treatment options and assessment of c-KIT mutational status. J Neurosurg. 2006;104(5):749–56.
42. Salas S, Dufresne A, Bui B, et al. Prognostic factors influencing progression-free survival determined from a series of sporadic desmoid tumors: a wait-and-see policy according to tumor presentation. J Clin Oncol. 2011;29(26):3553–8.
43. Crago AM, Denton B, Mezhir JJ, et al. A prognostic nomogram for prediction of recurrence in desmoid fibromatosis. Ann Surg. (2012, submitted).
44. Ballo MT, Zagars GK, Pollack A, et al. Desmoid tumor: prognostic factors and outcome after surgery, radiation therapy, or combined surgery and radiation therapy. J Clin Oncol. 1999;17(1):158–67.
45. Gronchi A, Casali PG, Mariani L, et al. Quality of surgery and outcome in extra-abdominal aggressive fibromatosis: a series of patients surgically treated at a single institution. J Clin Oncol. 2003;21(7):1390–7.
46. Stoeckle E, Coindre JM, Longy M, et al. A critical analysis of treatment strategies in desmoid tumours: a review of a series of 106 cases. Eur J Surg Oncol. 2009;35(2):129–34.

Chapter 11
Solitary Fibrous Tumor/Hemangiopericytoma

Solitary fibrous tumor (SFT) can occur at any age (Fig. 11.1) and any site (Fig. 11.2). As with vascular sarcomas, solitary fibrous tumor/hemangiopericytoma (SFT/HPC) represents a spectrum of tumors ranging from well-circumscribed tumors with bland spindle-shaped cells to histologically malignant tumors with a high mitotic rate and significant risk of metastatic disease. SFT/HPC arises in the pleura, pelvis, and in the dura, where it is termed hemangiopericytoma exclusively by neuropathologists. Even among neuropathologists, there is increasing appreciation that what has been termed HPC and SFT are indeed related [1].

In the pleura, an old name for solitary fibrous tumor was fibrous mesothelioma, but it has no relationship to mesothelial cells (or to asbestos exposure). The cell of origin or line of differentiation is most likely fibroblastic, since SFT/HPC lacks actin reactivity, typically found in the perivascular pericytic cells [1, 2]. SFT/HPC is CD34 immunoreactive and often stain positive for Bcl2 and CD99. No consistent genetic alterations have been observed in SFT/HPC. The common origin of SFT and HPC appears likely, given the related pattern of gene expression observed regardless of the primary site of the tumor [2] (Fig. 11.3).

SFT/HPC is typically a tumor that grows slowly over many years and raises few suspicions until it is large in size [3]. Those SFT/HPCs with a greater degree of aggressiveness microscopically ("malignant" SFT/HPC) have a higher risk of metastatic disease [4], while that risk is very low for tumors lacking overt malignant changes (Figs. 11.4 and 11.5).

Primary therapy remains surgical, and those tumors in the pleura arise on a stalk and thus prove easier to remove than expected for a tumor of large size at presentation. Radiation can be used for recurrent or metastatic disease but is not generally employed as part of primary therapy due to the relatively low risk of local-regional recurrence for tumors removed with an R0 resection.

Metastatic disease is often only appreciated 10–20 years after initial diagnosis, and bone, lung, and liver appear to be common sites of metastatic disease. In our experience, anthracyclines are inactive, but ifosfamide with or without cisplatin appears to have at least modest activity. Radiation therapy can be employed for particular painful sites of what are typically bony metastases.

M.F. Brennan et al., *Management of Soft Tissue Sarcoma*,   179
DOI 10.1007/978-1-4614-5004-7_11, © Springer Science+Business Media New York 2013

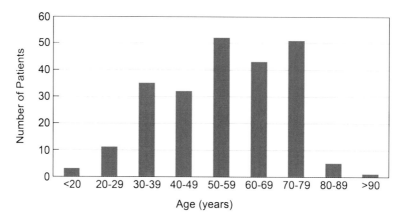

Fig. 11.1 Age distribution of adult patients with solitary fibrous tumor/hemangiopericytoma. MSKCC 7/1/11982–6/30/2010 n = 233

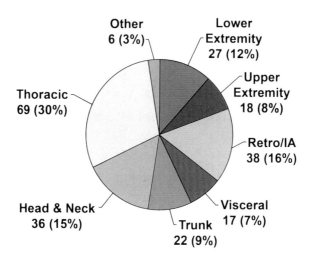

Fig. 11.2 Primary site distribution of adult patients with solitary fibrous tumor/hemangiopericytoma. MSKCC 7/1/1982–6/30/2010 n = 233 retro/IA = retroperitoneal/intra-abdominal

More interesting data have been generated recently with antiangiogenic compounds sunitinib, sorafenib [5], and bevacizumab (the latter with temozolomide) [6], which cause tumor devascularization detectable on scans, without much size change in tumor masses [7–9]. This phenomenon has also been seen with gastrointestinal stromal tumors (GIST) exposed to imatinib and other tyrosine kinase inhibitors [10], and progression of disease, like in GIST, is demonstrated by reactivation of the vasculature of the tumor. An angle on therapy recently brought to the fore is highlighted by Doege-Potter syndrome [10–12], in which SFT/HPC causes hypoglycemia on the basis of excessive production of an abnormal version of IGF-2.

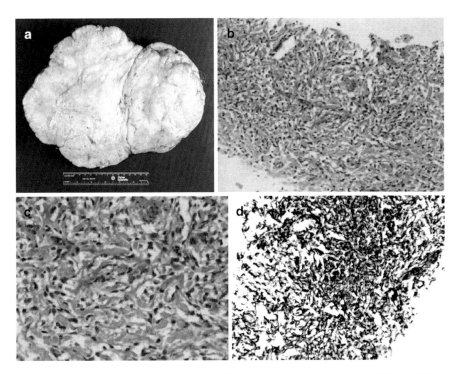

Fig. 11.3 Malignant solitary fibrous tumor – (**a**) gross pathology, (**b**) low power (100×), (**c**) high power (H&E, 400×), and (**d**) immunohistochemical staining for CD34 in a solitary fibrous tumor

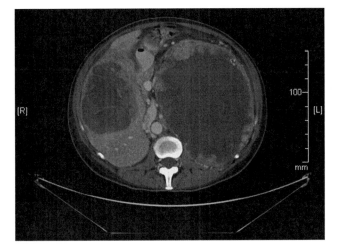

Fig. 11.4 Contrast-enhanced CT image of a large metastatic solitary fibrous tumor with liver metastasis. A substantial degree of central necrosis is observed in both large lesions

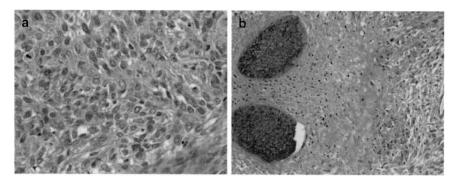

Fig. 11.5 Features differentiating malignant solitary fibrous tumor from a less aggressive lesion: (**a**) increased mitotic activity (5 mitoses/10 high-power fields), (**b**) focal necrosis

Table 11.1 Systemic therapy recommendations for patients with solitary fibrous tumor/ hemangiopericytoma

Clinical scenario	Comments	
Adjuvant chemotherapy		Not administered due to low risk of relapse and poor response to chemotherapy in the metastatic setting
Metastatic disease	First line	Sunitinib or other multi-targeted tyrosine kinase inhibitor; bevacizumab with temozolomide
	Second line	Insulin-like growth factor 1 inhibitor or combination, if available
	Third line	Ifosfamide-based therapy, clinical trial

Since IGF-2 binds IGF-1 receptor (IGF1R), one hypothesizes that IGF1R inhibitors could be active in SFT/HPC, and this appears to be the case for at least a minority of patients with metastatic disease from this diagnosis [13] (Table 11.1). It is unclear if there is any relationship between IGF-2 expression and markers of chromatin remodeling, such as histone 3 lysine 4 (H3K4) methylation status, a topic that requires further study [8].

Outcome

Local recurrence in 169 primary SFTs is shown in Fig. 11.6 with disease-specific survival for primary presentation in Fig. 11.7. Risk of recurrence/metastases is largely limited to those SFT/HPCs with malignant changes. The risk of recurrence of SFT/HPC without these changes is very low.

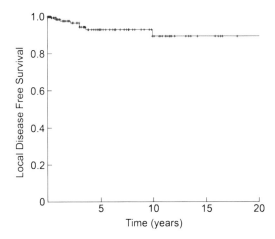

Fig. 11.6 Local disease-free survival for adult patients with adult primary solitary fibrous tumor of all sites. MSKCC 7/1/1982–6/30/2010 n = 169

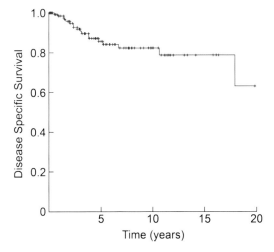

Fig. 11.7 Disease-specific survival for adult patients with adult primary solitary fibrous tumor of all sites. MSKCC 7/1/1982–6/30/2010 n = 169

References

1. Miettinen M. Antibody specific to muscle actins in the diagnosis and classification of soft tissue tumors. Am J Pathol. 1988;130(1):205–15.
2. Porter PL, Bigler SA, McNutt M, et al. The immunophenotype of hemangiopericytomas and glomus tumors, with special reference to muscle protein expression: an immunohistochemical study and review of the literature. Mod Pathol. 1991;4(1):46–52.
3. Hajdu M, Singer S, Maki RG, et al. IGF2 over-expression in solitary fibrous tumours is independent of anatomical location and is related to loss of imprinting. J Pathol. 2010;221(3):300–7.
4. Espat NJ, Lewis JJ, Leung D, et al. Conventional hemangiopericytoma: modern analysis of outcome. Cancer. 2002;95(8):1746–51.
5. Domont J, Massard C, Lassau N, et al. Hemangiopericytoma and antiangiogenic therapy: clinical benefit of antiangiogenic therapy (sorafenib and sunitinib) in relapsed malignant haemangiopericytoma/solitary fibrous tumour. Invest New Drugs. 2010;28(2):199–202.

6. Park MS, Patel SR, Ludwig JA, et al. Activity of temozolomide and bevacizumab in the treatment of locally advanced, recurrent, and metastatic hemangiopericytoma and malignant solitary fibrous tumor. Cancer. 2011;117(21):4939–47.

7. Gold JS, Antonescu CR, Hajdu C, et al. Clinicopathologic correlates of solitary fibrous tumors. Cancer. 2002;94(4):1057–68.

8. Stacchiotti S, Negri T, Palassini E, et al. Sunitinib malate and figitumumab in solitary fibrous tumor: patterns and molecular bases of tumor response. Mol Cancer Ther. 2010;9(5):1286–97.

9. George S, Merriam P, Maki RG, et al. Multicenter phase II trial of sunitinib in the treatment of nongastrointestinal stromal tumor sarcomas. J Clin Oncol. 2009;27(19):3154–60.

10. Choi H, Charnsangavej C, Faria SC, et al. Correlation of computed tomography and positron emission tomography in patients with metastatic gastrointestinal stromal tumor treated at a single institution with imatinib mesylate: proposal of new computed tomography response criteria. J Clin Oncol. 2007;25(13):1753–9.

11. Chamberlain MH, Taggart DP. Solitary fibrous tumor associated with hypoglycemia: an example of the Doege-Potter syndrome. J Thorac Cardiovasc Surg. 2000;119(1):185–7.

12. Roy TM, Burns MV, Overly DJ, et al. Solitary fibrous tumor of the pleura with hypoglycemia: the Doege-Potter syndrome. J Ky Med Assoc. 1992;90(11):557–60.

13. Baldwin RS. Hypoglycemia with Neoplasia (Doege-Potter syndrome). Wis Med J. 1965; 64:185–9.

Chapter 12
Fibrosarcoma and Its Variants

Fibrosarcoma can occur at all ages (Fig. 12.1) and in all sites (Fig. 12.2). Before the era of immunohistochemistry, fibrosarcoma was one of the most common diagnoses for a soft tissue sarcoma. With the development of immunohistochemical and molecular techniques, it is now rare for a sarcoma to be termed a fibrosarcoma, which by its name implies fibroblasts as the cell of origin. With increasing sophistication in diagnosis, more and more subtypes of fibroblastic sarcomas are now appreciated, all relatively rare tumors.

Accordingly, while surgery and radiation remain the standard of care for primary therapy for any of these soft tissue sarcomas, there has been less experience with each of these subtypes of tumors with respect to chemotherapy than with more common diagnoses. Beyond dermatofibrosarcoma protuberans, recommendations presented here are provisional and should be considered a starting point for prospective clinical trials including patients with these diagnoses.

Outcome

Local recurrence for all primary fibrosarcomas is shown in Fig. 12.3, and disease-specific survival in Fig. 12.4 for those with primary presentation. Metastatic disease is recognized but affects only a minority of patients with primary disease, although some of these recurrences can be very late.

Dermatofibrosarcoma Protuberans

Dermatofibrosarcoma protuberans (DFSP) presents in middle age (Fig. 12.5) and at essentially any anatomic site (Fig. 12.6). DFSP is a superficial sarcoma with a predilection for local recurrence. Rare DFSP will metastasize, usually after at least a decade of recurrences and degeneration to a fibrosarcomatous variant. Deaths from

M.F. Brennan et al., *Management of Soft Tissue Sarcoma*,
DOI 10.1007/978-1-4614-5004-7_12, © Springer Science+Business Media New York 2013

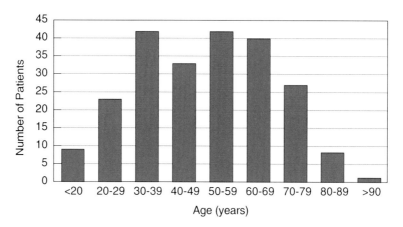

Fig. 12.1 Age distribution of adult patients with fibrosarcoma (all types except Dermato-fibrosarcoma protuberans). MSKCC 7/1/1982–6/30/2010 n = 225

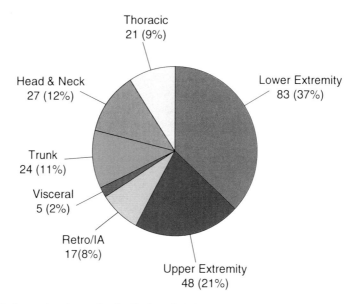

Fig. 12.2 Anatomic primary site distribution of adult patients with fibrosarcoma (all types except DFSP). MSKCC 7/1/1982 – 6/30/2010 n = 225 Retro/IA = retroperitoneal/intra-abdominal

disease are uncommon and limited to those people with the development of metastatic disease.

DFSP is characterized by CD34 positivity and the t(17;22) involving *COL1A1-PDGFB* [1], as well as giant ring and marker chromosomes that contain multiple copies of the translocation product [2]. It is typically plaque-like tumor at presentation and composed of long, monotonous spindle cells arranged in a storiform pattern.

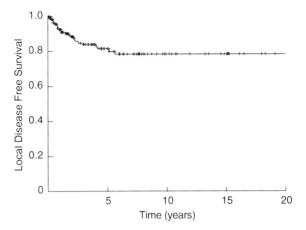

Fig. 12.3 Local disease-free survival for adult patients with primary fibrosarcomas (all types except DFSP). MSKCC 7/1/1982–6/30/2010 n = 164

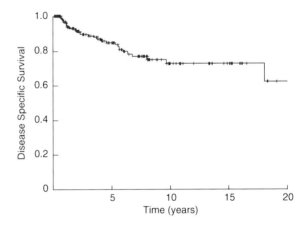

Fig. 12.4 Disease-specific survival for adult patients with primary fibrosarcomas (all types except DFSP). MSKCC 7/1/1982–6/30/2010 n = 164

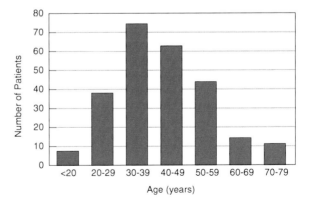

Fig. 12.5 Age distribution of adult patients with dermatofibrosarcoma protuberans. MSKCC 7/1/1982–6/30/2010 n = 252

The degeneration of DFSP to fibrosarcoma is seen in 10–15% of cases, and it is in this situation in which metastatic disease occurs [3]. A pigmented version (Bednar tumor) and a version found in children (giant cell fibroblastoma) are also

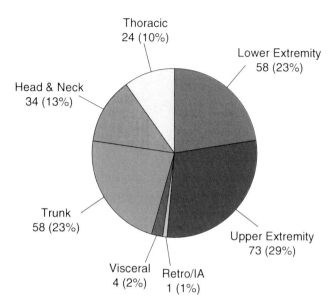

Fig. 12.6 Anatomic primary site distribution of adult patients with dermatofibrosarcoma protuberans. MSKCC 7/1/1982–6/30/2010 n = 252 Retro/IA = retroperitoneal/intra-abdominal

characterized by the same translocation and behave similarly biologically [4]. For unclear reasons, multifocal DFSP is observed in some patients with adenosine deaminase deficiency (ADA) [5], whose gene is located on chromosome 20, and thus not near either gene involved in the translocation product.

Primary surgery is the standard of care, without adjuvant radiation. There is a high risk of local recurrence of the tumor, and wide margins are generally advocated. One school of thought has led to use of Mohs micrographic surgery for this diagnosis, especially when the tumor occurs on the head and neck area as a primary site (Fig. 12.7); however, this surgical technique is often accompanied by local recurrence.

For recurrent disease, our experience is that standard doxorubicin or ifosfamide is not effective. In contrast, as with gastrointestinal stromal tumor (GIST), imatinib can be very useful for disease recurrence [6–9]. In our experience, the median time to progression is shorter than that seen for GIST, but important palliation can be achieved with imatinib. We have observed some benefit from other tyrosine kinase inhibitors in DFSP as well, but none that stands out as particularly meaningful in terms of durability of response (Tables 12.1 and 12.2).

Outcome

Outcome is predicted based on fibrosarcomatous presentation, margin status, and depth of invasion. Local disease-free survival is shown in Fig. 12.8, and disease-specific survival for those presenting with primary lesions in Fig. 12.9.

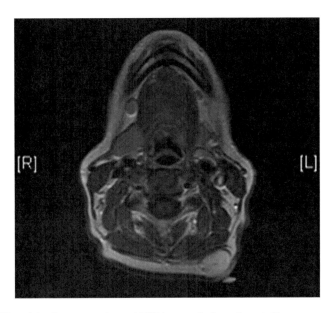

Fig. 12.7 T1-weighted contrast-enhanced MRI image of a 2-cm dermatofibrosarcoma protuberans of the superficial posterior left neck

Table 12.1 Systemic therapy recommendations for patients with dermatofibrosarcoma protuberans

Clinical scenario		Comments
Adjuvant chemotherapy		Not employed outside a clinical trial; the local–regional recurrence risk is low for patients who have adequate surgery
Recurrent or metastatic disease	First line	Imatinib
	Second line	Other tyrosine kinase inhibitor such as pazopanib, sunitinib or sorafenib. Clinical trials are appropriate

Low-Grade Fibromyxoid Sarcoma (Evans' Tumor)

Evans' tumor is uncommon and occurs in young patients (Fig. 12.10) involving the deep soft tissues of limbs or head and neck area (Figs. 12.11 and 12.12). Low-grade fibromyxoid sarcoma (LGFMS) was first described by Dr. Evans in 1987 as a deceptively bland low-grade tumor that has the ability to metastasize (Fig. 12.13). Metastases can be observed even decades after initial diagnosis. One histologic variant of this tumor has a characteristic appearance, the so-called hyalinizing spindle cell tumor with giant rosettes. The diagnosis is difficult and generally made by

Table 12.2 Patient and tumor characteristics of 240 patients treated for primary and recurrent dermatofibrosarcoma protuberans at MSKCC from 1982 to 2009 (Used with permission from Fields et al. [29])

Characteristic	Primary (n = 196) No.	%	Local recurrence (n = 44) No.	%	P value[a]
Median age (years)	39		46		0.03
Gender					1.00
Male	95	48	21	47	
Female	101	52	23	53	
Primary site					0.66
Extremity	101	52	25	57	
Trunk/thorax	63	32	13	29	
Head and neck	29	15	4	10	
Other	3	1	2	4	
Tumor size					0.27
<5 cm	152	78	36	81	
5–10 cm	36	19	5	11	
>10 cm	6	2	3	7	
Unknown	2	1	0	0	
Tumor depth					0.42
Deep	42	21	12	27	
Superficial	154	79	31	70	
Unknown	0	0	1	3	
Tumor histology					0.64
"Classic" DFSP	166	68	39	88	
FS-DFSP	30	32	5	12	
Surgical margin					0.24
R0 (negative)	169	86	35	80	
R1 (microscopically positive)	26	14	9	20	
Unknown	1	<1	0	0	
Recurrence events					NE[b]
Local recurrence	9	4	5	11	
Distant recurrence	1[c]	<1	1	<1	
Vital status[d]					NE[b]
No evidence of disease	185	94	37	84	
Alive with disease	3	2	3	7	
Died of other causes	8	4	3	7	
Died of disease	0	0	1	2	

DFSP dermatofibrosarcoma protuberans, *FS-DFSP* fibrosarcomatous DFSP, *LR* locally recurrent, *MSKCC* Memorial Sloan-Kettering Cancer Center, *NE* not evaluable
[a]Fisher exact test for all variables (except age, which was analyzed using Wilcoxon rank-sum test)
[b]Not evaluable. See text for explanation and Kaplan–Meyer analysis for comparison of disease-free survival
[c]Synchronous distant and local recurrence
[d]As of July 2009

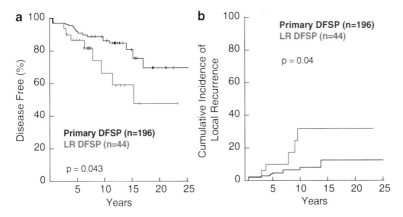

Fig. 12.8 (a) Disease-free survival and (b) cumulative incidence of local recurrence of DFSP in patients presenting with primary disease (*dark line*) or locally recurrent disease (*light line*) (Used with permission from Fields et al. [29])

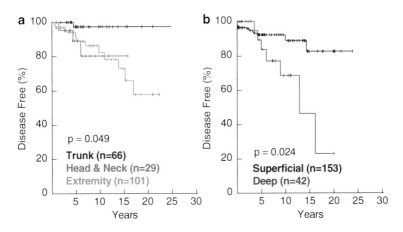

Fig. 12.9 Disease-free survival as a function of (a) anatomic primary site and (b) tumor depth at presentation (Used with permission from Fields et al. [29])

morphology, since there are no characteristic immunochemical features of the tumor. However, diagnosis can be confirmed by demonstrating the characteristic t(7;16)(q34;p11) involving *FUS-CREB3L2* (or *CREB3L1* in isolated cases) [10–12]. Mucin MUC4 appears characteristic of the tumor and can be used to distinguish from other histologic mimics [10]. There is some histologic and genetic overlap of these tumors with sclerosing epithelioid fibrosarcomas, which also may contain t(7;16) *FUS-CREB3L2* in a subset of cases (see below) [13].

Primary treatment is wide local excision with negative margins. Adjuvant radiation is reserved for positive margins or tumors with a high risk of local recurrence.

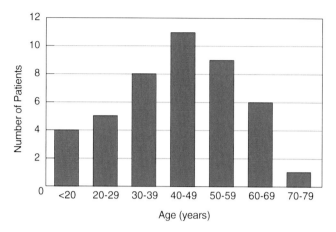

Fig. 12.10 Age distribution of adult patients with low grade fibromyxoid sarcoma. MSKCC 7/1/1982–/30/2010 n=45

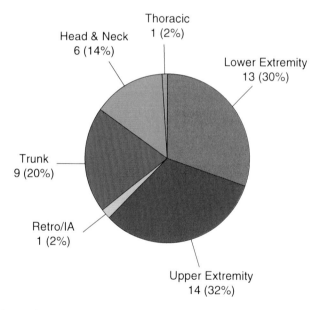

Fig. 12.11 Anatomic primary site distribution of adult patients with low grade fibromyxoid sarcoma. MSKCC 7/1/1982–6/30/2010 n=45 Retro/IA=retroperitoneal/intra-abdominal

Regarding systemic therapy for metastatic disease, the long survival of even those with metastatic disease makes it difficult to recommend doxorubicin-based therapy (e.g., pegylated liposomal doxorubicin), although we have seen at least minor responses in treated patients. Hopefully systemic agents that are less toxic that can be administered for a long period time can help achieve meaningful

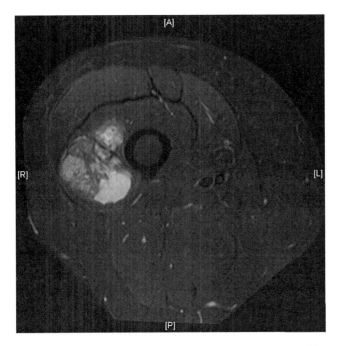

Fig. 12.12 T2-weighted MRI image of a 7-cm right thigh low grade fibromyxoid sarcoma

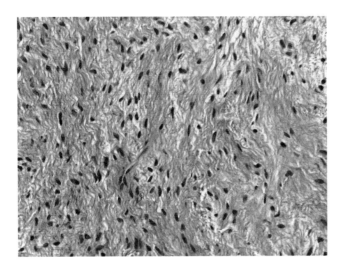

Fig. 12.13 Microscopic appearance of low grade fibromyxoid sarcoma showing deceptively bland spindle cells embedded in a loose fibrous and myxoid stroma (H&E, 200×)

Table 12.3 Systemic therapy recommendations for patients with low-grade fibromyxoid sarcoma

Clinical scenario	Comments	
Adjuvant chemotherapy		Not utilized due to slow rate of tumor growth and only modest responses in the metastatic setting
Metastatic disease	First line	Pegylated liposomal doxorubicin, metronomic (low daily dose) oral agent such as cyclophosphamide
	Second line and greater	Pazopanib; Clinical trial

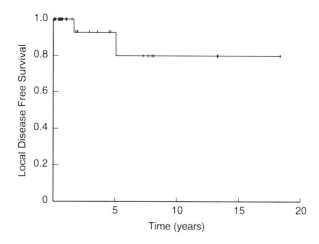

Fig. 12.14 Local disease-free survival for adult patients with primary fibromyxoid sarcoma. MSKCC 7/1/1982–6/30/2010 n = 36

palliation for patients (Table 12.3). As with other slowly progressing metastatic sarcomas, we suggest attempting to match toxicity of any proposed therapy to the aggressiveness of the metastatic disease.

Outcome

Local recurrence occurs (Fig. 12.14) but is uncommon, and death from such tumors is relatively uncommon.

Sclerosing Epithelioid Fibrosarcoma

Sclerosing epithelioid fibrosarcoma is another rare version of fibrosarcoma that may be related to low-grade fibromyxoid sarcoma on the basis of translocations shared in at least some of both types of tumor [13]. Histology shows monotonous

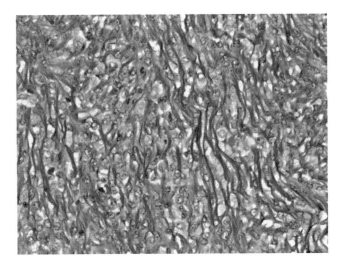

Fig. 12.15 Microscopic appearance of sclerosing epithelioid fibrosarcoma showing monotonous epithelioid cells with scant amphophilic cytoplasm arranged in cords, separated by refractile collagenous columns (H&E, 400×)

Table 12.4 Systemic therapy recommendations for patients with sclerosing epithelioid fibrosarcoma

Clinical scenario	Comments	
Adjuvant chemotherapy		Not administered (low response rate for people with metastatic disease)
Metastatic disease	First line	Pegylated liposomal doxorubicin, "metronomic" chemotherapy such as oral daily cyclophosphamide
	Second line	Pazopanib; Clinical trial

epithelioid cells with scant amphophilic cytoplasm, arranged in sheets or cords, separated by refractile collagenous columns (H&E, 400×) (Fig. 12.15). This is usually a sarcoma of deep soft tissues of the extremities, but paraspinal and intracranial locations have been also reported [14]. Compared to LGFMS, sclerosing epithelioid fibrosarcoma follows an aggressive clinical course, with a significantly higher metastatic rate and disease-related mortality [15]. Primary therapy is surgery alone; we have observed minor responses to anthracycline-based therapy (again typically pegylated liposomal doxorubicin, given the slow-changing nature of the tumor) (Table 12.4).

Inflammatory Myofibroblastic Tumor

Inflammatory myofibroblastic tumor (IMT) is another rare sarcoma that occurs in a younger population, affecting pleura and peritoneum, often in the pelvis. It also displays pathologic heterogeneity in that younger patients have tumors that express

Table 12.5 Systemic therapy recommendations for patients with inflammatory myofibroblastic tumor

Clinical scenario	Comments	
Adjuvant chemotherapy		Not administered
Metastatic disease	First line	ALK inhibitor for ALK (+) tumors
	Second line	Clinical trial

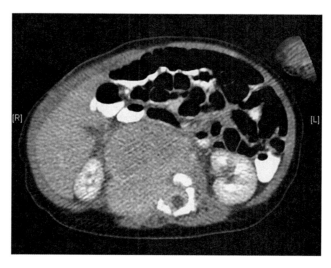

Fig. 12.16 Contrast-enhanced CT image of a patient with infantile fibrosarcoma of the right psoas musculature causing destruction of the spine and involvement of the spinal canal

anaplastic lymphoma kinase (ALK) and contain rearrangements of the *ALK* oncogene, while older patients typically lack this molecular finding [16]. ALK expression by immunohistochemistry correlates often, but not always, with ALK translocation. A case report of a patient with ALK(+) IMT responded to crizotinib, an inhibitor of MET and ALK, while a patient with an ALK(−) IMT did not respond, as proof of principle of the utility of ALK inhibitors in patients with this diagnosis [17]. Resistance in this responding patient to the ALK inhibitor crizotinib has already been identified in a manner similar to that seen with imatinib and KIT in GIST [18]. Glucocorticoids may be useful for the inflammatory component of this tumor [19], but there are only case reports of systemic therapy for this diagnosis (Table 12.5).

Infantile Fibrosarcoma

Infantile fibrosarcoma most commonly occurs before age 1 (Fig. 12.16). There is a characteristic translocation found in this sarcoma, t(12;15)(p13;q25), encoding *ETV6-NTRK3*, which is also found in congenital mesoblastic nephroma [20, 21].

Table 12.6 Systemic therapy recommendations for patients with infantile/congenital fibrosarcoma

Clinical scenario		Comments
Neoadjuvant/adjuvant chemotherapy		Vincristine/dactinomycin
Metastatic disease	First line	Agents for rhabdomyosarcoma or Ewing sarcoma
	Second line	Clinical trial

Table 12.7 Systemic therapy recommendations for patients with myxoinflammatory fibroblastic sarcoma/inflammatory myxohyaline tumor

Clinical scenario		Comments
Adjuvant chemotherapy		Not given, due to the low risk of recurrence
Metastatic disease	First line or greater	Not defined

Despite its very rapid growth, children can do well with complete resection alone, avoiding radiation and chemotherapy. Chemotherapy can be considered if resection would be particularly morbid, with good results with an anthracycline- and alkylating-free regimen [22] (Table 12.6).

Myxoinflammatory Fibroblastic Sarcoma/Inflammatory Myxohyaline Tumor of Distal Extremities

Myxoinflammatory fibroblastic sarcoma is recognized as a separate entity based on both histology and anatomic location, nearly always found from the wrists and ankles distally [23, 24]. A characteristic t(1;10)(p22;q24) translocation, sometimes unbalanced, involving translocations of genes *MGEA5* and *TGFBR3* has been identified [25, 26] and is also seen in the unusual benign hemosiderotic fibrolipomatous tumor [27, 28]. Both diagnoses also appear to have amplification of *VGLL3* and other genes from chromosome 3p12. Notably, the translocation attaches the genes head-to-head, so that they are not part of the same fusion gene product. Metastases are rare, so conservative management with complete resection is the standard of care (e.g., ray amputation). Chemotherapy is unknown in this tumor (Table 12.7).

Adult-Type Fibrosarcoma

The adult-type fibrosarcoma is now a diagnosis of exclusion, after other immuno-histochemical and/or molecular analyses have ruled out other sarcoma diagnoses (Fig. 12.17). Given the change in the diagnostic landscape for this tumor, it is hard to recommend adjuvant chemotherapy and anything other than standard chemotherapy agents or clinical trials for patients with metastatic disease (Table 12.8).

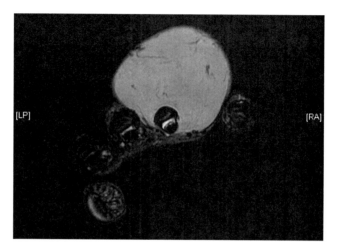

Fig. 12.17 T2-weighted MRI image of a 5-cm true fibrosarcoma of the fourth metatarsal soft tissues and extensor tendons of the right third, fourth, and fifth digits

Table 12.8 Systemic therapy recommendations for patients with (true) fibrosarcoma

Clinical scenario	Comments	
Adjuvant chemotherapy		Unknown, given the lack of perceived benefit for other types of fibrosarcoma adjuvant therapy is not generally recommended
Metastatic disease	First line	Anthracycline-based regimens
	Second line	Ifosfamide, pazopanib, clinical trial

References

1. Pedeutour F, Simon MP, Minoletti F, et al. Translocation, t(17;22)(q22;q13), in dermatofibrosarcoma protuberans: a new tumor-associated chromosome rearrangement. Cytogenet Cell Genet. 1996;72(2–3):171–4.
2. Pedeutour F, Coindre JM, Sozzi G, et al. Supernumerary ring chromosomes containing chromosome 17 sequences. A specific feature of dermatofibrosarcoma protuberans? Cancer Genet Cytogenet. 1994;76(1):1–9.
3. Bowne WB, Antonescu CR, Leung DH, et al. Dermatofibrosarcoma protuberans: A clinicopathologic analysis of patients treated and followed at a single institution. Cancer. 2000;88(12):2711–20.
4. Maire G, Martin L, Michalak-Provost S, et al. Fusion of COL1A1 exon 29 with PDGFB exon 2 in a der(22)t(17;22) in a pediatric giant cell fibroblastoma with a pigmented Bednar tumor component. Evidence for age-related chromosomal pattern in dermatofibrosarcoma protuberans and related tumors. Cancer Genet Cytogenet. 2002;134(2):156–61.
5. Kesserwan C, Sokolic R, Cowen EW, et al. Multicentric dermatofibrosarcoma protuberans in patients with adenosine deaminase-deficient severe combined immune deficiency. J Allergy Clin Immunol. 2012;129(3):762–9.

6. Rubin BP, Schuetze SM, Eary JF, et al. Molecular targeting of platelet-derived growth factor B by imatinib mesylate in a patient with metastatic dermatofibrosarcoma protuberans. J Clin Oncol. 2002;20(17):3586–91.

7. McArthur GA, Demetri GD, van Oosterom A, et al. Molecular and clinical analysis of locally advanced dermatofibrosarcoma protuberans treated with imatinib: imatinib target exploration consortium study B2225. J Clin Oncol. 2005;23(4):866–73.

8. Maki RG, Awan RA, Dixon RH, et al. Differential sensitivity to imatinib of 2 patients with metastatic sarcoma arising from dermatofibrosarcoma protuberans. Int J Cancer. 2002;100(6):623–6.

9. Heinrich MC, Joensuu H, Demetri GD, et al. Phase II, open-label study evaluating the activity of imatinib in treating life-threatening malignancies known to be associated with imatinib-sensitive tyrosine kinases. Clin Cancer Res. 2008;14(9):2717–25.

10. Doyle LA, Moller E, Dal Cin P, et al. MUC4 is a highly sensitive and specific marker for low-grade fibromyxoid sarcoma. Am J Surg Pathol. 2011;35(5):733–41.

11. Reid R, de Silva MV, Paterson L, et al. Low-grade fibromyxoid sarcoma and hyalinizing spindle cell tumor with giant rosettes share a common t(7;16)(q34;p11) translocation. Am J Surg Pathol. 2003;27(9):1229–36.

12. Mertens F, Fletcher CD, Antonescu CR, et al. Clinicopathologic and molecular genetic characterization of low-grade fibromyxoid sarcoma, and cloning of a novel FUS/CREB3L1 fusion gene. Lab Invest J Tech Method Pathol. 2005;85(3):408–15.

13. Guillou L, Benhattar J, Gengler C, et al. Translocation-positive low-grade fibromyxoid sarcoma: clinicopathologic and molecular analysis of a series expanding the morphologic spectrum and suggesting potential relationship to sclerosing epithelioid fibrosarcoma: a study from the French Sarcoma Group. Am J Surg Pathol. 2007;31(9):1387–402.

14. Bilsky MH, Schefler AC, Sandberg DI, et al. Sclerosing epithelioid fibrosarcomas involving the neuraxis: report of three cases. Neurosurgery. 2000;47(4):956–9. discussion 959–960.

15. Antonescu CR, Rosenblum MK, Pereira P, et al. Sclerosing epithelioid fibrosarcoma: a study of 16 cases and confirmation of a clinicopathologically distinct tumor. Am J Surg Pathol. 2001;25(6):699–709.

16. Coffin CM, Hornick JL, Fletcher CD. Inflammatory myofibroblastic tumor: comparison of clinicopathologic, histologic, and immunohistochemical features including ALK expression in atypical and aggressive cases. Am J Surg Pathol. 2007;31(4):509–20.

17. Butrynski JE, D'Adamo DR, Hornick JL, et al. Crizotinib in ALK-rearranged inflammatory myofibroblastic tumor. N Engl J Med. 2010;363(18):1727–33.

18. Sasaki T, Okuda K, Zheng W, et al. The neuroblastoma-associated F1174L ALK mutation causes resistance to an ALK kinase inhibitor in ALK-translocated cancers. Cancer Res. 2010;70(24):10038–43.

19. Dagash H, Koh C, Cohen M, et al. Inflammatory myofibroblastic tumor of the pancreas: a case report of 2 pediatric cases–steroids or surgery? J Pediatr Surg. 2009;44(9):1839–41.

20. Rubin BP, Chen CJ, Morgan TW, et al. Congenital mesoblastic nephroma t(12;15) is associated with ETV6-NTRK3 gene fusion: cytogenetic and molecular relationship to congenital (infantile) fibrosarcoma. Am J Pathol. 1998;153(5):1451–8.

21. Knezevich SR, McFadden DE, Tao W, et al. A novel ETV6-NTRK3 gene fusion in congenital fibrosarcoma. Nat Genet. 1998;18(2):184–7.

22. Orbach D, Rey A, Cecchetto G, et al. Infantile fibrosarcoma: management based on the European experience. J Clin Oncol. 2010;28(2):318–23.

23. Meis-Kindblom JM, Kindblom LG. Acral myxoinflammatory fibroblastic sarcoma: a low-grade tumor of the hands and feet. Am J Surg Pathol. 1998;22(8):911–24.

24. Montgomery EA, Devaney KO, Giordano TJ, et al. Inflammatory myxohyaline tumor of distal extremities with virocyte or Reed-Sternberg-like cells: a distinctive lesion with features simulating inflammatory conditions, Hodgkin's disease, and various sarcomas. Mod Pathol. 1998;11(4):384–91.

25. Lambert I, Debiec-Rychter M, Guelinckx P, et al. Acral myxoinflammatory fibroblastic sarcoma with unique clonal chromosomal changes. Virchows Arch. 2001;438(5):509–12.

26. Hallor KH, Sciot R, Staaf J, et al. Two genetic pathways, t(1;10) and amplification of 3p11-12, in myxoinflammatory fibroblastic sarcoma, haemosiderotic fibrolipomatous tumour, and morphologically similar lesions. J Pathol. 2009;217(5):716–27.
27. Wettach GR, Boyd LJ, Lawce HJ, et al. Cytogenetic analysis of a hemosiderotic fibrolipomatous tumor. Cancer Genet Cytogenet. 2008;182(2):140–3.
28. Antonescu CR, Zhang L, Nielsen GP, et al. Consistent t(1;10) with rearrangements of TGFBR3 and MGEA5 in both myxoinflammatory fibroblastic sarcoma and hemosiderotic fibrolipomatous tumor. Genes Chromosomes Cancer. 2011;50(10):757–64.
29. Fields RC, Hameed M, Qin L-X, Moraco N, Jia X, Maki RG, Singer S, Brennan MF. Dermatofibrosarcoma protuberans (DFSP): predictors of recurrence and the use of systemic therapy. Ann Surg Oncol. 2011;18:328–36.

Chapter 13
Vascular Sarcomas

Vascular tumors run the gamut from benign hemangiomas to intermediate grade of malignancy epithelioid hemangioendotheliomas, to highly aggressive angiosarcomas. We refrain in this section in discerning vascular sarcomas from similar tumors arising from lymphatics (lymphangiosarcomas) as there have not been good markers to definitively separate the two forms of tumors. Nonetheless, there is reason to believe VEGFR3 (also termed FLT4) is a good marker for lymphatics and lack of it leads to a congenital form of lymphedema (Milroy disease) [1, 2].

Epithelioid Hemangioendothelioma

Epithelioid hemangioendothelioma (EHE) is a rare vascular neoplasm with distinctive morphologic appearance, presenting as a deep painful soft tissue mass, although can be found primarily in lung, bone, and liver [3]. Multicentric presentation is often seen, particularly with visceral lesions (Fig. 13.1). The average age of presentation is 50 years, with no gender difference (Fig. 13.2).

The tumors are composed of epithelioid cells with densely eosinophilic cytoplasm, arranged in cords, strands, or nests and often with intracytoplasmic vacuoles (Fig. 13.3). Often there is a myxochondroid background and generally low mitotic rate. Mature vascular lumen formation is typically absent; this feature distinguishes EHE from other epithelioid vascular lesions, including epithelioid hemangioma and epithelioid angiosarcoma. Immunohistochemistry shows high factor VIII-related antigens, CD31, CD34, and FLI1 positivity [5]. The novel translocation t(1;3), resulting in *WWTR1-CAMTA1* fusion, has been identified in most if not all EHE samples [6, 7] and can be used as a very useful molecular test in challenging diagnosis. Various studies report local recurrence rates of approximately 15%, 30% with distal metastasis, and 50% involvement with regional lymph nodes.

Rare presentations such as in the heart can occur. The tumor is most commonly seen as multifocal disease affecting liver, lung, pleura, or several of these sites simultaneously (Fig. 13.4). Only a minority of these tumors progress over the course

M.F. Brennan et al., *Management of Soft Tissue Sarcoma*,
DOI 10.1007/978-1-4614-5004-7_13, © Springer Science+Business Media New York 2013

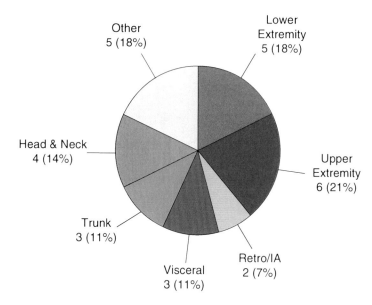

Fig. 13.1 Primary site distribution of adult patients with hemangioendothelioma. MSKCC 7/1/1982–6/30/2010 n = 28 *Retro/IA* retroperitoneal/intra-abdominal

Fig. 13.2 Age distribution of adult patients with hemangioendothelioma. MSKCC 7/1/1982–6/30/2010 n = 28

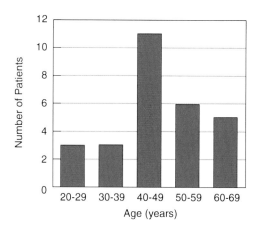

of 1–3 years with many appearing largely dominant for a decade or more, suggesting observation as a viable option for management of such patients with unresectable multifocal disease. Approximately 20% of EHE are more aggressive and thus may require intervention. Liver-only disease has been treated with chemotherapy, bland embolization, chemoembolization, or even liver transplant in those rare patients who develop liver failure from disease.

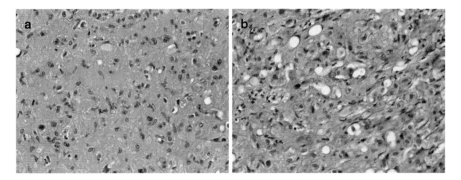

Fig. 13.3 (**a**) Microscopic appearance (H&E, 200×) of epithelioid hemangioendothelioma demonstrating bland, single epithelioid cells embedded in a distinctive myxochondroid stroma, (**b**) a second example demonstrating intracytoplasmic vacuoles with digested erythrocytes. In comparison to angiosarcoma, epithelioid hemangioendothelioma typically lacks the well-formed vascular channel formation and high degree of anaplasia

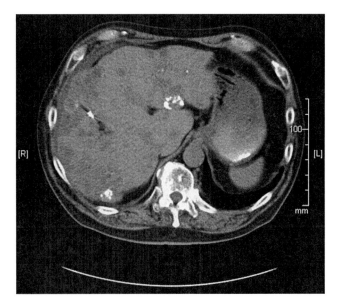

Fig. 13.4 Noncontrast CT image of multicentric epithelioid hemangioendothelioma affecting the liver. Heterotopic calcifications are demonstrated. The radiological abnormalities were essentially unchanged over 5 years of monitoring

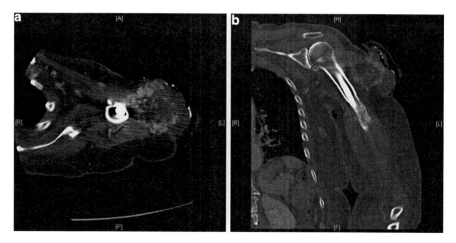

Fig. 13.5 CT images (a and b) of angiosarcoma of the humerus causing pathological fracture (s/p fixation) with demonstration of soft tissue metastases affecting the left upper extremity soft tissues

A high mitotic and profound nuclei atypia are independent predictors of survival, and the WHO classification suggests the use of "malignant EHE" terminology for this group of lesions, to distinguish from the more bland-appearing examples. The primary treatment is surgical excision with an uncertain role for radiation and chemotherapy.

Angiosarcoma/Lymphangiosarcoma

Angiosarcomas constitute a difficult family of tumors to manage, given both their local-regional failure and high risk of mortality from metastatic disease (Figs. 13.5 and 13.6). Angiosarcoma does present a unique profile of sensitivity to chemotherapy [8], and like leiomyosarcomas of different sites, there appears to be differential sensitivity to various chemotherapy agents based on the anatomic origin of the tumor (see above).

Angiosarcomas, like most sarcomas, tend to occur after age 50, and the head and neck are a common primary site (Figs. 13.7, 13.8, and 13.9) [9–13]. They have been observed in essentially every conceivable location and challenge surgeons and medical oncologists by their local-regional recurrence risk and convincing but brief responses to a variety of systemic agents. They can be found associated with radiation (Fig. 13.10) or lymphedema (Stewart-Treves syndrome) (Fig. 13.11) or lymphedema from other causes such as filariasis [14] (Fig. 13.12) and are particularly deadly in that setting, as are those that arise in bone as a primary site. Primary therapy, as for other sarcomas, includes excision with negative margins and consideration of irradiation for those tumors that did not arise after prior radiation. In

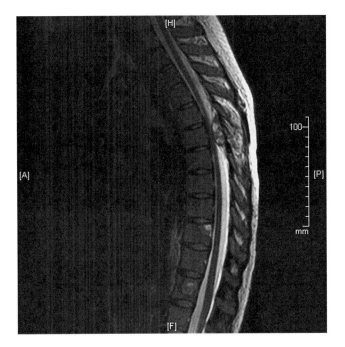

Fig. 13.6 T1-weighted MRI images of metastatic cardiac angiosarcoma with spinal metastases and invasion into the spinal canal

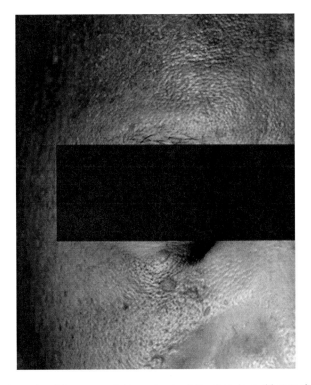

Fig. 13.7 Photograph of the upper right quadrant of the face in a 66-year-old Asian male demonstrating unresectable angiosarcoma involving the face, scalp, and neck

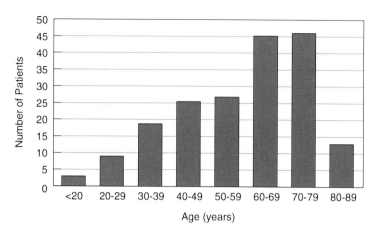

Fig. 13.8 Age distribution of adult patients with angiosarcoma. MSKCC 7/1/1982–6/30/2010 n = 188

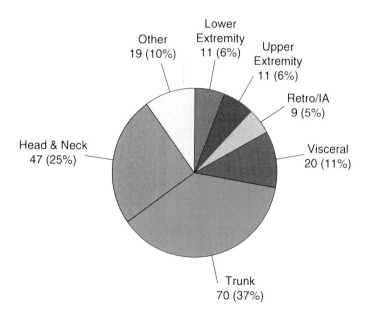

Fig. 13.9 Anatomic primary site distribution of adult patients with angiosarcoma. MSKCC 7/1/1982–6/30/2010 n = 187 Retro/IA = retroperitoneal/intra-abdominal

particular, the head and neck area requires both wide margins and even larger radiation port if local-regional control is to be achieved.

Tumors are typically CD31and ERG positive, as expected for a cell of endothelial origin, and about half are positive for CD34. Microscopic imaging of a radiation-induced angiosarcoma is shown in Fig. 13.13. VEGFR3/FLT4 is positive by

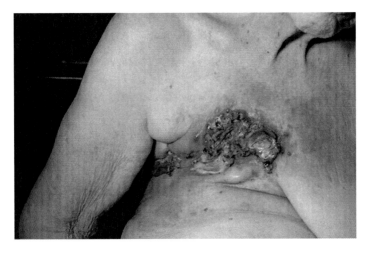

Fig. 13.10 Angiosarcoma of the right chest wall in a 77-year-old Caucasian woman 8 years after surgery and radiation therapy for infiltrating ductal adenocarcinoma of the breast

Fig. 13.11 Postmastectomy, postradiation lymphedema with multifocal lymphangiosarcoma (Stewart-Treves syndrome) (Used with permission from Brennan and Lewis [4])

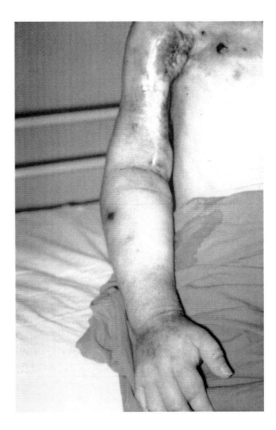

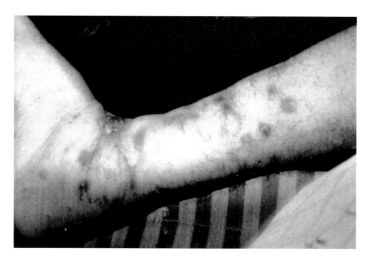

Fig. 13.12 Postfilarial lymphedema with multifocal angiosarcoma (Used with permission from Brennan and Lewis [4])

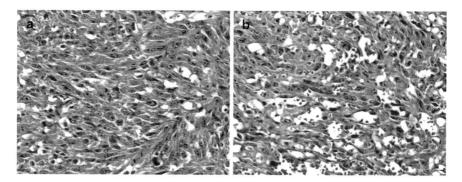

Fig. 13.13 Microscopic appearance (H&E, 200 X) of postradiation angiosarcoma of the breast, demonstrating (**a**) a solid undifferentiated component with high mitotic activity and (**b**) a vasoformative component with interanastomosing, slit-like channels. The images are from the same primary tumor specimen

immunohistochemistry in a majority of cases, and positivity for KIT or cytokeratins is occasionally found in angiosarcomas as well. There is no characteristic genetic change in angiosarcomas known to date, although ~10% of angiosarcomas (all breast primaries) harbor mutations in *VEGFR2/KDR* [15]. It is not clear in that setting if the mutation is a driver or passenger mutation, but the overexpressed gene can be inhibited with VEGFR inhibitors such as sunitinib or sorafenib.

Given a tumor that is chemotherapy sensitive but frequently progressing after a relatively short interval, adjuvant chemotherapy can be considered with active agents such as anthracyclines and taxanes [8, 16, 17]. However, it is not clear if adjuvant chemotherapy impacts survival in this disease. Ifosfamide is

Table 13.1 Systemic therapy recommendations for angiosarcoma

Clinical scenario		Comments
Adjuvant chemotherapy		To consider anthracycline with or without taxane or ifosfamide; may at least delay recurrence
Metastatic disease	First line	Anthracycline or taxane if not given, gemcitabine or combination, ifosfamide
	Second line	VEGF receptor active tyrosine kinase inhibitor (e.g. pazopanib, sorafenib, sunitinib) if breast primary angiosarcoma, clinical trials

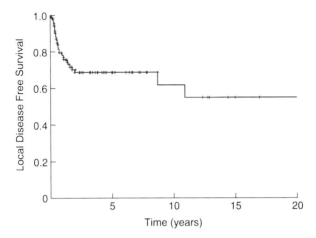

Fig. 13.14 Local disease-free survival for adult patients with primary angiosarcoma. MSKCC 7/1/1982–6/30/2010 n = 108

less active in angiosarcoma than in other sarcomas, in our experience. Agents such as bevacizumab, sorafenib, and sunitinib directed against VEGF receptors have some activity against angiosarcomas. We have observed the best responses in women with breast angiosarcomas, while for other sites such as head and neck, we have observed (at best) stable disease to blanching of extensive tumor lesions, but few if any overt partial responses [18, 19] (Table 13.1).

Outcome

Local disease-free survival is shown in Fig. 13.14 and those with primary presentation and disease-specific survival in Fig. 13.15, emphasizing the high risk of metastatic disease even in those with only a primary tumor at presentation.

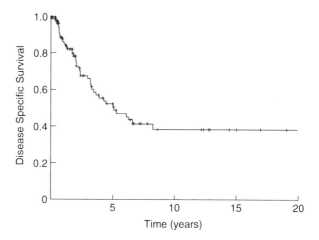

Fig. 13.15 Disease-specific survival for adult patients with primary angiosarcoma. MSKCC 7/1/1982–6/30/2010 n = 108

Kaposi Sarcoma

Kaposi sarcoma (KS) has "historically" been a complicating factor of HIV (human immunodeficiency virus) disease, although Kaposi first described it in 1872 [20, 21]. It is less well appreciated that it also arises endemically in a population with low CD4+ T cell counts in the Mediterranean basin and in Africa, where it is most commonly observed. A version of KS has been recognized more recently in people who are therapeutically immunosuppressed to prevent rejection of organ transplants. In each situation, human herpesvirus-8 (HHV8, also called Kaposi sarcoma herpesvirus, KSHV) is the etiological agent. What was once a devastating disease in the HIV population has been largely suppressed with the use of ART (antiretroviral therapy), such that cases of KS are now relatively uncommon in the HIV population. It is not clear if there are direct effects of HIV-directed therapy against HHV8 or if improvement in CD4+ T cell counts is most responsible for the improvement in such patients. In endemic cases and in HIV-related cases alike, local therapy can be active for skin lesions and systemic therapy can be used for visceral disease or when local therapies fail.

KS affects skin most commonly, but also involves lymph nodes and visceral organs, in particular the gastrointestinal tract. Since KS typically affects multiple sites of skin, surgery is usually not indicated. Local control of individual skin lesions can be achieved by a number of means, be it alitretinoin gel, which was proved effective in controlling the plaque form of the disease [22] compared with a placebo gel alone, and other agents with anti-KS activity include intralesional vinca alkaloids [23], intralesional sodium tetradecyl sulfate (a soap) [23], and other topical agents.

Table 13.2 Systemic therapy recommendations for Kaposi sarcoma

Clinical scenario		Comments
Primary therapy	First line	Depends on anatomic distribution; can involve topical or intralesional therapy for skin-only disease; taxanes or PLD is a good option for systemic therapy for disseminated disease
Persistent/metastatic disease	First line	Agent not used above; oral etoposide has activity; mTOR inhibitor such as sirolimus in patients not on retroviral therapy (pharmacodynamic interaction)
	Second line	Clinical trial; tyrosine kinase inhibitor – caution should be taken regarding interaction with anti-HIV medications

In terms of randomized studies involving actively used agents, pegylated liposomal doxorubicin (PLD, Caelyx®/Doxil®) has been shown superior to combination chemotherapy in at least two randomized studies and is a good standard of care for local disease refractory to other therapy, or for disseminated disease [24, 25], though paclitaxel appeared to have superior progression-free survival in one randomized study [26]. PLD is less toxic than liposomal daunorubicin, which was also shown useful in KS [27]. Taxanes are active against KS [26, 28], as are a variety of agents tested in phase II studies such as interferon-alfa [29], interleukin-12 [30], or etoposide [31]. Since the first publication of disappearance of KS lesions in solid tumor organ transplant patients after switching immunosuppression from cyclosporine to sirolimus [32], other case reports have supported the utility of mTOR inhibitors in Kaposi sarcoma. The use of sirolimus in the HIV + KS population has been limited by pharmacodynamic interaction between protease inhibitors and sirolimus [33]. (Table 13.2)

References

1. Dankaerts W, O'Sullivan PB, Burnett AF, et al. Reliability of EMG measurements for trunk muscles during maximal and sub-maximal voluntary isometric contractions in healthy controls and CLBP patients. J Electromyogr Kinesiol. 2004;14(3):333–42.
2. Randall MD, Kendall DA, O'Sullivan S. The complexities of the cardiovascular actions of cannabinoids. Br J Pharmacol. 2004;142(1):20–6.
3. Weiss SW, Enzinger FM. Epithelioid hemangioendothelioma: a vascular tumor often mistaken for a carcinoma. Cancer. 1982;50(5):970–81.
4. Brennan MF, Lewis JJ. Diagnosis and management of soft tissue sarcoma. London: Martin Dunitz; 1998.
5. Mentzel T, Beham A, Calonje E, et al. Epithelioid hemangioendothelioma of skin and soft tissues: clinicopathologic and immunohistochemical study of 30 cases. Am J Surg Pathol. 1997;21(4):363–74.
6. Errani C, Zhang L, Sung YS, et al. A novel WWTR1-CAMTA1 gene fusion is a consistent abnormality in epithelioid hemangioendothelioma of different anatomic sites. Genes Chromosomes Cancer. 2011;50(8):644–53.

7. Tanas MR, Sboner A, Oliveira AM, et al. Identification of a disease-defining gene fusion in epithelioid hemangioendothelioma. Sci Transl Med. 2011;3(98):98ra82.
8. Fury MG, Antonescu CR, Van Zee KJ, et al. A 14-year retrospective review of angiosarcoma: clinical characteristics, prognostic factors, and treatment outcomes with surgery and chemotherapy. Cancer J. 2005;11(3):241–7.
9. Meis-Kindblom JM, Kindblom LG. Angiosarcoma of soft tissue: a study of 80 cases. Am J Surg Pathol. 1998;22(6):683–97.
10. Fletcher CD, Beham A, Bekir S, et al. Epithelioid angiosarcoma of deep soft tissue: a distinctive tumor readily mistaken for an epithelial neoplasm. Am J Surg Pathol. 1991;15(10):915–24.
11. Mayer F, Aebert H, Rudert M, et al. Primary malignant sarcomas of the heart and great vessels in adult patients–a single-center experience. Oncologist. 2007;12(9):1134–42.
12. McGowan TS, Cummings BJ, O'Sullivan B, et al. An analysis of 78 breast sarcoma patients without distant metastases at presentation. Int J Radiat Oncol Biol Phys. 2000;46(2):383–90.
13. Espat NJ, Lewis JJ, Woodruff JM, et al. Confirmed angiosarcoma: prognostic factors and outcome in 50 prospectively followed patients. Sarcoma. 2000;4(4):173–7.
14. Stewart FW, Treves N. Lymphangiosarcoma in postmastectomy lymphedema; a report of six cases in elephantiasis chirurgica. Cancer. 1948;1(1):64–81.
15. Antonescu CR, Yoshida A, Guo T, et al. KDR activating mutations in human angiosarcomas are sensitive to specific kinase inhibitors. Cancer Res. 2009;69(18):7175–9.
16. Casper ES, Waltzman RJ, Schwartz GK, et al. Phase II trial of paclitaxel in patients with soft-tissue sarcoma. Cancer Invest. 1998;16(7):442–6.
17. Skubitz KM, Haddad PA. Paclitaxel and pegylated-liposomal doxorubicin are both active in angiosarcoma. Cancer. 2005;104(2):361–6.
18. Maki RG, D'Adamo DR, Keohan ML, et al. Phase II study of sorafenib in patients with metastatic or recurrent sarcomas. J Clin Oncol. 2009;27(19):3133–40.
19. Maguire LS, O'Sullivan SM, Galvin K, et al. Fatty acid profile, tocopherol, squalene and phytosterol content of walnuts, almonds, peanuts, hazelnuts and the macadamia nut. Int J Food Sci Nutr. 2004;55(3):171–8.
20. Kaposi M. Idiopathisches multiples pigmentsarkom der Haut. Arch Dermatol Syph. 1872;4:265–73.
21. Shiels RA. A history of Kaposi's sarcoma. J R Soc Med. 1986;79(9):532–4.
22. Bodsworth NJ, Bloch M, Bower M, et al. Phase III vehicle-controlled, multi-centered study of topical alitretinoin gel 0.1 % in cutaneous AIDS-related Kaposi's sarcoma. Am J Clin Dermatol. 2001;2(2):77–87.
23. Ramirez-Amador V, Esquivel-Pedraza L, Lozada-Nur F, et al. Intralesional vinblastine vs. 3 % sodium tetradecyl sulfate for the treatment of oral Kaposi's sarcoma. A double blind, randomized clinical trial. Oral Oncol. 2002;38(5):460–7.
24. Northfelt DW, Dezube BJ, Thommes JA, et al. Pegylated-liposomal doxorubicin versus doxorubicin, bleomycin, and vincristine in the treatment of AIDS-related Kaposi's sarcoma: results of a randomized phase III clinical trial. J Clin Oncol. 1998;16(7):2445–51.
25. Stewart S, Jablonowski H, Goebel FD, et al. Randomized comparative trial of pegylated liposomal doxorubicin versus bleomycin and vincristine in the treatment of AIDS-related Kaposi's sarcoma. International pegylated liposomal doxorubicin study group. J Clin Oncol. 1998;16(2):683–91.
26. Cianfrocca M, Lee S, Von Roenn J, et al. Randomized trial of paclitaxel versus pegylated liposomal doxorubicin for advanced human immunodeficiency virus-associated Kaposi sarcoma. Cancer. 2010;116(16):3969–77.
27. Uthayakumar S, Bower M, Money-Kyrle J, et al. Randomized cross-over comparison of liposomal daunorubicin versus observation for early Kaposi's sarcoma. AIDS. 1996;10(5):515–9.
28. Lim ST, Tupule A, Espina BM, et al. Weekly docetaxel is safe and effective in the treatment of advanced-stage acquired immunodeficiency syndrome-related Kaposi sarcoma. Cancer. 2005;103(2):417–21.

29. Krown SE, Lee JY, Lin L, et al. Interferon-alpha2b with protease inhibitor-based antiretroviral therapy in patients with AIDS-associated Kaposi sarcoma: an AIDS malignancy consortium phase I trial. J Acquir Immune Defic Syndr. 2006;41(2):149–53.
30. Little RF, Pluda JM, Wyvill KM, et al. Activity of subcutaneous interleukin-12 in AIDS-related Kaposi sarcoma. Blood. 2006;107(12):4650–7.
31. Evans SR, Krown SE, Testa MA, et al. Phase II evaluation of low-dose oral etoposide for the treatment of relapsed or progressive AIDS-related Kaposi's sarcoma: an AIDS clinical trials group clinical study. J Clin Oncol. 2002;20(15):3236–41.
32. Stallone G, Schena A, Infante B, et al. Sirolimus for Kaposi's sarcoma in renal-transplant recipients. N Engl J Med. 2005;352(13):1317–23.
33. Marfo K, Greenstein S. Antiretroviral and immunosuppressive drug-drug interactions in human immunodeficiency virus-infected liver and kidney transplant recipients. Transplant Proc. 2009;41(9):3796–9.

Chapter 14
Epithelioid Sarcoma

Epithelioid sarcomas tend to occur in young adults (Fig. 14.1) either in distal locations (classical form) or in the perineum/groin area (so-called proximal type) (Fig. 14.2). The classical form typically arises in the feet, lower extremity, digits, or forearms of younger men and can be sometimes difficult to distinguish from reactive processes, such as granuloma annulare or an ulcer base. In contrast, the proximal-type epithelioid sarcoma exhibits a high degree of cytologic atypia, sometimes displaying a rhabdoid morphology microscopically [1]. The classical form of epithelioid sarcoma is usually a slowly growing lesion that metastasizes relatively early to lymph nodes, which will be positive in 1/3 to 1/2 of cases [2, 3] (Fig. 14.3). The proximal type is often associated with a more aggressive clinical behavior.

In the case of proximal-type epithelioid sarcoma, the differential diagnosis typically includes other high-grade malignancies, such as metastatic carcinoma and melanoma. Epithelioid sarcomas are EMA+ and generally positive for keratins. Nuclear hSNF5/INI1 expression is distinctly lost in these tumors, which may help excluding other diagnostic considerations (Fig. 14.4) [4, 5].

Although the loss of hSNF5/INI1 expression is consistent and is similar to the pattern seen in the extrarenal rhabdoid tumors, the presence of a genetic mutation at this locus is documented only in a minority of cases [6]. Primary therapy is resection, and given the frequency of nodal disease, sentinel node mapping seems advisable, with more complete node dissection in appropriate cases. Adjuvant radiation is generally not given except in tumors with positive or close margins as may be found proximally, and it is not clear if it is helpful in this histology in preventing recurrence, since local-regional relapse despite radiation and surgery is common.

Chemotherapy is not given in the adjuvant situation for this tumor given its relatively slow evolution and at-best modest response to chemotherapy in the metastatic setting. The slow-moving nature of the tumor means that long exposures to chemotherapy (months) may be necessary to achieve evidence of tumor shrinking. We have observed at least minor responses to a variety of drugs used for epithelial tumors and sarcomas as well, such as doxorubicin, ifosfamide, vinorelbine, cisplatin, and others, but since people may need to be treated for many years for recurrence, parsimony is appropriate in patients with minimal symptoms (Table 14.1).

M.F. Brennan et al., *Management of Soft Tissue Sarcoma*,
DOI 10.1007/978-1-4614-5004-7_14, © Springer Science+Business Media New York 2013

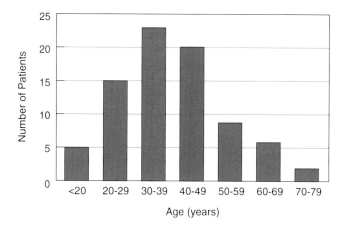

Fig. 14.1 Age distribution of adult patients with epithelioid sarcoma. MSKCC 7/1/1982–6/30/2010, n = 80

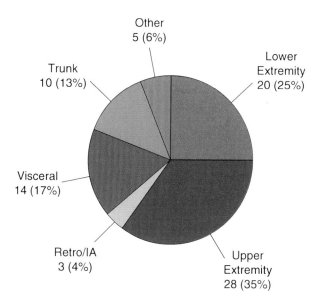

Fig. 14.2 Primary site distribution of adult patients with epithelioid sarcoma. MSKCC 7/1/1982–6/30/2010 n = 80 *Retro/IA* retroperitoneal/intra-abdominal

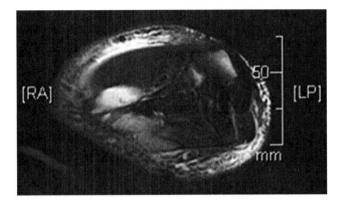

Fig. 14.3 T1 weighted MRI image of metastatic epithelioid sarcoma of the left upper extremity causing edema and multiple cutaneous and soft tissue implants

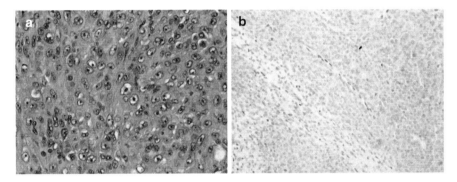

Fig. 14.4 Microscopic appearance of proximal-type epithelioid sarcoma. (**a**) Solid sheets of epithelioid cells are seen, having ill-defined cell borders, eosinophilic cytoplasm, and macronuclei (H&E, 400X). (**b**) BAF47 immunohistochemistry demonstrating complete loss of INI1 staining expression in the tumor cells; an internal positive control shows retained expression in blood vessels

Outcome

Local disease-free survival is shown in Fig. 14.5 and disease-specific survival in Fig. 14.6.

Table 14.1 Systemic therapeutic recommendations for patients with epithelioid sarcoma

Clinical scenario		Comments
Adjuvant chemotherapy		Not generally administered
Metastatic disease	First line	Ifosfamide ± doxorubicin
	Second line and greater	Platinum-based therapy or combinations, vinorelbine, taxanes, pazopanib, clinical trials

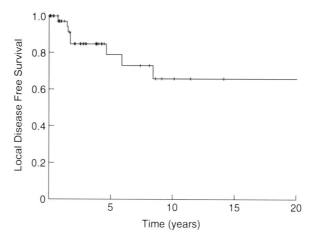

Fig. 14.5 Local disease-free survival for adult patients with primary epithelioid sarcoma (all types). MSKCC 7/1/1982–6/30/2010, n = 48

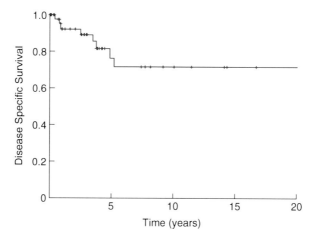

Fig. 14.6 Disease-specific survival for adult patients with primary epithelioid sarcoma (all types). MSKCC 7/1/1982–6/30/2010, n = 48

References

1. Guillou L, Wadden C, Coindre JM, et al. "Proximal-type" epithelioid sarcoma, a distinctive aggressive neoplasm showing rhabdoid features. Clinicopathologic, immunohistochemical, and ultrastructural study of a series. Am J Surg Pathol. 1997;21(2):130–46.
2. Chbani L, Guillou L, Terrier P, et al. Epithelioid sarcoma: a clinicopathologic and immunohistochemical analysis of 106 cases from the French sarcoma group. Am J Clin Pathol. 2009; 131(2):222–7.
3. Sakharpe A, Lahat G, Gulamhusein T, et al. Epithelioid sarcoma and unclassified sarcoma with epithelioid features: clinicopathological variables, molecular markers, and a new experimental model. Oncologist. 2011;16(4):512–22.
4. Modena P, Lualdi E, Facchinetti F, et al. SMARCB1/INI1 tumor suppressor gene is frequently inactivated in epithelioid sarcomas. Cancer Res. 2005;65(10):4012–9.
5. Hornick JL, Dal Cin P, Fletcher CD. Loss of INI1 expression is characteristic of both conventional and proximal-type epithelioid sarcoma. Am J Surg Pathol. 2009;33(4):542–50.
6. Kohashi K, Izumi T, Oda Y, et al. Infrequent SMARCB1/INI1 gene alteration in epithelioid sarcoma: a useful tool in distinguishing epithelioid sarcoma from malignant rhabdoid tumor. Hum Pathol. 2009;40(3):349–55.

Chapter 15
Sarcomas More Common in Children

Ewing sarcoma
Ewing sarcoma-like small round blue cell tumor
Rhabdomyosarcoma
Embryonal sarcoma
Calcifying nested stromal and epithelial tumor

Soft Tissue Sarcomas More Commonly Observed in Pediatric Patients

Several types of sarcomas are more common in children, the most common of which include osteogenic sarcoma, Ewing sarcoma, and rhabdomyosarcoma. While osteogenic sarcoma presents similarly in children and adults under age 40, there are a variety of differences in the presentation of Ewing sarcoma in adults versus pediatric patients. Ewing sarcoma is predominantly a bone tumor in children, while in adults it occurs much more commonly in soft tissue. As is also noted below, there is a new class of sarcomas that are similar in appearance to Ewing sarcoma but contain translocation products other than the classical t(11;22) *EWSR1-FLI1* translocation. Pleomorphic rhabdomyosarcoma is much more common in adults than in children, while alveolar rhabdomyosarcoma is rare in adults.

Regardless, pediatric randomized studies showing efficacy of chemotherapy for the sarcomas more common in children provide the standard by which adults receiving therapy for these rare sarcomas are treated. While it is not typically possible to treat adults with chemotherapy at the same intensity as children (using, e.g., the weekly administration of vincristine for rhabdomyosarcoma), these regimens provide a good basis by which adults with these diagnoses can be treated. Discussed below are treatments of two sarcomas more common in children than adults, i.e., the Ewing sarcoma family of tumors (EFT) and rhabdomyosarcoma.

M.F. Brennan et al., *Management of Soft Tissue Sarcoma*,   221
DOI 10.1007/978-1-4614-5004-7_15, © Springer Science+Business Media New York 2013

Ewing Sarcoma Family of Tumors (EFT)

The Ewing sarcoma family of tumors (EFT) includes Ewing sarcoma, primitive neuroectodermal tumor (PNET), and Askin tumor of the chest wall. In 1921, James Ewing described the tumor that now bears his name in a 14-year-old girl, calling it "diffuse endothelioma of bone" [1]. With the advent of karyotyping of different sarcomas, it became clear that all EFT members contain the defining chromosomal translocation t(11;22) *EWSR1-FLI1* or related translocations and that they should be treated in the same manner. Conversely, not all tumors positive for an *EWSR1* translocation should be treated like Ewing sarcoma. For example, clear cell sarcoma and extraskeletal myxoid chondrosarcoma contain *EWSR1* translocations, but involve different partners than those involved in Ewing sarcoma, and are essentially impervious to standard chemotherapy agents. Furthermore, *EWSR1* rearrangements have been more recently described in benign tumors, such as angiomatoid fibrous histiocytoma [2], and myoepithelial tumors [3].

While 80% or so of EFT in the pediatric population occurs in bone, some 75% or more of adult EFT occurs in soft tissues, an example of which is shown in Figs. 15.1, 15.2, 15.3, 15.4, 15.5, and 15.6. Surprisingly, extraskeletal Ewing sarcoma (EES) was not described until 1969 [4]. EES most commonly affects trunk and extremity, but unusual sites such as head and neck or retroperitoneum are also observed. There is no gender predominance of this form of the disease, and as expected from above, the median age of presentation is higher than for those patients with bone primaries.

In the present day, the primary management typically involves multidisciplinary treatment including chemotherapy, surgery, and occasionally radiation therapy.

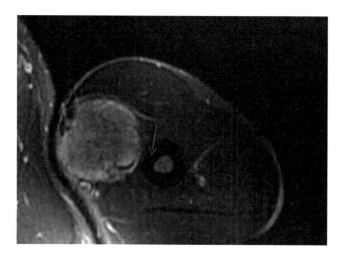

Fig. 15.1 T2 fat-saturated MRI image of a 9×4.5×4.5 cm bicipital Ewing sarcoma in a 34 year-old woman without other symptoms. *Red arrow*: possible local bony involvement with tumor. The patient had no evidence of viable tumor in the bone after neoadjuvant chemotherapy

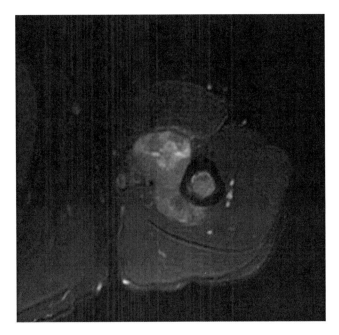

Fig. 15.2 T2 fat-saturated MRI image of a local-regional soft tissue and bone marrow recurrence Ewing sarcoma of the right upper extremity in a 50 year-old woman despite primary neoadjuvant chemotherapy, surgery, and radiation. The patient is without evidence of disease 6 years after surgery and further chemotherapy

Historical data demonstrate that survival for patients with primary EFT treated with local therapy alone is poor, on the range of 15%. The addition of systemic chemotherapy has increased the cure rate for EFT to ~75% in children with primary disease, but only ~50% in adults (Fig. 15.7). The addition of chemotherapy for the treatment of EFT provides among the most dramatic improvements in overall survival compared to primary treatment alone of any solid tumor.

Specific genetic events appear to affect patient outcome, e.g., type of *EWSR1-FLI1* fusion [5], though there remains controversy on this point. Adults appear to fare poorly compared to pediatric patients [6]. There appears to be a stronger relationship between *TP53* mutation or *INK4A* deletion and poorer prognosis [7]. These data do not presently impact upon the choice of chemotherapy agents for adjuvant treatment of primary disease. A new subset of *EWSR1*-negative small round blue cell tumors has been identified with novel translocations, e.g., *CIC-DUX4*, which we speculate accounts for a significant portion of the inferior outcomes with chemotherapy in this family of tumors in adults versus children [8–11].

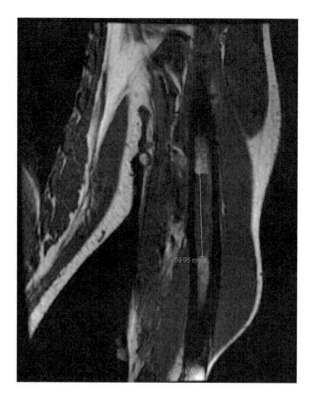

Fig. 15.3 T1-weighted MRI image of the patient of Fig. 15.2 after neoadjuvant chemotherapy. The soft tissue component has decreased in size, but the bony component has not changed significantly in size

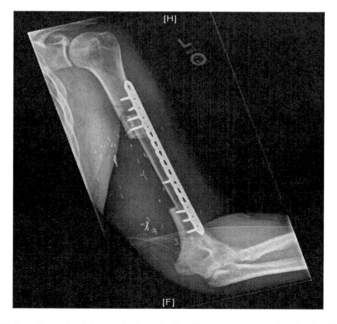

Fig. 15.4 Plain radiograph of the surgical result after limb-sparing operation for locally recurrent disease for the patient of Figs. 15.2 and 15.3

Fig. 15.5 Gross image of the
surgical specimen of the patient
in Figs. 15.2, 15.3, and 15.4 after
neoadjuvant chemotherapy and
surgery

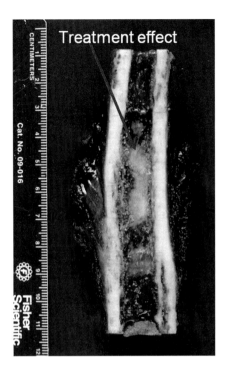

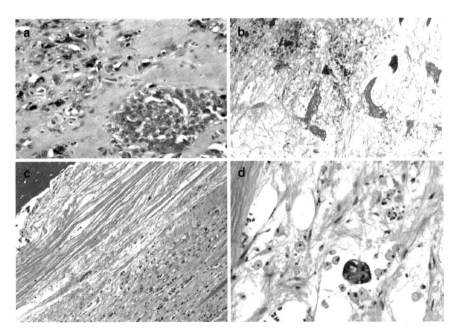

Fig. 15.6 Microscopic images of the surgical specimen of Fig. 15.5 demonstrating ~80% treatment
effect of tumor (H&E, 100–400X)

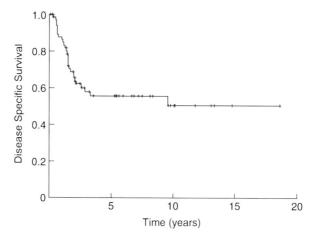

Fig. 15.7 Disease-specific survival for adults with primary soft tissue Ewing sarcoma. MSKCC 7/1/1982–6/30/2010 n = 70

Demographics

Even as the anatomic primary site changes from bone in children to soft tissue in adults, Ewing sarcoma is most common in younger patients, although we have treated rare patients over age 70 with this diagnosis (Fig. 15.8). The anatomic distribution is wide, with lower extremity the most common in adults (Fig. 15.9). Local disease control is on a par with other soft tissue sarcomas (Fig. 15.10), but survival in adults appears inferior to that of children (Fig. 15.7), although SEER data indicate soft tissue sites for Ewing sarcoma may have a superior prognosis to those arising in bone [12]. Patients with European ancestry have a higher incidence of Ewing sarcomas than patients with Asian or African ancestry, but in the USA, data outcomes are superior for white non-Hispanic patients, implicating access to care as a significant risk factor for outcomes for this type of sarcoma [13].

Primary Therapy

Surgery remains an integral portion of treatment for pediatric sarcomas such as Ewing sarcoma; however, it is common to use neoadjuvant chemotherapy in pediatric clinical trials before primary surgery, with radiation typically given only after several cycles of chemotherapy have been given. RT can be given safely in the extremities during cycles of ifosfamide-etoposide chemotherapy, or omitting the etoposide for concerns of increased risk of leukemia. In patients who have surgery first, adjuvant chemotherapy can be administered thereafter. In some patients with areas difficult to resect, definitive radiation therapy is the primary treatment of choice.

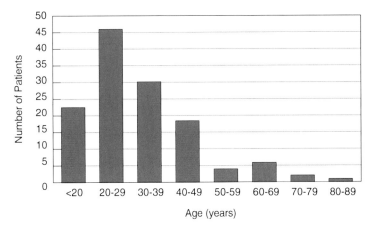

Fig. 15.8 Age distribution of adult patients with Ewing sarcoma of soft tissue. MSKCC 7/1/1982–6/30/2010 n = 129

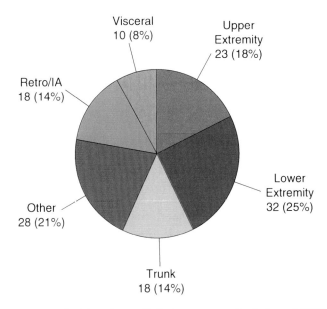

Fig. 15.9 Primary site of adult patients with Ewing sarcoma of soft tissue. MSKCC 7/1/1982–6/30/2010 n = 129 *Retro/IA* retroperitoneal/intra-abdominal

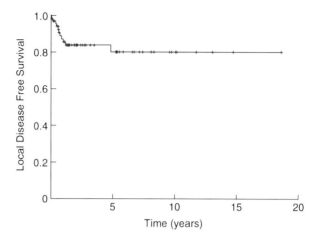

Fig. 15.10 Local disease-free survival for adult patients with primary soft tissue Ewing sarcoma. MSKCC 7/1/1982–6/30/2010 n = 70

Adjuvant Chemotherapy

Cyclophosphamide, doxorubicin, and dactinomycin were all found to be active in Ewing sarcoma in single-agent studies in the 1960s and 1970s [14, 15]. These studies led to performance of randomized studies that led to present-day adjuvant therapy. The randomized Intergroup Ewing's Sarcoma Study (IESS)-I showed that the inclusion of doxorubicin was associated with improved overall survival [16]; IESS-II showed that higher-dose therapy was superior to moderate-dose continuous infusion therapy [17].

In Europe, different approaches have been taken for adjuvant chemotherapy that have led to much the same synthesis of agents, albeit using different schedules and doses. The CESS-86 (Cooperative Ewing's Sarcoma Studies) showed that patients with high-risk Ewing sarcoma fared as well as patients with lower risk disease if they received ifosfamide as part of their treatment program [18]. In Italy, the results of the REN-3 study showed that the addition of ifosfamide to standard VACA (vincristine, dactinomycin, cyclophosphamide, doxorubicin) therapy was associated with an improved histological response compared to patients treated on prior studies. Use of ifosfamide (VAIA [vincristine, doxorubicin, ifosfamide, dactinomycin]) was associated with improved disease-free survival compared to VACA therapy for standard-risk patients in the European Intergroup Cooperative Ewing's Sarcoma Study (EICESS)-92, and addition of etoposide gave further benefit for high-risk patients compared to VAIA, although the difference did not reach statistical significance [19]. These studies have supported the utility of ifosfamide and etoposide in the primary therapy of Ewing sarcoma.

For most of the last 20 years, a large randomized clinical trial of the Pediatric Oncology Group/Children's Cancer Group (POG-9354/CCG-7942) defined the standard of care in the United States for primary EFT. In this trial, the standard arm was vincristine-doxorubicin-cyclophosphamide, and the experimental arm, the same combination alternating with cycles of ifosfamide-etoposide [20]. Although this decreased the dose density of each treatment combination by half, survival was improved for patients with nonmetastatic disease (from 61% to 72% at 5 years), but not with metastatic disease, presumably since the patients progressing on the standard three-drug arm could receive benefit from ifosfamide-etoposide after progression. Of note, 20–25% of patients with metastatic disease, typically with lung metastases as the only site of metastatic disease, were cured with this multimodality approach.

Two studies varying the intensity of the five-drug Ewing sarcoma regimen are very instructive regarding current approaches for adjuvant treatment of Ewing sarcoma. In the COG study from Granowetter et al. [21], the doses of cycles of therapy were increased to shorten the time of administration of standard CAV (cyclophosphamide, doxorubicin, and vincristine) and ifosfamide/etoposide regimens from 48 weeks to 30 weeks. There was no significant difference in 5-year event-free survival between the two arms (76% vs. 75%, respectively) [21].

Conversely, shortening the cycle length had an impact on overall survival in patients under 18 years old receiving CAV-IE (ifosfamide, etoposide). Patients who received cycles of therapy every 2 weeks instead of every 3 had improved overall survival (only in patients under 18 years of age) [22]. Median cycle length in the 2-week arm of the study was actually 18 days. This proof of principle of dose density as described by Norton and Simon [23, 24] defines a new standard of care for primary treatment of Ewing sarcoma in patients less than 18 years of age. Over age 18, the 3-week interval alternating CAV-IE combination remains a standard of care in the United States, since the data showing interval compression did not hold true in the subset of adult patients analyzed, although an attempt to more rapidly cycle chemotherapy in adults is equally valid given the overall results of the study. The lack of benefit seen with higher doses per cycle of chemotherapy used in the Granowetter COG study [21] argues against schedules of the P6 regimen (involving 4.2 g/m^2 cyclophosphamide per cycle) in the treatment of small round cell sarcomas.

High-Dose Systemic Therapy for Metastatic Disease

For metastatic EFT, cures remain uncommon, with a cure rate in the 20–25% range in the study by Grier et al. [20]. High-dose therapy with autologous stem cell transplant (ASCT) has been abandoned in most centers in the United States based on poor survival data from retrospective analyses [25].

Conversely, other data support the potential utility of high-dose therapy and ASCT in patients with metastatic Ewing sarcoma. A series of 33 EFT patients with relapsed or progressive disease treated with a variety of conditioning regimens and bone marrow or peripheral blood stem cells showed some promise for the modality, with 5-year EFS (event-free survival) of 38% [26]. In addition, a series of 97 patients with metastatic disease at diagnosis, 75% of whom received high-dose therapy and ASCT, had a 5-year EFS of 37% [27]. The ISG/SSG III study, closed in December 2006, also points to the potential viability of high-dose chemotherapy with ASCT in EFT. Preliminary data were reported at the ASCO 2007 [28]. With a median follow-up of 37 months, the 5-year overall survival and event-free survival were 74% and 66%, respectively. Importantly, the EFS for poor responders who received HDCT (high-dose chemotherapy) (68%) and the EFS for the good responders (71%) were similar [28].

The combination of vincristine, ifosfamide, doxorubicin, and etoposide (VIDE) is associated with significant responses in high-risk patients [29] and was used as the induction regimen before comparing high-dose therapy with autologous stem cell support versus vincristine, dactinomycin, and ifosfamide chemotherapy for patients with high-risk Ewing sarcoma (European Ewing Tumour Working Initiative of National Groups, Euro-E.W.I.N.G 99 study) (22). Two hundred eighty-one patients received six cycles of VIDE, one cycle of vincristine-dactinomycin-ifosf-amide, local treatment, followed by high-dose busulfan-melphalan supported by stem cell transplantation. Event-free survival (EFS) at 3 years was 27%, and overall survival (OS) at 3 years was 34%. A total of 169 patients (60%) received stem cell-based therapy. For children under age 14, the 3-year EFS was 45% (n=46). The authors were able to define risk factors that predicted for poor outcome (tumor volume over 200 mL, more than one bony metastatic site, bone marrow metastases, age over 14, and additional lung metastases), graded with a point system. Patients in group 1 (score 3 or lower) had 3-year EFS of 50%, those in group 2 (score=4) had 3-year EFS of 25%, and those in group 3 (score of 5 or more) had 3-year EFS of 10%. The study is the first to indicate the patients in whom more aggressive therapy may be warranted, but randomized data are lacking. These data are also used as a justification for bone marrow biopsy in all patients. However, since the bone marrow biopsy does not change therapy, it is difficult to justify in the evaluation of patients off study. It is also not clear that more aggressive therapy is better than standard-dose chemotherapy alone as the cure rate in metastatic disease in the CCG-POG Ewing sarcoma study was 22%. Randomized data will be the best way to address this issue. Another approach undergoing evaluation presently is use of allo-geneic transplant in appropriate high-risk patients.

Standard Cytotoxic Chemotherapy After Disease Relapse

While they are not useful in other adult sarcomas, topoisomerase I inhibitors demonstrate activity in Ewing sarcoma (as well as rhabdomyosarcoma). For metastatic disease, temozolomide-irinotecan has activity but is associated with a relatively brief duration of benefit and diarrhea from the protracted irinotecan schedule typically employed (5 days of treatment 20 mg/m^2, 2 weeks on, 1 off) [30]. The authors question the use of temozolomide since there are no single-agent data to indicate that either dacarbazine or temozolomide is active in Ewing sarcoma, while conversely there are good data to support the use of irinotecan in EFT and rhabdomyosarcoma [31–33]. Adjustments in the dose or schedule are necessary in adult patients treated with the pediatric regimen of 20 mg/m2 IV daily x 5, 2 weeks on, one off. Cyclophosphamide-topotecan is another active combination with greater myelotoxicity and less gastrointestinal toxicity than temozolomide-irinotecan [34–37]. There are no data comparing these two regimens.

A variety of other agents have been examined in Ewing sarcoma in metastatic disease without significant success.

Investigational Approaches

The finding of patients with responses to insulin-like growth factor 1 receptor (IGF1R) inhibitors in 2007 has led to a flurry of interest in using such agents in patients with refractory Ewing sarcoma. However, only modest but consistent RECIST response rates of 10–15% have been observed in a series of phase I–II studies of a variety of monoclonal antibodies, all directed against IGF1R [38–43]. The biological basis/bases of responding tumors remain unknown, but could involve specific translocation subtypes or variations in IGF-binding proteins in one patient to another. We note that very few responses in other sarcomas have been seen with IGF1R inhibitors, save for occasional patients with solitary fibrous tumor and desmoplastic small round cell tumor responding. Perhaps, part of the reason for this finding is the genuine dependence of the cell on one signaling pathway. In one study, there was an association with high serum IGF1 level and longer survival [41], but it is not known if this is a feature of the therapy, patient, or the tumor itself.

Although EFT is usually positive for the marker KIT, like small cell lung carcinoma and seminoma, there appears to be no activity of the KIT inhibitor imatinib in Ewing sarcoma, based on data from one prospective phase II study [44]. A variety of other agents have been investigated with little benefit clinically. Thus, it is hoped that new approaches, based on the biology of activation of downstream effectors of the EWSR1-FLI1 translocation product, immunological or other approaches, will yield data that will yield new avenues for clinical trials in the near future. One of the most promising recent avenues is the use of poly(ADP-ribose) polymerase (PARP) inhibitors in the treatment of Ewing sarcoma, found in two very different sets of investigations of Ewing sarcoma cell lines [45, 46] (suggestions for therapy – Table 15.1).

Table 15.1 Systemic therapy recommendations for patients with Ewing sarcoma

Clinical scenario		Comments
Adjuvant chemotherapy		Enrollment of clinical trials: pediatric studies are often open to adult patients. Off trial, chemotherapy includes agents with a doxorubicin backbone, e.g., VAdrC-ifosfamide-etoposide (VACIE) alternating cycles, or VIDE. For VACIE in patients under age 18, every 2-week therapy, when feasible, is superior to every 3-week therapy. In adults, every 3-week therapy remains a standard of care on the basis of one randomized study, but an attempt to compress cycle length appears prudent
Metastatic disease	1st line	Irinotecan, irinotecan-temozolomide, or cyclophosphamide-topotecan
	2nd line	IGF1R inhibitor if available; PARP inhibitors, other clinical trials

VActC vincristine + dactinomycin + cyclophosphamide, *VAdrC* vincristine + doxorubicin + cyclophosphamide, *VIDE* vincristine + ifosfamide + doxorubicin + etoposide, *PARP* poly(ADP-ribose) polymerase

Ewing Sarcoma-Like Small Round Cell Tumors

The finding of small round blue cell tumors that do not contain translocations seen in Ewing sarcoma, synovial sarcoma, round cell liposarcoma, or alveolar rhabdomyosarcoma has caused consternation regarding their management. Are such tumors to be treated like Ewing sarcoma or as another sarcoma, perhaps undifferentiated pleomorphic sarcoma?

Classification of translocation-negative small round blue cell tumors is now made somewhat easier with the finding of a consistent morphology and translocations found in a significant percentage of these sarcomas [8, 47–56]. Initial reports described individual cases of such tumors [8, 47, 48, 51–55], and subsequently two papers identified groups of patients with consistent *CIC-DUX4* translocations [49, 50]. The assessment of these translocations has been made both difficult and intriguing with the finding of *DUX4* in more than one copy, as the result of duplication events over evolution at the ends of chromosomes 4 and 10, yielding either t(4;19) *CIC-DUX4* (4q35;19q13) or t(10;19)(10q26.3;19q13). Notably, defective splicing in *DUX4* is found in a form of muscular dystrophy, specifically fascioscapular muscular dystrophy [57], highlighting as with other sarcoma oncogenes the need for the proper cellular context for transformation rather than apoptosis in a given cell type.

Microscopically, *CIC-DUX4*-positive sarcomas demonstrate small- to medium-sized round to oval cells, packed in solid sheets with minimal or absent intervening collagen [50]. Distinct areas of spindle-shaped cells are seen only infrequently. Most tumor cells had an ill-defined cell border, with scant amount of amphophilic or lightly eosinophilic cytoplasm, and contained vesicular nuclei, with distinct, often enlarged nucleoli. Although the presence of larger, pleomorphic cells was not seen, there was a higher degree of heterogeneity in nuclear shape and size compared with the rather consistent appearance seen in Ewing sarcoma. Geographic areas of necrosis are commonly seen, as is individual cell necrosis with "starry sky" appearance. A high mitotic rate of >10 mitotic figures per 10 HPFs was observed in all cases. There does not appear to be a difference in morphology between the tumors that do and do not have *CIC* rearrangements. Approximately two-thirds of *EWSR1* rearrangement-negative small round blue cell tumors in one series appear to contain a *CIC-DUX4* rearrangement [50].

The clinical features of this new sarcoma entity are still somewhat unclear given the small number of cases characterized to date. The series of 15 patients from Italiano et al. [50] combined with 9 other cases reported from other investigators indicate a male predominance (male to female gender ratio 1.4), median age at diagnosis of 24 years (range 6–62), frequent primary tumor location in the limb (50%), and high rate of metastatic relapse (11 cases out of 22 with available follow-up, 50%). Therefore, besides similar histological patterns, these tumors share with the Ewing family of tumors an aggressive clinical course.

Shortly thereafter, the publication of the cases containing *CIC-DUX4* translocations, a novel intrachromosomal X-chromosome fusion *BCOR-CCNB3*, was described in Ewing-like sarcomas of bone and soft tissue in a screen of 594 sarcomas lacking *EWSR1* or other known sarcoma fusion products [56]. Notably, these tumors could also be identified uniquely with simple CCNB3 immunohistochemistry. BCOR is a gene encoding a ubiquitously expressed transcriptional corepressor that binds BCL6 and proteins involved in chromatin dynamics, while CCNB3 encodes an otherwise testis-specific meiotic cyclin.

These data will inform us on new approaches to manage these tumors, as there may be continued commonalities between these tumors and hematological and other malignancies. There is little doubt that the use of newer generations of sequencing techniques will rapidly give us new data to both characterize and treat these tumors over the next few years.

In terms of clinical outcomes for these patients, there are few data to provide guidance as of early 2012. Preliminary data regarding neoadjuvant therapy and response in metastatic disease indicate that the *CIC-DUX4* Ewing sarcoma subtype is less sensitive than Ewing sarcoma to standard chemotherapy agents (doxorubicin-ifosfamide or combination 5-drug therapy with vincristine-doxorubicin-cyclophosphamide with ifosfamide-etoposide) [50], while data are yet to be published on the clinical behavior of *BCOR-CCNB3* Ewing-like sarcomas. Thus, it is presently not clear from these data if this new tumor category should be considered enough like a Ewing sarcoma to mandate systemic chemotherapy.

Rhabdomyosarcoma

Rhabdomyosarcomas (RMS) are a family of rare tumors with evidence of skeletal muscle differentiation, of which there are perhaps 300–350 cases a year in the United States (incidence ~1 per million). It qualifies as the most common soft tissue

Table 15.2 Histological classification of rhabdomyosarcoma

Superior prognosis
Botryoid rhabdomyosarcoma
Spindle cell rhabdomyosarcoma
Intermediate prognosis
Embryonal rhabdomyosarcoma
Poor prognosis
Alveolar rhabdomyosarcoma
Undifferentiated sarcoma
Subtypes whose prognosis is not presently evaluable
Rhabdomyosarcoma with rhabdoid features

sarcoma in the pediatric population and has led pediatric oncologists to coin the term non-rhabdomyosarcoma soft tissue sarcomas (NRSTS) for diagnoses other than rhabdomyosarcoma, though this makes little sense to the oncologist caring for adult patients who treats patients with a panoply of soft tissue tumors.

Rhabdomyosarcoma, *sui generis* even among sarcomas, is made complex due to several factors. Multiple classification systems have been developed, but the most recent recognizes subtypes based on prognosis (Table 15.2), including a slight modification of the classically recognized subtypes of alveolar, embryonal, botryoid, and pleomorphic RMS.

Demographics

As with Ewing sarcoma, rhabdomyosarcoma remains a primary sarcoma of patients under age 21 (Fig. 15.11), with most patients presenting in their first 5 years of life having embryonal rhabdomyosarcoma and a second peak around age 15 of alveolar rhabdomyosarcoma [58]. In adults, the pleomorphic variety is most common with a peak incidence in the sixth decade. It is notable that RMS is one class of sarcomas (as well as, e.g., differentiated/**de**differentiated liposarcoma and gastrointestinal stromal tumor) in which primary site is an important factor in clinical outcome. There is a wide anatomic distribution (Fig. 15.12). The anatomic site of presentation (not accounting for age) is most commonly head and neck (the orbit and other parameningeal sites are classic primary sites of disease), or trunk (with paratesticular disease being common), more than extremities or other sites [59]. The histologic subtype also varies by primary site [60], with alveolar RMS most common in the extremities and embryonal RMS most common in the head and neck, genitourinary, and retroperitoneal sites [60].

Males are more frequently affected than females (approximately 4:3 ratio), and Caucasians appear to be affected somewhat more commonly than people of other

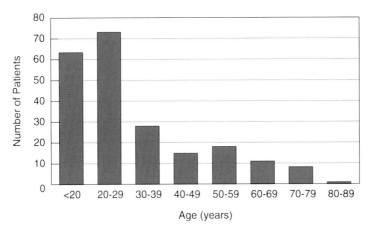

Fig. 15.11 Age distribution of adult patients with rhabdomyosarcoma (all types). MSKCC 7/1/1982–6/30/2010 n = 217

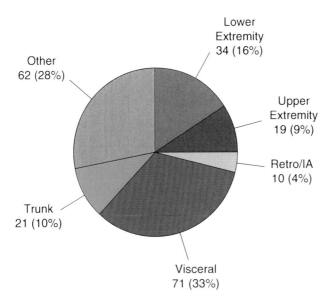

Fig. 15.12 Primary site of adult patients with rhabdomyosarcoma (all types). MSKCC 7/1/1982–6/30/2010 n = 217 *Retro/IA* retroperitoneal intra-abdominal

ethnicities. As with Ewing sarcoma and other primary soft tissue sarcomas, there is usually very good local control independent of histology (Fig. 15.13), but patients frequently die of metastatic disease. Even patients with embryonal rhabdomyosarcoma, a "favorable" histology, have only a 50% 10-year disease-specific survival rate (Fig. 15.14).

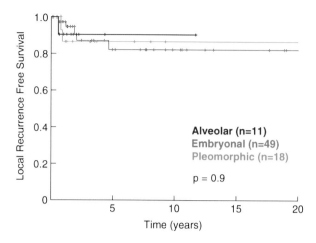

Fig. 15.13 Local disease-free survival for adult patients with primary rhabdomyosarcoma, distinguished by histology. MSKCC 7/1/1982–6/30/2010 n = 78

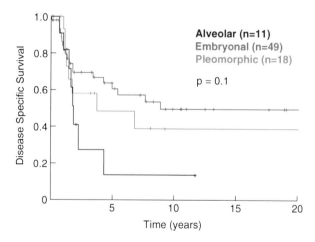

Fig. 15.14 Disease-specific survival for adult patients with primary rhabdomyosarcoma distinguished by histology. MSKCC 7/1/1982–6/30/2010 n = 78

Molecular Biology

The molecular biology of each form of RMS is distinct, in keeping with their different biological behavior and risk of recurrence (Figs. 15.15 and 15.16).

Alveolar RMS has a characteristic translocation t(2;13), with a minority of cases involving a variant translocation t(1;13) [61–63]. The translocation fuses the *PAX3* gene (which regulates a transcriptional program for neuromuscular development)

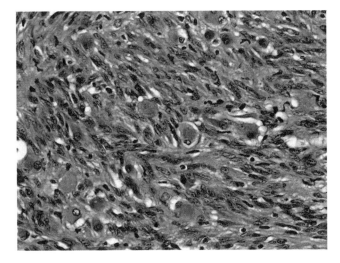

Fig. 15.15 Microscopic appearance of embryonal rhabdomyosarcoma, demonstrating large rhab-domyoblasts with abundant cytoplasm filled with eosinophilic whorls of myosin fibrils (H&E, 200X)

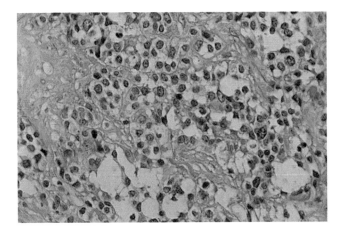

Fig. 15.16 Microscopic appearance of alveolar rhabdomyosarcoma, demonstrating nests of cells typical for the histology (H&E, 200X)

with the *FOXOA1* (a member of the forkhead family of transcription factors). The fusion transcription factor appears to activate both transforming and differentiation gene programs. The variant t(1;13) fuses the *PAX7* gene located on chromosome 1 with *FOXOA1*. Translocation-containing tumors tend to occur in the extremity and appear to occur in somewhat younger patients than translocation-negative tumors.

Embryonal RMS frequently have loss of heterozygosity (LOH) at chromosome 11p15.5; [64, 65] the target of this inactivation is still not well defined, but may

Table 15.3 Intergroup Rhabdomyosarcoma Study Group IRS-V tumor classification

Group I:	Localized disease, completely resected; regional nodes not involved – lymph node biopsy or sampling is highly advised/required, except for head and neck lesions
	(a) Confined to muscle or organ of origin
	(b) Contiguous involvement – infiltration outside the muscle or organ of origin, as through fascial planes
Group II:	Total gross resection with evidence of regional spread
	(a) Grossly resected tumor with microscopic residual disease
	(b) Regional disease with involved nodes, completely resected with microscopic residual
	(c) Regional disease with involved nodes, grossly resected, but with evidence of microscopic residual and/or histologic involvement of the most distal regional node (from the primary site) in the dissection
Group III:	Incomplete resection with gross residual disease
	(a) After biopsy only
	(b) After gross or major resection of the primary (>50%)
Group IV:	Distant metastatic disease present at onset (lung, liver, bones, bone marrow, brain, and distant muscle and "nodes")

involved *GOK* [66–68], a gene that can control growth of RMS cell lines. Trisomy 8 is also common in embryonal RMS.

Pleomorphic RMS most typically has an aneuploid karyotype, most similar to other forms of high-grade undifferentiated pleomorphic sarcoma, formerly termed malignant fibrous histiocytoma.

Risk Stratification

An expanded classification system is used for the present randomized study of patients with RMS, based on risk categories of tumors, denoted in Table 15.3. This staging system includes anatomy and histology and differentiates patients fairly well in terms of outcome, given that stage III patients (Table 15.4 and 15.5) have a ~50% survival rate and there are presently no standardized criteria as to how to better risk stratify such patients. With the new classification system, low-risk patients have an estimated 3-year failure-free survival (FFS) rate of 88%; for intermediate-risk patients, 3-year FFS is ~65%; and for high-risk patients, it is under 30%.

Staging

In addition to routine staging with physical exam, routine laboratory data, and the like, a few other tests that are useful in the patient workup include assessment of lactate dehydrogenase, which can be an indicator of tumor bulk, magnetic resonance

Table 15.4 Pretreatment staging of rhabdomyosarcoma

Stage	Sites	T	Size	N	M
1	Orbit, head and neck, (excluding paramen-ingeal) GU – non-bladder/non-prostate, biliary tract/liver	T1 or T2	a or b	N0 or N1 or Nx	M0
2	Bladder/prostate, extremity, cranial, parameningeal, other (includes trunk, retroperitoneum, etc.) except biliary tract/liver	T1 or T2	a	N0 or Nx	M0
3	Bladder/prostate, extremity, cranial, parameningeal, other (includes trunk, retroperitoneum, etc.) except biliary tract/liver	T1 or T2	a	N1	M0
			b	N0 or N1 or Nx	M0
4	All	T1 or T2	a or b	N0 or N1	M1

Tumor

T (site)1: confined to anatomic site of origin
　a. ≤5 cm in diameter in size
　b. >5 cm in diameter in size
T (site)2: extension and/or fixative to surrounding tissue
　a. ≤5 cm in diameter in size
　b. >5 cm in diameter in size

Regional nodes

N0 regional nodes not clinically involved
N1 regional nodes *clinically* involved by neoplasm
Nx clinical status of regional nodes unknown (especially sites that preclude lymph node valuation)

Metastasis

M0 no distant metastasis
M1 metastasis present

Table 15.5 Simplified rhabdomyosarcoma risk categories, based on Intergroup Rhabdomyosarcoma and Children's Oncology Group studies

Risk category	Histology	Clinical group	Stage
Low	Embryonal and variants	I–III	1
	Embryonal and variants	I–II	2–3
Intermediate	Embryonal and variants	III	2–3
	Alveolar	I–III	1–3
High	Any	IV	4

imaging (MRI) or computed tomography (CT) of the primary site, and CT of the chest to rule out metastatic disease. For tumors of the head and neck, CT or MRI of the head/brain is indicated. A bone scan will help to rule out bony metastatic disease, and cerebrospinal fluid (CSF) cytology assessment for tumor cells is appropriate for patients with parameningeal tumors. Oncologists treating adult patients at our institutions do not routinely obtain bone marrow biopsies or aspirates given the very low yield of such tests and lack of impact on therapeutic decision-making, although it is still performed as part of many clinical trials of therapy for RMS.

Imaging

Rhabdomyosarcomas are radiologically indistinguishable from other soft tissue sarcoma (Fig. 15.17). They also behave similar to other soft tissue sarcomas other than their sometimes explosive growth as well as risk of lymph node metastatic disease that occurs more commonly than with other sarcomas.

Primary Therapy

In the era before chemotherapy, the mortality rate from RMS was high, except in patients with favorable subtypes in favorable locations in which the tumor could be controlled with surgery and radiation. The mortality rate in older series varies from 30% to over 90%, depending on the stage, anatomic site, and treatment [69]. Chemotherapy, which was recognized as active in RMS in the early 1960s [70], quickly became a standard of care, as did radiation therapy to the primary site [69]. Details of adjuvant chemotherapy and treatment of metastatic disease are indicated below.

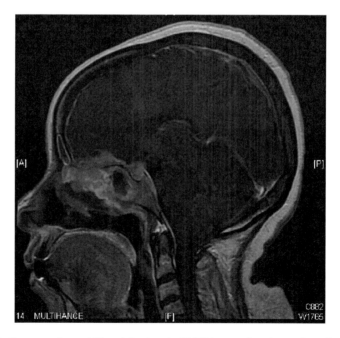

Fig. 15.17 Contrast-enhanced T1-weighted sagittal MRI image of a primary sinus alveolar rhabdomyosarcoma in a child

Multidisciplinary care is the present standard for patients with RMS, as it is for patients with Ewing sarcoma. While surgery, radiation, and chemotherapy are all employed for patients with RMS, the effects on growth and long-term effects of radiation make one more circumspect about the use of radiation for younger pediatric patients with RMS. The intensity of the therapy and need for multidisciplinary expertise make this one diagnosis where referral to expert centers is appropriate for most patients [71].

Adults with RMS benefit from a high proportion of pediatric patients being enrolled on clinical trials which have advanced the standard of care over the last 35 years doubling the cure rate over that time [72–76]. The full details of these studies are beyond the scope of this chapter, but several important findings of these studies help to direct care for all patients with RMS.

In Intergroup Rhabdomyosarcoma Study (IRS)-I, three randomized studies were performed within one larger study, based on clinical risk categories (clinical groups 1, 2, or 3–4) [74]. Patients with low-stage disease (clinical group 1, those with local disease and complete resections) did not benefit from radiation added to vincristine, dactinomycin, and cyclophosphamide (VActC). Those with regional disease but gross complete resection (clinical group 2) who received radiation did not benefit from the addition of cyclophosphamide to vincristine and dactinomycin. Those with more extensive disease (clinical groups 3 [gross residual disease after surgery] and 4 [metastatic disease]) did not benefit from the addition of doxorubicin to aggressive VActC plus irradiation. Distant metastatic recurrence was more common than local recurrence, and overall survival was 55% for all patients involved. Tumors of the orbit and gastrointestinal tract had the best prognosis.

IRS-II also addressed several questions regarding optimal care for patients in different clinical groups, enrolling 999 patients [75, 77]. VActC and VAct gave similar results for patients in clinical group 1. Patients in group 2, excluding extremity alveolar RMS, received radiation and were randomized to VAct or repetitive-pulse VActC, and DFS and survival were similar. Thus, it became feasible to use less intense therapy for patients with group 1–2 disease. Patients in groups 3 and 4 received radiation and were randomized to repetitive-pulse VActC or repetitive-pulse VAct alternating with CAV (vincristine, doxorubicin, cyclophosphamide). Complete remission (CR) rates were similar, as were survival rates, indicating that doxorubicin did not add to dactinomycin in the cure rate for such patients. Central nervous system prophylaxis with radiation for group 3 patients with cranial parameningeal sarcoma demonstrated a long-term survival rate to 67%, compared to 45% in IRS-I.

Over 1,000 patients were enrolled in IRS-III, in which patients were stratified by risk factors in addition to clinical groupings [72]. Like IRS-II, VAct was found as useful as VActC for patients with favorable group 1 patients. The addition of doxorubicin did not significantly alter the outcome for patients with favorable group 2 patients over those who received VAct alone. The addition of cisplatin-etoposide did not improve outcomes over VActC alone for patients with group 3–4 tumors.

IRS-IV examined multiple subgroups in detail and developed a new risk-based staging system integrating the stage and clinical groupings of IRS I–III [73]. Younger patients with group 1 paratesticular embryonal primary tumors and patients with group 1 or 2 orbit or eyelid tumors had a >90% cure rate with vincristine and dactinomycin, with the addition of radiation for patients with group 2 disease. For group 3 patients, patients could be randomized to hyperfractionated radiotherapy compared to conventional radiotherapy, but no benefit was noted. Most notably, VActC, VAct+ifosfamide, and vincristine-ifosfamide-etoposide with surgery (with or without RT) were equally effective for patients with local or regional rhabdomyosarcoma, indicating that the standard of care remained VActC, since it was less myelotoxic than other regimens.

A follow-up study to IRS-IV is a study of VActC versus alternating VActC/vincristine-topotecan-cyclophosphamide for intermediate-risk rhabdomyosarcomas (group 3) [76]. This study showed no advantage to the more complex regimen in comparison to VActC, which for this intermediate-risk group of tumors remains the standard of care.

Attempts have been made to decrease chemotherapy intensity in the lowest-risk patients. In Children's Oncology Group study D9602, radiotherapy doses were reduced and cyclophosphamide was eliminated for the lowest-risk patients, with survival rates similar for the lower radiation therapy dose patients but the suggestion of slightly inferior outcome for the patients not receiving cyclophosphamide. The follow-up study for patients with low-risk ERMS (ARST0331) uses data from IRS-IV and D9602. The ideas for the new study being tested include decreasing the duration of vincristine-dactinomycin chemotherapy to 22 weeks for subset 1 patients (stages 1/2 groups I/II, stage 1 group III orbit) and adding a total cumulative dose of 4.8 g/m^2 of cyclophosphamide. For patients with orbital and group IIA tumors, decreased RT doses will be used, and they will receive vincristine-dactinomycin and 4.8 g/m^2 of cyclophosphamide. Finally, cyclophosphamide cumulative dose will be reduced to 4.8 gm/m^2 for subset 2 patients, i.e., those with stage 1 group III nonorbital primaries and stage 3 groups I/II primaries [78].

Chemotherapy for Metastatic Disease

For metastatic RMS, a variety of agents show at least modest activity, depending on the subtype. For alveolar and embryonal RMS, as with Ewing sarcoma, single-agent topoisomerase inhibitors using topotecan [35, 79–82], irinotecan [31–33, 83, 84], or combinations involving them [35, 84] have activity. Best studied of these agents include irinotecan, irinotecan-temozolomide, and cyclophosphamide-topotecan.

In a few patients treated in a randomized study as well as anecdotally, gemcitabine and combinations (e.g., with docetaxel) have significant activity for patients with pleomorphic rhabdomyosarcoma [85]. The activity of gemcitabine and combinations in other forms of rhabdomyosarcoma is unknown, though apparently single-agent activity of gemcitabine against RMS in general is relatively low [86].

IGF1 receptor (IGF1R) inhibitors, mostly monoclonal antibodies, block IGF1R signaling thought to be critical in permitting the *PAX3* or *PAX7-FOXO1* translocation of alveolar RMS to transform cells and cause RMS [87–92]. However, responses to

Table 15.6 Systemic therapy recommendations for patients with rhabdomyosarcoma

Clinical scenario		Comments
Primary treatment		Clinical trial enrollment is preferred since pediatric studies often now accrue adult patients. In an off-study setting, primary treatment usually involves surgery and often radiation as well. Polychemotherapy is administered whenever feasible. ((a) VDactino Act C, (b) VAdrC-ifosfamide-etoposide regimen as for Ewing sarcoma, and (c) VIDE are all treatment options in the absence of adult-specific data)
Metastatic disease	1st line	Irinotecan, irinotecan-temozolomide, or cyclophosphamide-topotecan
	2nd line	IGF1R inhibitor or combination if available on study; gemcitabine combinations (in particular for pleomorphic rhabdomyosarcoma); clinical trial

VActC vincristine + dactinomycin + cyclophosphamide, *VAdrC* vincristine + doxorubicin + cyclophosphamide, *VIDE* vincristine + ifosfamide + doxorubicin + etoposide

IGF1R inhibitors appear to be low [93], although it is not clear how much of this low rate of activity is related to treating particular subtypes of rhabdomyosarcoma, age, and other factors, research that continues presently. Given the biological distinctiveness of each of the primary forms of rhabdomyosarcoma, it is clear that one treatment may not be appropriate for all RMS subtypes. There are data to support the idea that rhabdomyosarcomas may continue signaling through AKT [91, 94] and other proteins by switching from IGF1R signaling to another kinase [95]. This finding appears consistent with the transient benefit seen in genetically engineered mouse models of rhabdomyosarcoma treated with IGF1R inhibitors [96] as well as in humans with recurrent rhabdomyosarcoma treated with anti-IGF1R monoclonal antibodies.

Future directions are examining IGF1R inhibitors and temozolomide in high-risk RMS, while for embryonal RMS, given the number of interesting oncogenes involved in an area of loss of heterozygosity in these tumors, perhaps more cell cycle-specific therapeutics will prove more useful; that being said, embryonal RMS is more sensitive to standard therapy than alveolar or pleomorphic RMS. For pleomorphic RMS, hopefully future therapeutics can be built from the few anecdotes of patients responding well to known gemcitabine-based combinations, suggesting another sarcoma that will benefit from more careful analysis of cell cycle-specific compounds (Table 15.6, treatment recommendations).

Embryonal Sarcoma

Embryonal sarcoma is a rare sarcoma unique to the liver, typically occurring in children around the age of 10, akin to other small round blue cell tumors. It can be difficult to distinguish histologically from rhabdomyosarcoma or Wilms tumor, in

Table 15.7 Systemic therapy recommendations for patients with embryonal sarcoma

Primary therapy	Surgery and neoadjuvant or adjuvant chemotherapy. Regimens used for Ewing sarcoma or rhabdomyosarcoma. We have opted to use the 5-drug VAdrC-IE regimen; VIDE would be used more commonly in Europe
Recurrent disease	Surgery and or chemotherapy as directed toward small round blue cell sarcoma. Clinical trials are appropriate

particular the former, since rhabdomyosarcoma can affect the biliary tree [97]. However, in comparison to rhabdomyosarcoma, embryonal sarcoma does not express the classic rhabdomyosarcoma MyoD or myogenin. Embryonal sarcoma does not bear the chromosomal translocation involving *PAX3* or *PAX7* and the *FOXO1* (*FKHR*) gene. Given its rarity, it is not clear that chemotherapy is necessary in primary treatment of such tumors. However, given (1) poor outcomes with surgery alone from older studies [98], (2) the outcomes such patients experienced on chemotherapy when included in International Rhabdomyosarcoma Study (IRS) groups, as well as (3) the response of patients with unresectable disease to chemotherapy [99], we advocate for the use of neoadjuvant or adjuvant chemotherapy using a Ewing sarcoma regimen such as VAdrC-IE 5-drug therapy as used in the United States or VIDE, more commonly employed in Europe. Given the data with IRS studies, a dactinomycin regimen could be considered as well (suggestions for therapy – Table 15.7).

Calcifying Nested Stromal and Epithelial Tumor

Calcifying nested stromal and epithelial tumor, also called desmoplastic nested spindle cell tumor or nested stromal-epithelial tumor, was proposed as a new tumor entity that affected the liver in children in 2005. These tumors were described as well-circumscribed, intrahepatic, lobular white-colored masses. By immunohistochemistry, they were positive in the cytoplasm for vimentin, pancytokeratin, and CD57, and there was nuclear staining for WT1. In the four cases described, there was no evidence of recurrence [100], but in other series, recurrent disease has been observed [101]. Since this initial description, cases have been described in adults [102], two cases in boys with fragile X syndrome [103]. Calcifying nested stromal and epithelial tumor can be responsive to standard agents used for soft tissue sarcoma when recurrent in the rare instances where such treatment is necessary (suggestions for therapy – Table 15.8)

Table 15.8 Systemic therapy recommendations for patients with calcifying nested stromal and epithelial tumor

Primary therapy	Surgery alone
Recurrent disease	Surgery if possible; radiofrequency ablation can be used on isolated unresectable recurrence. Chemotherapy with anthracycline or ifosfamide-based therapy is active in anecdotal experience

References

1. Ewing J. Diffuse endothelioma of bone. Proc New York Pathol Soc. 1921;21:17–24.
2. Antonescu CR, Dal Cin P, Nafa K, et al. EWSR1-CREB1 is the predominant gene fusion in angiomatoid fibrous histiocytoma. Genes Chromosomes Cancer. 2007;46(12):1051–60.
3. Antonescu CR, Zhang L, Chang NE, et al. EWSR1-POU5F1 fusion in soft tissue myoepithelial tumors. A molecular analysis of sixty-six cases, including soft tissue, bone, and visceral lesions, showing common involvement of the EWSR1 gene. Genes Chromosomes Cancer. 2010;49(12):1114–24.
4. Stuart-Harris R, Wills EJ, Philips J, et al. Extraskeletal Ewing's sarcoma: a clinical, morphological and ultrastructural analysis of five cases with a review of the literature. Eur J Cancer Clin Oncol. 1986;22(4):393–400.
5. de Alava E, Kawai A, Healey JH, et al. EWS-FLI1 fusion transcript structure is an independent determinant of prognosis in Ewing's sarcoma. J Clin Oncol. 1998;16(4):1248–55.
6. Lee J, Hoang BH, Ziogas A, et al. Analysis of prognostic factors in Ewing sarcoma using a population-based cancer registry. Cancer. 2010;116(8):1964–73.
7. Huang HY, Illei PB, Zhao Z, et al. Ewing sarcomas with p53 mutation or p16/p14ARF homozygous deletion: a highly lethal subset associated with poor chemoresponse. J Clin Oncol. 2005;23(3):548–58.
8. Yoshimoto M, Graham C, Chilton-MacNeill S, et al. Detailed cytogenetic and array analysis of pediatric primitive sarcomas reveals a recurrent CIC-DUX4 fusion gene event. Cancer Genet Cytogenet. 2009;195(1):1–11.
9. Kawamura-Saito M, Yamazaki Y, Kaneko K, et al. Fusion between CIC and DUX4 up-regulates PEA3 family genes in Ewing-like sarcomas with t(4;19)(q35;q13) translocation. Hum Mol Genet. 2006;15(13):2125–37.
10. Italiano A, Sung YS, Zhang L, et al. High prevalence of CIC fusion with double-homeobox (DUX4) transcription factors in EWSR1-negative undifferentiated small blue round cell sarcomas. Genes Chromosomes Cancer. 2012;51(3):207–18.
11. Graham C, Chilton-Macneill S, Zielenska M, et al. The CIC-DUX4 fusion transcript is present in a subgroup of pediatric primitive round cell sarcomas. Hum Pathol. 2012;43(2):180–9.
12. Applebaum MA, Worch J, Matthay KK, et al. Clinical features and outcomes in patients with extraskeletal Ewing sarcoma. Cancer. 2011;117(13):3027–32.
13. Worch J, Matthay KK, Neuhaus J, et al. Ethnic and racial differences in patients with Ewing sarcoma. Cancer. 2010;116(4):983–8.
14. Holcomb TM, Haggard ME, Windmiller J. Cyclophosphamide (Nsc-26271)-1 in uncommon malignant neoplasms in children. Cancer Chemother Rep. 1964;36:73–5.
15. Oldham RK, Pomeroy TC. Treatment of Ewing's sarcoma with adriamycin (NSC-123127). Cancer Chemother Rep. 1972;56(5):635–9.
16. Nesbit Jr ME, Gehan EA, Burgert Jr EO, et al. Multimodal therapy for the management of primary, nonmetastatic Ewing's sarcoma of bone: a long-term follow-up of the first intergroup study. J Clin Oncol. 1990;8(10):1664–74.

17. Burgert Jr EO, Nesbit ME, Garnsey LA, et al. Multimodal therapy for the management of nonpelvic, localized Ewing's sarcoma of bone: intergroup study IESS-II. J Clin Oncol. 1990;8(9):1514–24.
18. Paulussen M, Ahrens S, Dunst J, et al. Localized Ewing tumor of bone: final results of the cooperative Ewing's Sarcoma Study CESS 86. J Clin Oncol. 2001;19(6):1818–29.
19. Paulussen M, Craft AW, Lewis I, et al. Results of the EICESS-92 Study: two randomized trials of Ewing's sarcoma treatment–cyclophosphamide compared with ifosfamide in standard-risk patients and assessment of benefit of etoposide added to standard treatment in high-risk patients. J Clin Oncol. 2008;26(27):4385–93.
20. Grier HE, Krailo MD, Tarbell NJ, et al. Addition of ifosfamide and etoposide to standard chemotherapy for Ewing's sarcoma and primitive neuroectodermal tumor of bone. N Engl J Med. 2003;348(8):694–701.
21. Granowetter L, Womer R, Devidas M, et al. Dose-intensified compared with standard chemotherapy for nonmetastatic Ewing sarcoma family of tumors: a Children's Oncology Group Study. J Clin Oncol. 2009;27(15):2536–41.
22. Womer RB, West DC, Krailo MD, et al. Randomized comparison of every-two-week v. every-three-week chemotherapy in Ewing sarcoma family tumors. J Clin Oncol. 2008;26(20 suppl):Abstr 10504.
23. Norton L, Simon R. Tumor size, sensitivity to therapy, and design of treatment schedules. Cancer Treat Rep. 1977;61(7):1307–17.
24. Norton L, Simon R, Brereton HD, et al. Predicting the course of Gompertzian growth. Nature. 1976;264(5586):542–5.
25. Kushner BH, Meyers PA. How effective is dose-intensive/myeloablative therapy against Ewing's sarcoma/primitive neuroectodermal tumor metastatic to bone or bone marrow? The memorial sloan-kettering experience and a literature review. J Clin Oncol. 2001;19(3): 870–80.
26. McTiernan AM, Cassoni AM, Driver D, et al. Improving outcomes after relapse in Ewing's sarcoma: analysis of 114 patients from a single institution. Sarcoma. 2006;2006:83548.
27. Oberlin O, Rey A, Desfachelles AS, et al. Impact of high-dose busulfan plus melphalan as consolidation in metastatic Ewing tumors: a study by the Societe Francaise des Cancers de l'Enfant. J Clin Oncol. 2006;24(24):3997–4002.
28. Ferrari S, Alvegard T, Luksch R, et al. Non-metastatic Ewing's family tumors: high-dose chemotherapy with stem cell rescue in poor responder patients. Preliminary results of the Italian/Scandinavian ISG/SSG III protocol. J Clin Oncol. 2007;25(18S):Abstr 10014.
29. Strauss SJ, McTiernan A, Driver D, et al. Single center experience of a new intensive induction therapy for Ewing's family of tumors: feasibility, toxicity, and stem cell mobilization properties. J Clin Oncol. 2003;21(15):2974–81.
30. Wagner LM, McAllister N, Goldsby RE, et al. Temozolomide and intravenous irinotecan for treatment of advanced Ewing sarcoma. Pediatr Blood Cancer. 2007;48(2):132–9.
31. Bomgaars LR, Bernstein M, Krailo M, et al. Phase II trial of irinotecan in children with refractory solid tumors: a Children's Oncology Group Study. J Clin Oncol. 2007;25(29):4622–7.
32. Vassal G, Couanet D, Stockdale E, et al. Phase II trial of irinotecan in children with relapsed or refractory rhabdomyosarcoma: a joint study of the French Society of Pediatric Oncology and the United Kingdom Children's Cancer Study Group. J Clin Oncol. 2007;25(4):356–61.
33. Bisogno G, Riccardi R, Ruggiero A, et al. Phase II study of a protracted irinotecan schedule in children with refractory or recurrent soft tissue sarcoma. Cancer. 2006;106(3):703–7.
34. Bernstein M, Kovar H, Paulussen M, et al. Ewing's sarcoma family of tumors: current management. Oncologist. 2006;11(5):503–19.
35. Walterhouse DO, Lyden ER, Breitfeld PP, et al. Efficacy of topotecan and cyclophosphamide given in a phase II window trial in children with newly diagnosed metastatic rhabdomyosarcoma: a Children's Oncology Group study. J Clin Oncol. 2004;22(8):1398–403.
36. Saylors 3rd RL, Stine KC, Sullivan J, et al. Cyclophosphamide plus topotecan in children with recurrent or refractory solid tumors: a Pediatric Oncology Group phase II study. J Clin Oncol. 2001;19(15):3463–9.

37. Saylors 3rd RL, Stewart CF, Zamboni WC, et al. Phase I study of topotecan in combination with cyclophosphamide in pediatric patients with malignant solid tumors: a Pediatric Oncology Group Study. J Clin Oncol. 1998;16(3):945–52.

38. Tolcher AW, Sarantopoulos J, Patnaik A, et al. Phase I, pharmacokinetic, and pharmacodynamic study of AMG 479, a fully human monoclonal antibody to insulin-like growth factor receptor 1. J Clin Oncol. 2009;27(34):5800–7.

39. Olmos D, Postel-Vinay S, Molife LR, et al. Safety, pharmacokinetics, and preliminary activity of the anti-IGF-1R antibody figitumumab (CP-751,871) in patients with sarcoma and Ewing's sarcoma: a phase 1 expansion cohort study. Lancet Oncol. 2010;11(2):129–35.

40. Pappo AS, Patel SR, Crowley J, et al. R1507, a monoclonal antibody to the insulin-like growth factor 1 receptor, in patients with recurrent or refractory Ewing sarcoma family of tumors: results of a phase II sarcoma alliance for research through collaboration study. J Clin Oncol. 2011;29(34):4541–7.

41. Juergens H, Daw NC, Geoerger B, et al. Preliminary efficacy of the anti-insulin-like growth factor type 1 receptor antibody figitumumab in patients with refractory Ewing sarcoma. J Clin Oncol. 2011;29(34):4534–40.

42. Malempati S, Weigel B, Ingle AM, et al. Phase I/II trial and pharmacokinetic study of cixutumumab in pediatric patients with refractory solid tumors and Ewing sarcoma: a report from the Children's Oncology Group. J Clin Oncol. 2012;30(3):256–62.

43. Tap WD, Demetri G, Barnette P, et al. Phase II study of Ganitumab, a fully human anti-type-1 insulin-like growth factor receptor antibody, in patients with metastatic ewing family tumors or desmoplastic small round cell tumors. J Clin Oncol 2012;30(15):1849–56.

44. Chugh R, Wathen JK, Maki RG, et al. Phase II multicenter trial of imatinib in 10 histologic subtypes of sarcoma using a bayesian hierarchical statistical model. J Clin Oncol. 2009;27(19):3148–53.

45. Garnett MJ, Edelman EJ, Heidorn SJ, et al. Systematic identification of genomic markers of drug sensitivity in cancer cells. Nature. 2012;483(7391):570–5.

46. Brenner JC, Feng FY, Han S, et al. PARP-1 inhibition as a targeted strategy to treat Ewing's sarcoma. Cancer Res. 2012;72(7):1608–13.

47. Richkind KE, Romansky SG, Finklestein JZ. t(4;19)(q35;q13.1): a recurrent change in primitive mesenchymal tumors? Cancer Genet Cytogenet. 1996;87(1):71–4.

48. Kawamura-Saito M, Yamazaki Y, Kaneko K, et al. Fusion between CIC and DUX4 up-regulates PEA3 family genes in Ewing-like sarcomas with t(4;19)(q35;q13) translocation. Hum Mol Genet. 2006;15(13):2125–37.

49. Graham C, Chilton-Macneill S, Zielenska M, et al. The CIC-DUX4 fusion transcript is present in a subgroup of pediatric primitive round cell sarcomas. Hum Pathol. 2011;43:180–9.

50. Italiano A, Sung YS, Zhang L, et al. High prevalence of CIC fusion with double-homeobox (DUX4) transcription factors in EWSR1-negative undifferentiated small blue round cell sarcomas. Genes Chromosomes Cancer 2012;51(3):207–18.

51. Rakheja D, Goldman S, Wilson KS, et al. Translocation (4;19)(q35;q13.1)-associated primitive round cell sarcoma: report of a case and review of the literature. Pediatr Dev Pathol. 2008;11(3):239–44.

52. Alaggio R, Bisogno G, Rosato A, et al. Undifferentiated sarcoma: does it exist? A clinicopathologic study of 7 pediatric cases and review of literature. Hum Pathol. 2009;40(11):1600–10.

53. Sirvent N, Trassard M, Ebran N, et al. Fusion of EWSR1 with the DUX4 facioscapulohumeral muscular dystrophy region resulting from t(4;22)(q35;q12) in a case of embryonal rhabdomyosarcoma. Cancer Genet Cytogenet. 2009;195(1):12–8.

54. Roberts P, Browne CF, Lewis IJ, et al. 12q13 abnormality in rhabdomyosarcoma. A nonrandom occurrence? Cancer Genet Cytogenet. 1992;60(2):135–40.

55. Riccardi GF, Stein C, de la Roza G, et al. Newly described translocation (18;19)(q23;q13.2) in abdominal wall soft-tissue tumor resembling Ewing sarcoma/primitive neuroectodermal tumor. Cancer Genet Cytogenet. 2010;201(1):1–5.

56. Pierron G, Tirode F, Lucchesi C, et al. A new subtype of bone sarcoma defined by BCOR-CCNB3 gene fusion. Nat Genet. 2012;44(4):461–6.
57. Lemmers RJ, van der Vliet PJ, Klooster R, et al. A unifying genetic model for facioscapulohumeral muscular dystrophy. Science. 2010;329(5999):1650–3.
58. Ragab AH, Heyn R, Tefft M, et al. Infants younger than 1 year of age with rhabdomyosarcoma. Cancer. 1986;58(12):2606–10.
59. Hayes-Jordan A, Andrassy R. Rhabdomyosarcoma in children. Curr Opin Pediatr. 2009;21(3):373–8.
60. Newton Jr WA, Soule EH, Hamoudi AB, et al. Histopathology of childhood sarcomas, Intergroup rhabdomyosarcoma studies I and II: clinicopathologic correlation. J Clin Oncol. 1988;6(1):67–75.
61. Turc-Carel C, Lizard-Nacol S, Justrabo E, et al. Consistent chromosomal translocation in alveolar rhabdomyosarcoma. Cancer Genet Cytogenet. 1986;19(3–4):361–2.
62. Douglass EC, Valentine M, Etcubanas E, et al. A specific chromosomal abnormality in rhabdomyosarcoma. Cytogenet Cell Genet. 1987;45(3–4):148–55.
63. Biegel JA, Meek RS, Parmiter AH, et al. Chromosomal translocation t(1;13)(p36;q14) in a case of rhabdomyosarcoma. Genes Chromosomes Cancer. 1991;3(6):483–4.
64. Gallego Melcon S, Sanchez de Toledo Codina J. Molecular biology of rhabdomyosarcoma. Clin Transl Oncol 2007;9(7):415–419.
65. Davicioni E, Anderson MJ, Finckenstein FG, et al. Molecular classification of rhabdomyosarcoma–genotypic and phenotypic determinants of diagnosis: a report from the Children's Oncology Group. Am J Pathol. 2009;174(2):550–64.
66. Sabbioni S, Veronese A, Trubia M, et al. Exon structure and promoter identification of STIM1 (alias GOK), a human gene causing growth arrest of the human tumor cell lines G401 and RD. Cytogenet Cell Genet. 1999;86(3–4):214–8.
67. Hu RJ, Lee MP, Connors TD, et al. A 2.5-Mb transcript map of a tumor-suppressing subchromosomal transferable fragment from 11p15.5, and isolation and sequence analysis of three novel genes. Genomics. 1997;46(1):9–17.
68. Sabbioni S, Barbanti-Brodano G, Croce CM, et al. GOK: a gene at 11p15 involved in rhabdomyosarcoma and rhabdoid tumor development. Cancer Res. 1997;57(20):4493–7.
69. Sutow WW, Sullivan MP, Ried HL, et al. Prognosis in childhood rhabdomyosarcoma. Cancer. 1970;25(6):1384–90.
70. Sutow WW, Sullivan MP. Successful chemotherapy for childhood rhabdomyosarcoma. Tex Med. 1970;66(4):78–81.
71. Wolden SL, Alektiar KM. Sarcomas across the age spectrum. Semin Radiat Oncol. 2010;20(1):45–51.
72. Crist W, Gehan EA, Ragab AH, et al. The third intergroup rhabdomyosarcoma study. J Clin Oncol. 1995;13(3):610–30.
73. Crist WM, Anderson JR, Meza JL, et al. Intergroup rhabdomyosarcoma study-IV: results for patients with nonmetastatic disease. J Clin Oncol. 2001;19(12):3091–102.
74. Maurer HM, Beltangady M, Gehan EA, et al. The intergroup rhabdomyosarcoma study-I. A final report. Cancer. 1988;61(2):209–20.
75. Maurer HM, Gehan EA, Beltangady M, et al. The intergroup rhabdomyosarcoma study-II. Cancer. 1993;71(5):1904–22.
76. Arndt CA, Stoner JA, Hawkins DS, et al. Vincristine, actinomycin, and cyclophosphamide compared with vincristine, actinomycin, and cyclophosphamide alternating with vincristine, topotecan, and cyclophosphamide for intermediate-risk rhabdomyosarcoma: children's oncology group study D9803. J Clin Oncol. 2009;27(31):5182–8.
77. Maurer HM. The intergroup rhabdomyosarcoma study II: objectives and study design. J Pediatr Surg. 1980;15(3):371–2.
78. Beverly Raney R, Walterhouse DO, Meza JL, et al. Results of the intergroup rhabdomyosarcoma study group D9602 protocol, using vincristine and dactinomycin with or without cyclophosphamide and radiation therapy, for newly diagnosed patients with low-risk embryonal

rhabdomyosarcoma: a report from the soft tissue sarcoma committee of the children's oncology group. J Clin Oncol. 2011;29(10):1312–8.

79. Blaney SM, Needle MN, Gillespie A, et al. Phase II trial of topotecan administered as 72-hour continuous infusion in children with refractory solid tumors: a collaborative pediatric branch, National Cancer Institute, and Children's Cancer Group Study. Clin Cancer Res. 1998;4(2): 357–60.

80. Lager JJ, Lyden ER, Anderson JR, et al. Pooled analysis of phase II window studies in children with contemporary high-risk metastatic rhabdomyosarcoma: a report from the Soft Tissue Sarcoma Committee of the Children's Oncology Group. J Clin Oncol. 2006;24 (21):3415–22.

81. Nitschke R, Parkhurst J, Sullivan J, et al. Topotecan in pediatric patients with recurrent and progressive solid tumors: a pediatric oncology group phase II study. J Pediatr Hematol Oncol. 1998;20(4):315–8.

82. Pappo AS, Lyden E, Breneman J, et al. Up-front window trial of topotecan in previously untreated children and adolescents with metastatic rhabdomyosarcoma: an intergroup rhabdomyosarcoma study. J Clin Oncol. 2001;19(1):213–9.

83. Cosetti M, Wexler LH, Calleja E, et al. Irinotecan for pediatric solid tumors: the memorial sloan-kettering experience. J Pediatr Hematol Oncol. 2002;24(2):101–5.

84. Pappo AS, Lyden E, Breitfeld P, et al. Two consecutive phase II window trials of irinotecan alone or in combination with vincristine for the treatment of metastatic rhabdomyosarcoma: the Children's Oncology Group. J Clin Oncol. 2007;25(4):362–9.

85. Maki RG, Wathen JK, Patel SR, et al. Randomized phase II study of gemcitabine and docetaxel compared with gemcitabine alone in patients with metastatic soft tissue sarcomas: results of sarcoma alliance for research through collaboration study 002 [corrected]. J Clin Oncol. 2007;25(19):2755–63.

86. Wagner-Bohn A, Paulussen M, Vieira Pinheiro JP, et al. Phase II study of gemcitabine in children with solid tumors of mesenchymal and embryonic origin. Anticancer Drugs. 2006;17(7):859–64.

87. Minniti CP, Helman LJ. IGF-II in the pathogenesis of rhabdomyosarcoma: a prototype of IGFs involvement in human tumorigenesis. Adv Exp Med Biol. 1993;343:327–43.

88. LeRoith D, Werner H, Neuenschwander S, et al. The role of the insulin-like growth factor-I receptor in cancer. Ann N Y Acad Sci. 1995;766:402–8.

89. Kalebic T, Blakesley V, Slade C, et al. Expression of a kinase-deficient IGF-I-R suppresses tumorigenicity of rhabdomyosarcoma cells constitutively expressing a wild type IGF-I-R. Int J Cancer. 1998;76(2):223–7.

90. Wan X, Harkavy B, Shen N, et al. Rapamycin induces feedback activation of Akt signaling through an IGF 1R dependent mechanism. Oncogene. 2007;26(13):1932 40.

91. Cao L, Yu Y, Darko I, et al. Addiction to elevated insulin-like growth factor I receptor and initial modulation of the AKT pathway define the responsiveness of rhabdomyosarcoma to the targeting antibody. Cancer Res. 2008;68(19):8039–48.

92. Rikhof B, de Jong S, Suurmeijer AJ, et al. The insulin-like growth factor system and sarcomas. J Pathol. 2009;217(4):469–82.

93. Patel S, Pappo A, Crowley J, et al. A SARC global collaborative phase II trial of R1507, a recombinant human monoclonal antibody to the insulin-like growth factor-1 receptor in patients with recurrent or refractory sarcomas. J Clin Oncol. 2009;27(15s):Abstract 10503.

94. Mayeenuddin LH, Yu Y, Kang Z, et al. Insulin-like growth factor 1 receptor antibody induces rhabdomyosarcoma cell death via a process involving AKT and Bcl-x(L). Oncogene. 2010;29(48):6367–77.

95. Huang F, Greer A, Hurlburt W, et al. The mechanisms of differential sensitivity to an insulin-like growth factor-1 receptor inhibitor (BMS-536924) and rationale for combining with EGFR/HER2 inhibitors. Cancer Res. 2009;69(1):161–70.

96. Soundararajan A, Abraham J, Nelon LD, et al. (18) F-FDG microPET imaging detects early transient response to an IGF1R inhibitor in genetically engineered rhabdomyosarcoma models. Pediatr Blood Cancer 2012;59(3):485–92.

97. Nicol K, Savell V, Moore J, et al. Distinguishing undifferentiated embryonal sarcoma of the liver from biliary tract rhabdomyosarcoma: a Children's Oncology Group study. Pediatr Dev Pathol. 2007;10(2):89–97.
98. Stocker JT, Ishak KG. Undifferentiated (embryonal) sarcoma of the liver: report of 31 cases. Cancer. 1978;42(1):336–48.
99. Kim DY, Kim KH, Jung SE, et al. Undifferentiated (embryonal) sarcoma of the liver: combination treatment by surgery and chemotherapy. J Pediatr Surg. 2002;37(10):1419–23.
100. Hill DA, Swanson PE, Anderson K, et al. Desmoplastic nested spindle cell tumor of liver: report of four cases of a proposed new entity. Am J Surg Pathol. 2005;29(1):1–9.
101. Makhlouf HR, Abdul-Al HM, Wang G, et al. Calcifying nested stromal-epithelial tumors of the liver: a clinicopathologic, immunohistochemical, and molecular genetic study of 9 cases with a long-term follow-up. Am J Surg Pathol. 2009;33(7):976–83.
102. Oviedo Ramirez MI, Bas Bernal A, Ortiz Ruiz E, et al. Desmoplastic nested spindle cell tumor of the liver in an adult. Ann Diagn Pathol. 2010;14(1):44–9.
103. Wirojanan J, Kraff J, Hawkins DS, et al. Two boys with fragile X syndrome and hepatic tumors. J Pediatr Hematol Oncol. 2008;30(3):239–41.

Chapter 16
Radiation-Induced Sarcomas

One of the few known causes of sarcomas is therapeutic irradiation. Therapeutic radiation has also been associated with development of breast cancer, lung cancer, and accelerated coronary artery disease in patients receiving thoracic radiation [1, 2]. With the increased recognition of second cancers as a long-term side effect of radiation therapy, some attempts have been made to use radiation more sparingly; however, for reasons unclear to the authors, use of therapeutic radiation is even more widespread than in the past, with the use of tylectomy and radiation therapy, a recognized standard of care for ductal carcinoma in situ of the breast, despite the ability to obtain negative margins in at least 95% of patients with surgery alone [3, 4]. The incidence of a sarcoma after radiation is not precisely known and may vary from one part of the body to the next. In a series of patients treated for cancer of all sites in Finland, for example, the crude risk was of the order of 0.05% [5].

In the prospectively collected series from MSKCC, consistent patterns have arisen regarding the types of diseases treated with radiation and the forms of sarcoma that arise after radiation. The most recent MSKCC update comes from Gladdy et al. from 2010 [6]. A total of 130 radiation-induced soft tissue sarcomas (RIS) were examined in over 7,600 patients treated surgically for sarcoma at MSKCC. A total of 34% of patients with RIS were treated for breast cancer, 18% for leukemia or lymphoma, and 17% for genitourinary tumors. In this most recent update, the median latency for development of the RIS was 10 years; however, the median latency varied based on the type of sarcoma involved, with the shortest median latency for liposarcomas (median 4.3 years) and longest for leiomyosarcoma (23 years).

Common RIS histologies included high-grade undifferentiated pleomorphic sarcoma (26%), angiosarcoma (21%), leiomyosarcoma (12%), and fibrosarcoma not otherwise specified (12%). Median age at presentation was 58.5 years (range 18–86). The trunk was the most common primary site (61%) highlighting secondary sarcomas of the breast. Five-year disease-specific survival was 58%, and independent predictors of poor outcome were large size > 5 cm, margin status, and RIS histology.

Primary management of RIS remains surgical. Given the difficulty in administering radiation to control these tumors and given the nature of the field to be operated

M.F. Brennan et al., *Management of Soft Tissue Sarcoma*,
DOI 10.1007/978-1-4614-5004-7_16, © Springer Science+Business Media New York 2013

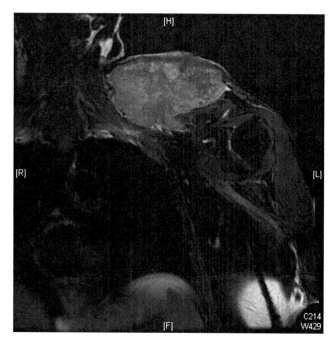

Fig. 16.1 Sagittal T2-weighted fat-saturated MRI image of a radiation-induced high-grade myofibroblastic sarcoma of the left trapezius/supraspinatus

upon, it is not surprising that there is a significant local-regional recurrence risk postoperatively and survival appears inferior to patient with similar sarcomas that are not radiation-induced [6–9] (Fig. 16.1). Radiation therapy, in particular the use of brachytherapy to deliver highly localized radiation therapy, can be entertained in some patients, despite prior use of radiation as a treatment for the initial clinical problem.

The development of RIS begs the question of whether less radiation therapy can be employed to decrease the risk of such malignancies. For example, can surgery without radiation therapy be employed for primary treatment of sarcomas? Given the low local recurrence risk of tumors under 5 cm in size in the MSKCC series, surgery alone is a good standard of care for sarcomas removed with negative margins, if there is a follow-up operation that can still be limb sparing. However, if there is a question of a margin, in particular in regions of the body such as the head and neck, where a second operation is less likely to achieve a good margin, then adjuvant or neoadjuvant radiation therapy should be considered.

As for chemotherapy for RIS, there are no specific guidelines, other than to use agents appropriate for the histology at hand. For example, angiosarcomas are responsive to anthracyclines and taxanes, and recent clinical data suggest that agents targeting VEGF (vascular endothelial growth factor) receptors can be active in radiation-induced angiosarcoma of the breast [10], although at present it is unclear if this is due to presence of KDR/VEGFR2 mutations in some breast angiosarcomas [11] or not. It should be noted that limb perfusion with tumor necrosis factor and chemotherapy such as melphalan is a possible option for patients with recurrent

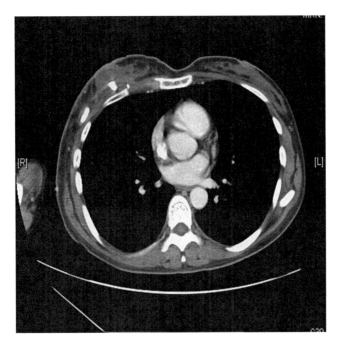

Fig. 16.2 Contrast-enhanced CT image of a radiation-induced sarcoma of the right chest wall after surgery and radiation therapy for ductal carcinoma in situ

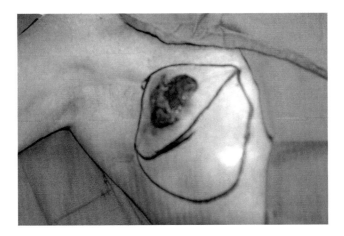

Fig. 16.3 Preoperative image of the right chest wall radiation-induced sarcoma from Fig. 16.2

disease despite attempts at local control, if the tumor site can be isolated for such therapy [12].

An example of a radiation-induced sarcoma is shown in Figs. 16.2, 16.3, 16.4, 16.5, 16.6, and 16.7, a 48-year-old woman treated with radiation therapy following excision of ductal carcinoma in situ of the breast. Two years later, she presented

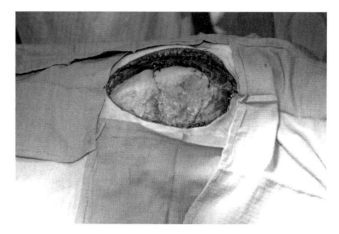

Fig. 16.4 Post-resection image of the chest wall resection of the patient in Figs. 16.2 and 16.3

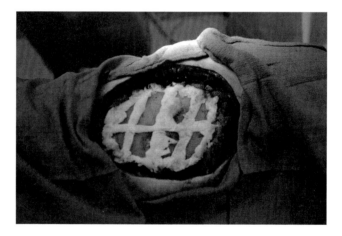

Fig. 16.5 Reconstruction of the chest wall after resection of the tumor from Figs. 16.2, 16.3, and 16.4

with an undifferentiated pleomorphic high-grade sarcoma. She was treated by local resection, and she then presented 2 years later (Fig. 16.2) with a fungating mass (Fig. 16.3) involving the chest wall with multiple foci. This was resected with the chest wall (Fig. 16.4) with reconstruction using methyl methacrylate for the rib cage (Fig. 16.5) and a rotational flap to cover the defect (Fig. 16.6). All margins were negative at the time. Within 2 years, she had further recurrence of a left anterior chest wall nodule and received chemotherapy. She progressed to demise within 1 year with extensive intrathoracic and chest wall recurrence (Fig. 16.7).

A similar lesion in the right groin of a radiation-induced extraskeletal osteogenic sarcoma is demonstrated (Fig. 16.8), requiring a tissue flap for reconstruction of the defect.

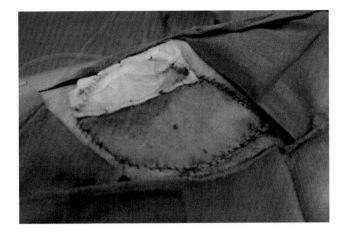

Fig. 16.6 Final surgical result for the patient from Figs. 16.2, 16.3, 16.4, and 16.5

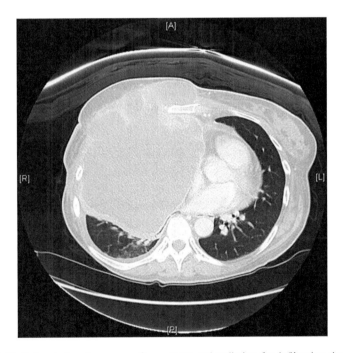

Fig. 16.7 Radiation-induced sarcoma after surgery and radiation for infiltrating ductal breast adenocarcinoma

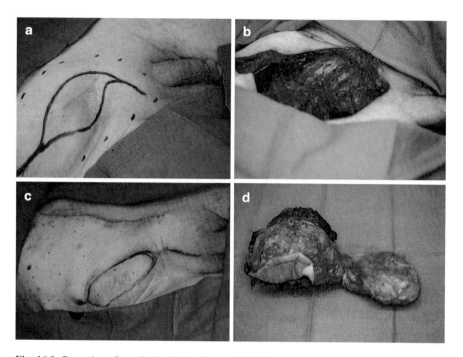

Fig. 16.8 Resection of a radiation-induced extraskeletal osteosarcoma of the right groin: (**a**) pre-operative, (**b**) intraoperative, and (**c**) postoperative images, and (**d**) an image of the resection specimen

References

1. Friedman DL, Whitton J, Leisenring W, et al. Subsequent neoplasms in 5-year survivors of childhood cancer: the childhood cancer survivor study. J Natl Cancer Inst. 2010;102(14):1083–95.
2. Oeffinger KC, Mertens AC, Sklar CA, et al. Chronic health conditions in adult survivors of childhood cancer. N Engl J Med. 2006;355(15):1572–82.
3. Motwani SB, Goyal S, Moran MS, et al. Ductal carcinoma in situ treated with breast-conserving surgery and radiotherapy: a comparison with ECOG study 5194. Cancer. 2011;117(6): 1156–62.
4. Virnig BA, Tuttle TM, Shamliyan T, et al. Ductal carcinoma in situ of the breast: a systematic review of incidence, treatment, and outcomes. J Natl Cancer Inst. 2010;102(3):170–8.
5. Virtanen A, Pukkala E, Auvinen A. Incidence of bone and soft tissue sarcoma after radiotherapy: a cohort study of 295,712 finnish cancer patients. Int J Cancer. 2006;118(4):1017–21.
6. Gladdy RA, Qin LX, Moraco N, et al. Do radiation-associated soft tissue sarcomas have the same prognosis as sporadic soft tissue sarcomas? J Clin Oncol. 2010;28(12):2064–9.
7. Bjerkehagen B, Smeland S, Walberg L, et al. Radiation-induced sarcoma: 25-year experience from the Norwegian Radium hospital. Acta Oncol. 2008;47(8):1475–82.
8. Riad S, Biau D, Holt GE, et al. The clinical and functional outcome for patients with radiation-induced soft tissue sarcoma. Cancer 2012;118(10):2682–92.
9. Bjerkehagen B, Smastuen MC, Hall KS, et al. Why do patients with radiation-induced sarcomas have a poor sarcoma-related survival? Br J Cancer 2012;106(2):297–306.

10. Maki RG, D'Adamo DR, Keohan ML, et al. Phase II study of sorafenib in patients with metastatic or recurrent sarcomas. J Clin Oncol. 2009;27(19):3133–40.
11. Antonescu CR, Yoshida A, Guo T, et al. KDR activating mutations in human angiosarcomas are sensitive to specific kinase inhibitors. Cancer Res. 2009;69(18):7175–9.
12. Bonvalot S, Rimareix F, Causeret S, et al. Hyperthermic isolated limb perfusion in locally advanced soft tissue sarcoma and progressive desmoid-type fibromatosis with TNF 1 mg and melphalan (T1-M HILP) is safe and efficient. Ann Surg Oncol. 2009;16(12):3350–7.

Chapter 17
Alveolar Soft Part Sarcoma

Alveolar soft part sarcoma (ASPS) is a rare sarcoma that typically arises in the lower extremity in adolescents and young adults between 15 and 40 years of age. Distribution by age and site in adults is shown in Figs. 17.1 and 17.2 for all adult ASPS. In children, a number of cases arise from the tongue and orbit, where it can be confused to some degree with embryonal rhabdomyosarcoma. ASPS is extremely rare, even at referral centers, which have been hard pressed to identify more than one to two patients a year per center in published series [1–3]. It frequently presents with innumerable small, round metastatic lesions in the lungs and shows a very slow rate of progression, one reason for the late presentation of what is often a primary >10 cm in greatest dimension. Progression is typically slow, but ultimately taking the patient's life after 10–15 years of metastatic disease. Brain metastases are a particular feature of ASPS, with an incidence at least thrice of that of other sarcomas in one series and documentation in other series [4–7].

Imaging

ASPS characteristically presents with a slow-growing primary mass (over years) as well as innumerable, round lung metastases. Bony metastases are seen with this diagnosis as well (Figs. 17.3 and 17.4).

Diagnosis/Molecular Pathology

ASPS has a highly characteristic microscopic appearance by H&E (hematoxylin and eosin) staining, with nests of tumor cells separated by thin fibrous septae (Fig. 17.5). It contains an equally characteristic unbalanced chromosomal translocation, t(X;17), involving *ASPL-TFE3* [7, 8]. The same, but balanced t(X;17), translocation is found in a proportion of (mostly pediatric) papillary renal cell

M.F. Brennan et al., *Management of Soft Tissue Sarcoma*,
DOI 10.1007/978-1-4614-5004-7_17, © Springer Science+Business Media New York 2013

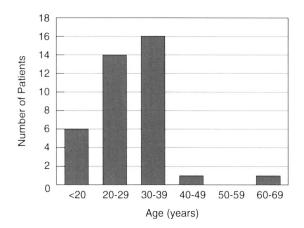

Fig. 17.1 Age distribution of adult patients with alveolar soft part sarcoma. MSKCC 7/1/1982–6/30/2010 n = 37

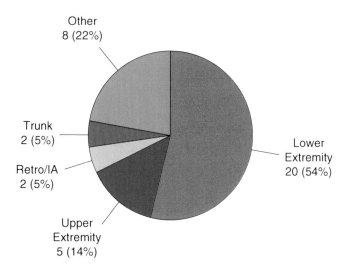

Fig. 17.2 Primary site of adult patients with alveolar soft part sarcoma. MSKCC 7/1/1982–6/30/2010 n = 37 *Retro/IA* retroperitoneal/intra-abdominal

cancers [9], indicating the context dependence of the oncogene in the development of the tumor in question. By electron microscopy, cytoplasmic granules of specific proteins, monocarboxylate transporter 1 and CD147, correlate with the eosinophilic deposits seen in the endoplasmic reticulum of ASPS cells by H&E staining (Fig. 17.5) [10].

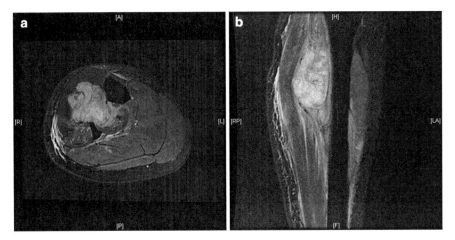

Fig. 17.3 T2 contrast-enhanced fat-saturated MRI images of a primary alveolar soft part sarcoma of the calf. Tumor extends through the interosseous membrane

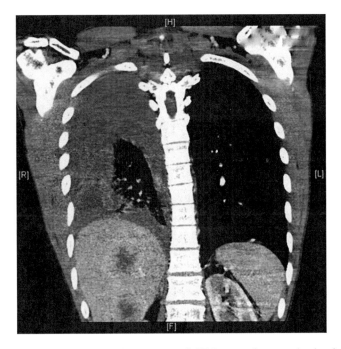

Fig. 17.4 Reconstructed contrast-enhanced coronal CT images of metastatic alveolar soft part sarcoma with substantial pleural-based and liver metastatic disease. A more typical pattern involves bilateral innumerable round lung metastases

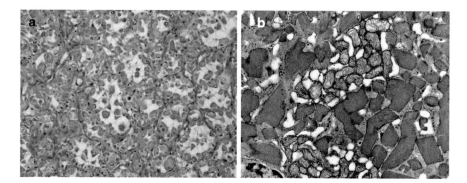

Fig. 17.5 Microscopic and ultrastructural detail of alveolar soft part sarcoma. (**a**) Microscopic appearance demonstrating well-defined alveolar structures lined by large epithelioid cells with abundant eosinophilic cytoplasm and eccentric nuclei with small nucleoli (H&E, 100X). (**b**) An electron micrograph demonstrates characteristic large rhomboid crystals as well as abundant mitochondria

Table 17.1 Systemic therapy recommendations for patients with alveolar soft part sarcoma

Clinical scenario	Suggested therapy
Primary disease	Surgery, radiation
First line for metastatic disease	Sunitinib, or similar multitargeted tyrosine kinase inhibitor, such as pazopanib
Second line for metastatic disease	Clinical trial, trabectedin, other VEGF-directed therapy; the activity of bevacizumab or other supposedly antiangiogenic agents is unknown

Primary Treatment

Primary surgery is appropriate for patients with both primary only disease and in our opinion also for patients with metastatic disease, since most symptoms can at least initially be related to the large primary, although metastatic lung disease typically dictates the late course of the tumor. Usually so many nodules are observed as metastatic disease in the lungs that surgery cannot be contemplated rationally (Table 17.1).

Treatment of Metastatic Disease

Systemic therapy for sarcomas continues to evolve and has affected the treatment of ASPS, although not to the degree of tyrosine kinase inhibitors for GIST. Systemic cytotoxic chemotherapy is essentially useless against ASPS in our experience, although there are isolated reports of responses in patients with metastatic disease [6]. There are also case reports of interferon-alfa2a being active in metastatic

ASPS [11, 12], suggesting an antiangiogenic approach for treatment of ASPS. This idea has been developed further with newer antiangiogenic agents. The striking activity of cediranib against ASPS in one prospective clinical trial reinvigorated interest in systemic therapy for ASPS [13]. Sunitinib, commercially available unlike cediranib as of the time of publication, has activity against metastatic ASPS [14]. How the ASPS translocation leads to signaling or dependence on VEGF (vascular endothelial growth factor)-related pathways remains unknown. In the setting of resistance to a VEGFR (VEGF receptor) tyrosine kinase inhibitor, other agents that target VEGF signaling, be it bevacizumab or other agents affecting downstream signaling steps from the VEGFRs, would appear to make most sense to investigate. The rarity of the diagnosis mandates coordinated efforts to determine activity of novel agents.

Outcome

Because these tumors are rare and prolonged survival occurs despite metastatic disease, long follow-up (10 years or more) is necessary. Overall survival for all patients is shown in Fig. 17.6, and the influence of metastatic disease highlighted in Fig. 17.7. A recent single institution study of 47 patients confirmed the high metastatic rate (72%), predominantly to lung, but with relatively long overall survival compared to other soft tissue sarcoma [15].

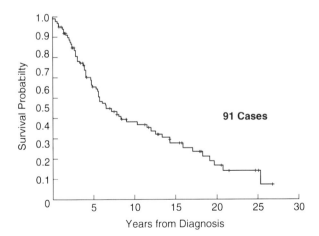

Fig. 17.6 Overall survival of 91 patients with alveolar soft part sarcoma. (Used with permission from: Lieberman et al. [1])

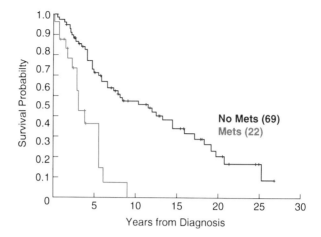

Fig. 17.7 Overall survival of 91 patients with alveolar soft part sarcoma, distinguishing primary from metastatic disease *Mets* metastases (Used with permission from: Lieberman et al. [1])

References

1. Lieberman PH, Brennan MF, Kimmel M, et al. Alveolar soft-part sarcoma. A clinico-pathologic study of half a century. Cancer. 1989;63(1):1–13.
2. Pennacchioli E, Fiore M, Collini P, et al. Alveolar soft part sarcoma: clinical presentation, treatment, and outcome in a series of 33 patients at a single institution. Ann Surg Oncol. 2010:17(12):3229–33.
3. Kayton ML, Meyers P, Wexler LH, et al. Clinical presentation, treatment, and outcome of alveolar soft part sarcoma in children, adolescents, and young adults. J Pediatr Surg. 2006;41(1):187–93.
4. Haga Y, Kusaka G, Mori S, et al. A case of alveolar soft-part sarcoma with cerebral metastases. No To Shinkei. 1996;48(3):269–74.
5. Postovsky S, Ash S, Ramu IN, et al. Central nervous system involvement in children with sarcoma. Oncology. 2003;65(2):118–24.
6. Reichardt P, Lindner T, Pink D, et al. Chemotherapy in alveolar soft part sarcomas. What do we know? Eur J Cancer. 2003;39(11):1511–6.
7. Pennacchioli E, Fiore M, Collini P, et al. Alveolar soft part sarcoma: clinical presentation, treatment, and outcome in a series of 33 patients at a single institution. Ann Surg Oncol. 2010;17(12):3229–33.
8. Ladanyi M, Lui MY, Antonescu CR, et al. The der(17)t(X;17)(p11;q25) of human alveolar soft part sarcoma fuses the TFE3 transcription factor gene to ASPL, a novel gene at 17q25. Oncogene. 2001;20(1):48–57.
9. Argani P, Antonescu CR, Illei PB, et al. Primary renal neoplasms with the ASPL-TFE3 gene fusion of alveolar soft part sarcoma: a distinctive tumor entity previously included among renal cell carcinomas of children and adolescents. Am J Pathol. 2001;159(1):179–92.
10. Ladanyi M, Antonescu CR, Drobnjak M, et al. The precrystalline cytoplasmic granules of alveolar soft part sarcoma contain monocarboxylate transporter 1 and CD147. Am J Pathol. 2002;160(4):1215–21.
11. Kuriyama K, Todo S, Hibi S, et al. Alveolar soft part sarcoma with lung metastases. Response to interferon alpha-2a? Med Pediatr Oncol. 2001;37(5):482–3.

12. Bisogno G, Rosolen A, Carli M. Interferon alpha for alveolar soft part sarcoma. Pediatr Blood Cancer. 2005;44(7):687–8.
13. Gardner K, Leahy M, Alvarez-Gutierrez M, et al. Activity of the VEGFR/KIT tyrosine kinase inhibitor cediranib (AZD2171) in alveolar soft part sarcoma. Proc Connect Tissue Oncol Soc (www.ctos.org). 2008;14:Abstr 34936
14. Stacchiotti S, Tamborini E, Marrari A, et al. Response to sunitinib malate in advanced alveolar soft part sarcoma. Clin Cancer Res. 2009;15(3):1096–104.
15. Rekhi B, Ingle A, Agarwal M, et al. Alveolar soft part sarcoma 'revisited': clinicopathological review of 47 cases from a tertiary cancer referral centre, including immunohistochemical expression of TFE3 in 22 cases and 21 other tumours. Pathology. 2012;44(1):11–7.

Chapter 18
Clear Cell Sarcoma/Melanoma of Soft Parts

Is it a sarcoma or is it a melanoma? Clear cell sarcoma (CCS), also called clear cell sarcoma of tendons and aponeuroses [1, 2], has features of both. CCS represents perhaps 1% of all sarcomas. Since it starts in soft tissue and usually does not affect skin [3], CCS is anatomically distinct from melanoma. Patients are typically younger, between 15 and 45 years of age, and women are more commonly affected than men. The foot and ankle are common primary locations for this rare sarcoma. Age and site distribution for adult patients are shown in Figs. 18.1 and 18.2.

Imaging

The appearance of clear cell sarcoma of the ankle, knee, and gastrointestinal tract is not distinguishable from other sarcomas, except for the higher risk of lymph node metastases compared to other sarcomas (Figs. 18.3 and 18.4).

Diagnosis: Molecular Pathology

Soft tissue CCS contains a characteristic translocation [4], typically t(12;22), *EWSR1-ATF1*, and much less commonly t(2;22), *EWSR1-CREB1* [5]. The reversed pattern is seen in the gastrointestinal tract CCS, where *EWSR1-CREB1* fusion is the most common abnormality. Both translocations also can be found in angiomatoid fibrous histiocytoma (AFH) [6, 7], suggesting the same translocation creates a tumor that is context-dependent upon the affected precursor cell, as with the *ASPL-TFE3* translocation of papillary renal cell cancer and alveolar soft part sarcoma. CCS does not contain mutation in *BRAF*, commonly detected in melanoma.

Unlike most sarcomas, CCS can metastasize to locoregional lymph nodes, and it is typically positive for markers commonly observed in melanoma, such as S100, MiTF, HMB45, melan-A, and tyrosinase, making diagnosis without the clinical history

M.F. Brennan et al., *Management of Soft Tissue Sarcoma*,
DOI 10.1007/978-1-4614-5004-7_18, © Springer Science+Business Media New York 2013

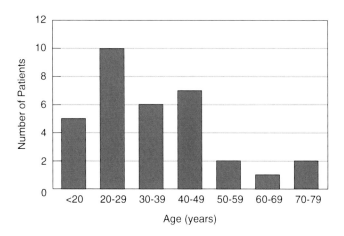

Fig. 18.1 Age distribution for adult patients with clear cell sarcoma. MSKCC 7/1/1982–6/30/2010 n = 33

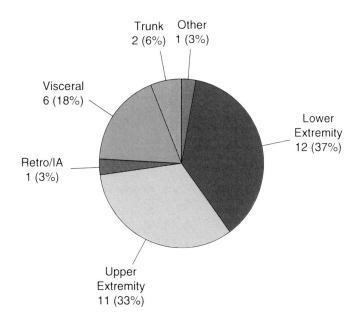

Fig. 18.2 Primary site distribution of adult patients with clear cell sarcoma. MSKCC 7/1/1982–6/30/2010 n = 33 *Retro/IA* retroperitoneal/intra-abdominal

difficult (Fig. 18.5). The tumor frequently invades dense connective tissue of tendons, where nests of tumor cells are separated by fibrous septa. The differential diagnosis includes MPNST and epithelioid sarcoma, while in the GI location also includes GIST and carcinoid tumor. It is worth noting that melanocytic markers are often negative in the gastrointestinal CCS [5]. Gastrointestinal CCS typically follows a much more aggressive clinical course with early lymph nodes and liver metastases [5].

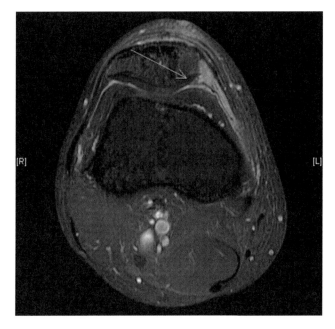

Fig. 18.3 Contrast-enhanced T2-weighted fat-saturated MRI image of a clear cell sarcoma of the knee with patellar invasion. The tumor was confirmed to have an *EWSR1* rearrangement

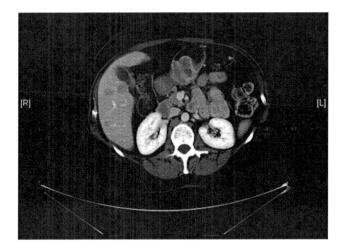

Fig. 18.4 Contrast-enhanced CT image of a gastric clear cell sarcoma with evidence of liver metastatic disease

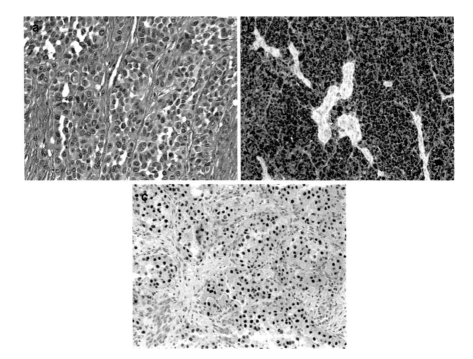

Fig. 18.5 Microscopic images of clear cell sarcoma demonstrating characteristic features. (**a**) High-power image of clear cell sarcoma demonstrating cords of loosely arranged small cells with eosinophilic cytoplasm separated by refractile collagen bundles, H&E, 200×. (**b**) Immunohistochemical staining showing strong S100 staining, 100X. (**c**) Strong nuclear staining for MiTF by immunohistochemistry, 100×

Treatment

Surgery remains the mainstay of primary treatment for this diagnosis. Given the ability of at least some CCS to metastasize to lymph nodes, we argue that sentinel lymph node biopsy is a reasonable standard of care as part of staging, similar to melanoma, with completion lymphadenectomy if positive. Primary surgery is often made difficult given the anatomy of the ankle and foot. As lymph node metastasis is relatively common compared to other soft tissue sarcomas (hence the name melanoma of soft parts), therapeutic lymph node dissection should be performed when lymph node metastasis is present [8, 9].

For recurrent disease, the chemotherapy sensitivity pattern of CCS is perhaps more consistent with melanoma, with occasional responses to platinum-based chemotherapy [10]. Ifosfamide may be active in the occasional patient [11]. Like other sarcomas involving *ATF1/CREB1* rearrangements, CCS can express MET, sug-

Table 18.1 Suggestions for therapy for clear cell sarcoma[a]

Clinical scenario	Treatment
Primary disease	Surgical excision; radiation when anatomically feasible without functional loss. Sentinel lymph node sampling may aid in staging, as may PET scans. Chemotherapy is not recommended
Recurrent/metastatic disease	Clinical trial, ifosfamide, platinum-based chemotherapy
Chemotherapy-refractory disease	Multitargeted tyrosine kinase inhibitor, such as pazopanib

[a]A clinical trial is appropriate when available

gesting an antiangiogenic approach to treat these tumors. However, a recent study of a MET inhibitor showed but one RECIST (Response Evaluation Criteria In Solid Tumors) partial response, implying that MET signaling, at least as can be blocked by the agent, is not the sole survival pathway for CCS [12]. A patient with CCS has responded to sunitinib, giving hope that receptor tyrosine kinase-specific agents could have activity in CCS [13]. Future studies will focus on signaling pathways activated or interacting in this tumor by the translocation product, similar to Ewing sarcoma and the EWSR1-FLI1 translocation product and IGF1R signaling [14].

Chemotherapy for Ewing sarcoma is inactive against clear cell sarcoma; the presence of an *EWSR1* translocation positive tumor does not predict sensitivity to cytotoxic chemotherapy in and of itself (Table 18.1).

Outcome

Local recurrence is uncommon but numbers in the various series are small. Our local recurrence in 13 patients is shown in Fig. 18.6, but systemic recurrence and death from disease is likely (Fig. 18.7) [15]. Unfortunately, even in large institutions, the experience is limited, and metastasis frequent, with demise within 2 years of appearance of metastatic disease. Only initial tumor size over 5 cm appears to be a predictor of poor outcome [16].

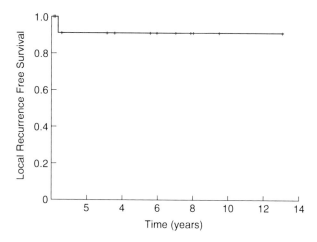

Fig. 18.6 Local disease-free survival for adult patients with primary clear cell sarcoma. MSKCC 7/1/1982–6/30/2010 n = 13

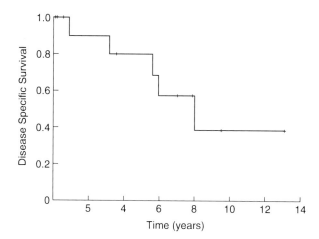

Fig. 18.7 Disease-specific survival for adult patients with primary clear cell sarcoma. MSKCC 7/1/1982–6/30/2010 n = 13

References

1. Enzinger FM. Clear-cell sarcoma of tendons and aponeuroses. An analysis of 21 cases. Cancer. 1965;18:1163–74.
2. Chung EB, Enzinger FM. Malignant melanoma of soft parts. A reassessment of clear cell sarcoma. Am J Surg Pathol. 1983;7(5):405–13.
3. Hantschke M, Mentzel T, Rutten A, et al. Cutaneous clear cell sarcoma: a clinicopathologic, immunohistochemical, and molecular analysis of 12 cases emphasizing its distinction from dermal melanoma. Am J Surg Pathol. 2010;34(2):216–22.

4. Bridge JA, Borek DA, Neff JR, et al. Chromosomal abnormalities in clear cell sarcoma. Implications for histogenesis. Am J Clin Pathol. 1990;93(1):26–31.
5. Antonescu CR, Nafa K, Segal NH, et al. EWS-CREB1: a recurrent variant fusion in clear cell sarcoma–association with gastrointestinal location and absence of melanocytic differentiation. Clin Cancer Res. 2006;12(18):5356–62.
6. Antonescu CR, Dal Cin P, Nafa K, et al. EWSR1-CREB1 is the predominant gene fusion in angiomatoid fibrous histiocytoma. Genes Chromosomes Cancer. 2007;46(12):1051–60.
7. Rossi S, Szuhai K, Ijszenga M, et al. EWSR1-CREB1 and EWSR1-ATF1 fusion genes in angiomatoid fibrous histiocytoma. Clin Cancer Res. 2007;13(24):7322–8.
8. Clark MA, Johnson MB, Thway K, et al. Clear cell sarcoma (melanoma of soft parts): The Royal Marsden hospital experience. Eur J Surg Oncol. 2008;34(7):800–4.
9. Daigeler A, Kuhnen C, Moritz R, et al. Lymph node metastases in soft tissue sarcomas: a single center analysis of 1,597 patients. Langenbecks Arch Surg. 2009;394(2):321–9.
10. Kawai A, Hosono A, Nakayama R, et al. Clear cell sarcoma of tendons and aponeuroses: a study of 75 patients. Cancer. 2007;109(1):109–16.
11. Jones RL, Constantinidou A, Thway K, et al. Chemotherapy in clear cell sarcoma. Med Oncol. 2011;28(3):859–63.
12. Goldberg J, Demetri GD, Choy E, et al. Preliminary results from a phase II study of ARQ197 in patients with microphthalmia transcription factor family-associated tumors. J Clin Oncol. 2009;27(15S):Abstr 10502.
13. Stacchiotti S, Grosso F, Negri T, et al. Tumor response to sunitinib malate observed in clear-cell sarcoma. Ann Oncol. 2010;21(5):1130–1.
14. Toretsky JA, Kalebic T, Blakesley V, et al. The insulin-like growth factor-I receptor is required for EWS/FLI-1 transformation of fibroblasts. J Biol Chem. 1997;272(49):30822–7.
15. Blazer 3rd DG, Lazar AJ, Xing Y, et al. Clinical outcomes of molecularly confirmed clear cell sarcoma from a single institution and in comparison with data from the surveillance, epidemiology, and end results registry. Cancer. 2009;115(13):2971–9.
16. Ipach I, Mittag F, Kopp HG, et al. Clear-cell sarcoma of the soft tissue – a rare diagnosis with a fatal outcome. Eur J Cancer Care (Engl). 2012;21(3):412–20.

Chapter 19
Desmoplastic Small Round Cell Tumor

Desmoplastic small round cell tumor (DSRCT) is a somewhat chemotherapy-sensitive, but highly lethal, sarcoma diagnosis. Distribution by age for adults is shown in Fig. 19.1, emphasizing that it is an uncommon tumor, seen mainly in adolescents and young adults (age 15–30). There is a strong male predominance (~5:1) and nearly always affects the peritoneum as multifocal/metastatic disease (Fig. 19.2). The best outcomes from therapy are those who have both a good response to chemotherapy (using agents typically employed for Ewing sarcoma) and successful surgical debulking [1]. Rare patients will present with disease elsewhere; if disease is localized, the cure rate is expected to be higher than the 5–15% typically encountered for those patients with primary abdominal disease [1, 2].

Imaging

The CT or MR scans of patients with DSRCT reflect tumor biology, with multiple typically large, dense masses in the abdomen, sometimes with central necrosis (Fig. 19.3). Those patients who develop lung metastases show signs of similar fibrotic patterns consistent with desmoplastic changes in the lung.

Diagnosis

DSRCT characteristically presents as multiple firm fibrous masses with significant vascularity that contain nests of small round blue cells surrounded by dense fibrous (desmoplastic) stroma on microscopic examination (Fig. 19.4). Mesothelial markers are negative, distinguishing DSRCT from mesothelioma. The tumor shows a polyphenotypic expression by IHC, showing both cytokeratin and desmin reactivity. While NSE (neuron-specific enolase) can be positive in many tumors, other neuroendocrine markers are typically negative [3, 4]. C-terminal WT1 (Wilms'

M.F. Brennan et al., *Management of Soft Tissue Sarcoma*,   275
DOI 10.1007/978-1-4614-5004-7_19, © Springer Science+Business Media New York 2013

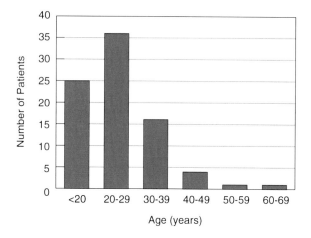

Fig. 19.1 Age distribution of adult patients with desmoplastic small round cell tumor. MSKCC 7/1/1982–6/30/2010 n = 83

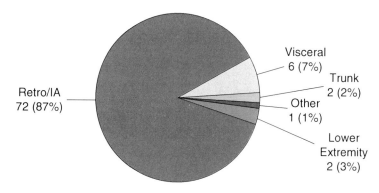

Fig. 19.2 Primary site distribution of adult patients with desmoplastic small round cell tumor. MSKCC 7/1/1982–6/30/2010 n = 83 *Retro/IA* retroperitoneal/intra-abdominal

tumor gene) staining is positive, on the basis of its characteristic t(11;22) translocation [5–8]. The *EWSR1-WT1* fusion product appears to upregulate PDGF, apparently accounting at least in part for the densely fibrotic nature of the tumor [9, 10].

Treatment

Combined modality therapy with chemotherapy and surgery is standard of care, but is clearly inadequate based on the poor overall survival rate. Combinations of drugs used for Ewing sarcoma are typically employed, i.e., vincristine-doxorubicin-cyclophosphamide, ifosfamide-etoposide, or the AIM (doxorubicin, ifosfamide, and mesna) or VIDE (vincristine, ifosfamide, doxorubicin, etoposide) regimens [11–13].

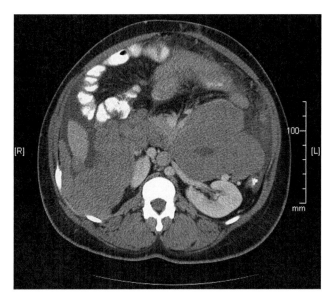

Fig. 19.3 Evidence of multiple abdominal implants from desmoplastic small round cell tumor on contrast-enhanced CT imaging of the abdomen

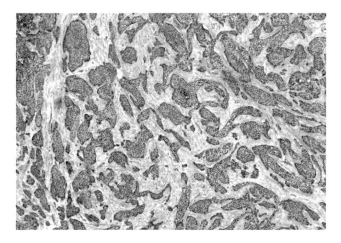

Fig. 19.4 Microscopic appearance of desmoplastic small round cell tumor. Nests of small round blue cells are seen, separated by a bland, desmoplastic fibrous stroma. The diagnosis is confirmed by expression of cytokeratins, desmin, and WT1, or at the molecular level by demonstration of the *EWSR1-WT1* fusion transcript

In the pediatric setting, the P6 regimen of very high-dose VAC/IE (cyclophosphamide, doxorubicin, vincristine/etoposide, ifosfamide) therapy has been employed [14], but is next to impossible to successfully administer to adults beyond 1–2 cycles of therapy, owing to the cyclophosphamide dose of 4.2 $g/m^2/cycle$. There are no published data that these high doses are superior to standard dose VAC/IE as given to patients with Ewing sarcoma. In fact, higher doses of chemotherapy administered to patients with Ewing sarcoma as part of a randomized clinical trial were associated with no better outcome than standard doses, in this more chemotherapy-sensitive disease (at least compared to desmoplastic small round cell tumor) [15]. It therefore stands to argue that standard Ewing sarcoma dosing should be employed as part of management of this diagnosis outside of the setting of a study.

Out of desperation from treating this diagnosis with poor outcomes, some clinicians employ intraperitoneal chemotherapy after optimal debulking surgery as treatment. One obvious difficulty with this diagnosis is that it does not spread in a superficial manner as ovarian or appendiceal carcinoma, but rather forms (even subclinical) masses or aggregates that intraperitoneal chemotherapy would not be expected to penetrate. In the authors' opinion, the use of intraperitoneal chemotherapy for DSRCT remains highly investigational [16], given the selection bias inherent in treatment series and lack of randomized data, as are high-dose therapy with stem cell support [17, 18] and therapy with WT1-directed immunotherapy [19–22], another avenue in which one would hope for eradication of metastatic disease.

A patient on a phase II clinical trial of sunitinib demonstrated reduction in tumor size, but increase in 18 F-FDG PET (18-fluorodeoxyglucose positron emission tomography) avidity, suggestive of a tumor whose desmoplastic reaction improved without direct effects on the tumor [23], a hypothesis that remains to be tested. Combinations of PDGFR-directed agents with cytotoxic chemotherapy, if technically feasible, may be one way forward for primary therapy for such patients. Regimens used for relapse of Ewing sarcoma, e.g., cyclophosphamide-topotecan [24], are often used for disease progression refractory to anthracycline-ifosfamide-based therapy (Table 19.1).

Outcome

Outcome of adult patients primarily treated by us is shown in Fig. 19.5, with few long-term survivors in our experience. Given improved supportive care and imaging, a randomized study will be necessary to confirm the benefit of any new therapy that shows promise in phase II.

Table 19.1 Suggestions for therapy for desmoplastic sarcoma

Clinical scenario	Suggested treatment
Initial presentation	Chemotherapy as used for Ewing sarcoma; surgery when feasible (debulking). Treatment with high-dose chemotherapy and stem cell rescue, abdominal radiation, or intraperitoneal chemotherapy remains investigational
Disease progression	Clinical trial, temozolomide-irinotecan, cyclophosphamide-topotecan

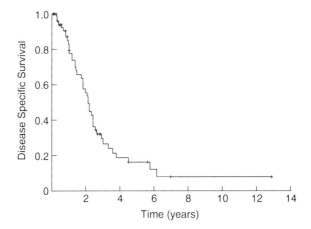

Fig. 19.5 Disease-specific survival for adult patients with a primary diagnosis of desmoplastic small round cell tumor. Most patients present with metastatic disease. MSKCC 7/1/1982–6/30/2010 n=69

References

1. La Quaglia MP, Brennan MF. The clinical approach to desmoplastic small round cell tumor. Surg Oncol. 2000;9(2):77–81.
2. Lal DR, Su WT, Wolden SL, et al. Results of multimodal treatment for desmoplastic small round cell tumors. J Pediatr Surg. 2005;40(1):251–5.
3. Gerald WL, Ladanyi M, de Alava E, et al. Clinical, pathologic, and molecular spectrum of tumors associated with t(11;22)(p13;q12): desmoplastic small round-cell tumor and its variants. J Clin Oncol. 1998;16(9):3028–36.
4. Ordonez NG. Desmoplastic small round cell tumor: II: an ultrastructural and immunohistochemical study with emphasis on new immunohistochemical markers. Am J Surg Pathol. 1998;22(11):1314–27.
5. Gerald WL, Rosai J, Ladanyi M. Characterization of the genomic breakpoint and chimeric transcripts in the EWS-WT1 gene fusion of desmoplastic small round cell tumor. Proc Natl Acad Sci USA. 1995;92(4):1028–32.
6. Ladanyi M, Gerald W. Fusion of the EWS and WT1 genes in the desmoplastic small round cell tumor. Cancer Res. 1994;54(11):2837–40.
7. Biegel JA, Conard K, Brooks JJ. Translocation (11;22)(p13;q12): primary change in intraabdominal desmoplastic small round cell tumor. Genes Chromosomes Cancer. 1993;7(2):119–21.
8. Sawyer JR, Tryka AF, Lewis JM. A novel reciprocal chromosome translocation t(11;22)(p13;q12) in an intraabdominal desmoplastic small round-cell tumor. Am J Surg Pathol. 1992;16(4):411–6.
9. Zhang PJ, Goldblum JR, Pawel BR, et al. PDGF-A, PDGF-Rbeta, TGFbeta3 and bone morphogenic protein-4 in desmoplastic small round cell tumors with EWS-WT1 gene fusion product and their role in stromal desmoplasia: an immunohistochemical study. Mod Pathol. 2005;18(3):382–7.
10. Froberg K, Brown RE, Gaylord H, et al. Intra-abdominal desmoplastic small round cell tumor: immunohistochemical evidence for up-regulation of autocrine and paracrine growth factors. Ann Clin Lab Sci. 1998;28(6):386–93.
11. Marina NM, Pappo AS, Parham DM, et al. Chemotherapy dose-intensification for pediatric patients with Ewing's family of tumors and desmoplastic small round-cell tumors: a feasibility study at St. Jude Children's Research Hospital. J Clin Oncol. 1999;17(1):180–90.

12. Kretschmar CS, Colbach C, Bhan I, et al. Desmoplastic small cell tumor: a report of three cases and a review of the literature. J Pediatr Hematol Oncol. 1996;18(3):293–8.
13. Farhat F, Culine S, Lhomme C, et al. Desmoplastic small round cell tumors: results of a four-drug chemotherapy regimen in five adult patients. Cancer. 1996;77(7):1363–6.
14. Kushner BH, LaQuaglia MP, Wollner N, et al. Desmoplastic small round-cell tumor: prolonged progression-free survival with aggressive multimodality therapy. J Clin Oncol. 1996;14(5):1526–31.
15. Granowetter L, Womer R, Devidas M, et al. Dose-intensified compared with standard chemotherapy for nonmetastatic Ewing sarcoma family of tumors: a Children's Oncology Group Study. J Clin Oncol. 2009;27(15):2536–41.
16. Hayes-Jordan A, Green H, Fitzgerald N, et al. Novel treatment for desmoplastic small round cell tumor: hyperthermic intraperitoneal perfusion. J Pediatr Surg. 2010;45(5):1000–6.
17. Al Balushi Z, Bulduc S, Mulleur C, et al. Desmoplastic small round cell tumor in children: a new therapeutic approach. J Pediatr Surg. 2009;44(5):949–52.
18. Bertuzzi A, Castagna L, Nozza A, et al. High-dose chemotherapy in poor-prognosis adult small round-cell tumors: clinical and molecular results from a prospective study. J Clin Oncol. 2002;20(8):2181–8.
19. Guo Y, Niiya H, Azuma T, et al. Direct recognition and lysis of leukemia cells by WT1-specific CD4+ T lymphocytes in an HLA class II-restricted manner. Blood. 2005;106(4): 1415–8.
20. Hashii Y, Sato E, Ohta H, et al. WT1 peptide immunotherapy for cancer in children and young adults. Pediatr Blood Cancer. 2010;55(2):352–5.
21. Maslak PG, Dao T, Krug LM, et al. Vaccination with synthetic analog peptides derived from WT1 oncoprotein induces T-cell responses in patients with complete remission from acute myeloid leukemia. Blood. 2010;116(2):171–9.
22. Tsuji T, Yasukawa M, Matsuzaki J, et al. Generation of tumor-specific, HLA class I-restricted human Th1 and Tc1 cells by cell engineering with tumor peptide-specific T-cell receptor genes. Blood. 2005;106(2):470–6.
23. George S, Merriam P, Maki RG, et al. Multicenter phase II trial of sunitinib in the treatment of nongastrointestinal stromal tumor sarcomas. J Clin Oncol. 2009;27(19):3154–60.
24. Kushner BH, Kramer K, Meyers PA, et al. Pilot study of topotecan and high-dose cyclophosphamide for resistant pediatric solid tumors. Med Pediatr Oncol. 2000;35(5):468–74.

Chapter 20
Extraskeletal Myxoid Chondrosarcoma

Extraskeletal myxoid chondrosarcoma (EMC) is a relatively slow-growing soft tissue sarcoma that often presents with metastatic disease, typically innumerable round lung nodules of varying sizes that also grow slowly but relentlessly [1, 2]. It is different in all genetic and histopathological aspects from skeletal chondrosarcoma [3]. EMC typically affects people between ages 30 and 60 [1, 4] (Fig. 20.1) and occurs most commonly in the lower extremity (Fig. 20.2). Men are affected more commonly than women, but there does not appear to be a difference in incidence based on race [5]. Tumors present as painless, slow-growing multi-lobulated masses and are soft, gelatinous in consistency, and often hemorrhagic.

Imaging

Radiology easily demonstrates the primary mass lesion (Fig. 20.3), which is indistinguishable from other sarcomas. However, metastases are usually noted early in the lungs (Fig. 20.4) as innumerable round marble-like lesions, which can develop central necrosis as they increase in size (Fig. 20.5).

Diagnosis

EMC demonstrates a broad group of morphological patterns, with bland epithelioid to oval cells arranged in a reticular pattern within a rich myxoid background consistent with expression of chondroitin sulfates (perhaps the only true link to skeletal chondrosarcoma) and relatively infrequent mitoses (Fig. 20.6). Histologic grading remains controversial, some authors suggesting that regardless of morphologic features, it should be regarded as a low-grade sarcoma. We and others have shown that histologic grade (based on nuclear pleomorphism, mitoses, necrosis) correlates with outcome [3]. In the high-grade lesions, a predominantly solid, non-myxoid pattern with rhabdoid morphology may occur.

M.F. Brennan et al., *Management of Soft Tissue Sarcoma*,
DOI 10.1007/978-1-4614-5004-7_20, © Springer Science+Business Media New York 2013

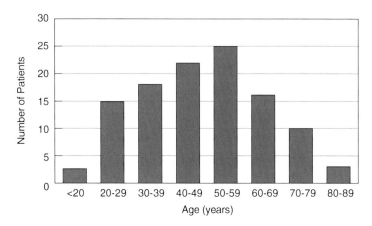

Fig. 20.1 Age distribution for adult patients with extraskeletal myxoid chondrosarcoma. MSKCC 7/1/82–6/30/10 n = 111

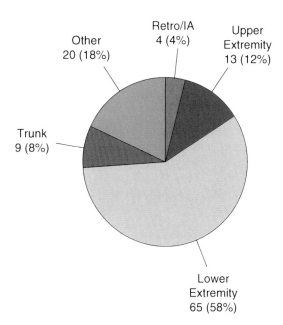

Fig. 20.2 Primary anatomic site for adult patients with extraskeletal myxoid chondrosarcoma. MSKCC 7/1/82–6/30/10 n = 111 *Retro/IA* retroperitoneal/intra-abdominal

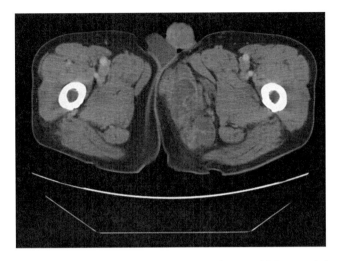

Fig. 20.3 Contrast-enhanced CT image of a peroneal/upper thigh extraskeletal myxoid chondrosarcoma

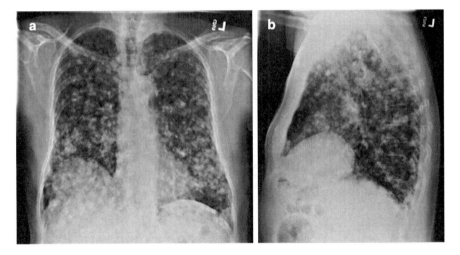

Fig. 20.4 Chest radiographs of the patient in Fig. 20.3; there is widespread lung metastasis in the setting of a relatively small primary tumor

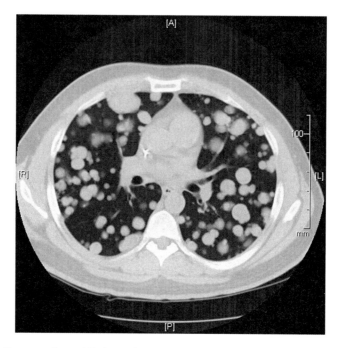

Fig. 20.5 Contrast-enhanced CT image from a patient with metastatic extraskeletal myxoid chondrosarcoma, alive over 7/1/1982-6/30/2010 er diagnosis of metastatic disease

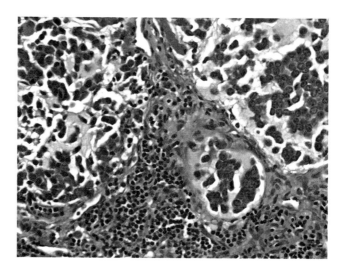

Fig. 20.6 Microscopic appearance of extraskeletal myxoid chondrosarcoma, in this demonstrating tumor metastatic to lymph node, with uniform epithelioid cells with scant eosinophilic cytoplasm, embedded in a myxoid stroma (H&E, 200X)

EMC usually contains the characteristic chromosomal translocation t(9;22), resulting in *EWSR1-NR4A3* fusion [6–9], although other translocation partners with *NR4A3* are also observed.

Treatment

Primary therapy is surgery; given the local recurrence risk over many years in the primary site, it is not clear that radiation therapy adds to surgery for this particular diagnosis [4]. Even with metastatic disease, the primary site is relatively large, and symptom relief could be anticipated for resection of the primary site in that setting since patients can often live for years despite metastatic disease. For recurrent disease, responses have been few [2], making this a diagnosis looking for a targeted agent that is responsible for the survival of EMC cells based on the tumor's specific translocation.

There is no well-defined standard of care for chemotherapy, since standard agents are inactive [2]. The presence of an *EWSR1*-containing translocation does not predict for sensitivity to chemotherapy used for Ewing sarcoma. However, the metastases are typically slow growing, and as a result periods of observation are frequently observed. It is conjecture if one form of kinase-directed or DNA-modifying agent would any more be effective than chemotherapy. Although the NR4A3-related pathway biological function is largely unknown, it is a potential target for future therapy [10], given its relationship to steroid-binding nuclear receptors. Given the understanding that the translocation product may suppress rather than promote gene expression in a general fashion, thus decreasing expression of pro-apoptotic proteins, DNA-modifying agents may merit further investigation (Table 20.1).

Outcome

Local recurrence-free survival for patients with primary adult EMC is shown in Fig. 20.7, and for disease-specific survival in Fig. 20.8. Relatively long-term survival following the development of metastatic disease is not unusual (Fig. 20.5).

Table 20.1 Therapeutic recommendations for patients with extraskeletal myxoid chondrosarcoma

Primary disease	Surgical resection; radiation therapy controversial. Resection can be contemplated for larger tumors even in setting of metastatic disease
Recurrent/metastatic disease	Clinical trials, no clear guidance, given very low response rate to standard chemotherapy

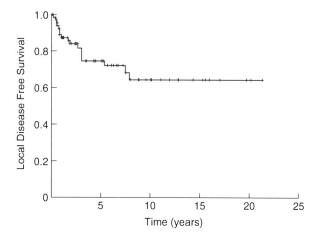

Fig. 20.7 Local recurrence-free survival for adult patients with primary extraskeletal myxoid chondrosarcoma. MSKCC 7/1/1982–6/30/2010 n = 71

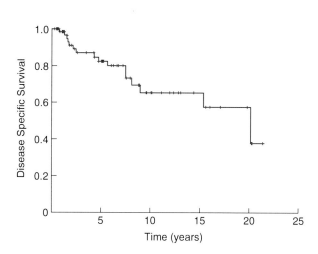

Fig. 20.8 Disease-specific survival for adult patients with primary extraskeletal myxoid chondrosarcoma. MSKCC 7/1/1982–6/30/2010 n = 71

References

1. Enzinger FM, Shiraki M. Extraskeletal myxoid chondrosarcoma. An analysis of 34 cases. Hum Pathol. 1972;3(3):421–35.
2. Drilon AD, Popat S, Bhuchar G, et al. Extraskeletal myxoid chondrosarcoma: a retrospective review from 2 referral centers emphasizing long-term outcomes with surgery and chemotherapy. Cancer. 2008;113(12):3364–71.

3. Antonescu CR, Argani P, Erlandson RA, et al. Skeletal and extraskeletal myxoid chondrosarcoma: a comparative clinicopathologic, ultrastructural, and molecular study. Cancer. 1998;83(8): 1504–21.

4. Meis-Kindblom JM, Bergh P, Gunterberg B, et al. Extraskeletal myxoid chondrosarcoma: a reappraisal of its morphologic spectrum and prognostic factors based on 117 cases. Am J Surg Pathol. 1999;23(6):636–50.

5. Worch J, Cyrus J, Goldsby R, et al. Racial differences in the incidence of mesenchymal tumors associated with EWSR1 translocation. Cancer Epidemiol Biomarkers Prev. 2011;20(3): 449–53.

6. Brody RI, Ueda T, Hamelin A, et al. Molecular analysis of the fusion of EWS to an orphan nuclear receptor gene in extraskeletal myxoid chondrosarcoma. Am J Pathol. 1997;150(3): 1049–58.

7. Sciot R, Dal Cin P, Fletcher C, et al. t(9;22)(q22-31;q11-12) is a consistent marker of extraskeletal myxoid chondrosarcoma: evaluation of three cases. Mod Pathol. 1995;8(7):765–8.

8. Turc-Carel C, Dal Cin P, Rao U, et al. Recurrent breakpoints at 9q31 and 22q12.2 in extraskeletal myxoid chondrosarcoma. Cancer Genet Cytogenet. 1988;30(1):145–50.

9. Turc-Carel C, Dal Cin P, Sandberg AA. Nonrandom translocation in extraskeletal myxoid chondrosarcoma. Cancer Genet Cytogenet. 1987;26(2):377.

10. Hisaoka M, Hashimoto H. Extraskeletal myxoid chondrosarcoma: updated clinicopathological and molecular genetic characteristics. Pathol Int. 2005;55(8):453–63.

Chapter 21
Other Uterine Sarcomas

Beyond leiomyosarcoma, uterine sarcomas and tumors that contain "sarcoma" in the name (i.e., carcinosarcoma) are well-recognized biological entities. The three non-leiomyosarcoma tumors, (low-grade) endometrial stromal sarcoma, high-grade undifferentiated stromal sarcoma, and malignant mixed Müllerian tumors including carcinosarcoma, are all very different from one another biologically. They are often omitted in discussions of soft tissue pathology as different groups of pathologists generally review such cases in expert centers than those who review soft tissue or bone tumors. Age distribution for adult uterine endometrial stromal tumors is shown in Fig. 21.1.

Endometrial Stromal Sarcoma

Endometrial stromal sarcoma (ESS) resembles proliferating endometrial stroma. The tumor is relatively indolent but can be associated with locoregional (Fig. 21.2) as well as lung metastatic disease (Fig. 21.3) over the course of many years (not uncommonly a decade or more) in as many as a third of patients [1, 2]. It is the one sarcoma in which hormonal therapy reproducibly controls disease in a manner not dissimilar from estrogen-receptor-positive (ER+) breast adenocarcinoma. ESS is usually both ER + and progesterone receptor positive (PR+).

Diagnosis

Genetically ESS is interesting as it contains a unique translocation t(7;17)(p15;q21) involving *JAZF1* at 7p15 and *SUZ12* at 17q21 as the most common change, although t(6;7) and t(6;10) and others have been described [3–6]. What has been called in the past high-grade endometrial stromal sarcoma may represent a separate entity and thus is a diagnosis in transition that may disappear with the observation of a separate group of translocations for what is now frequently termed undifferentiated endometrial sarcoma (see below).

M.F. Brennan et al., *Management of Soft Tissue Sarcoma*,
DOI 10.1007/978-1-4614-5004-7_21, © Springer Science+Business Media New York 2013

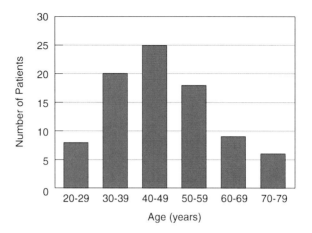

Fig. 21.1 Age distribution of adult patients with uterine endometrial sarcomas, all grades. MSKCC 7/1/1982 to 6/30/2010 n = 86

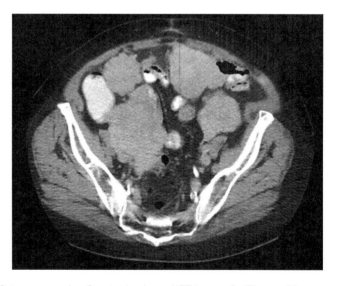

Fig. 21.2 Intravenous and oral contrast-enhanced CT image of a 71-year-old woman with metastatic endometrial stromal sarcoma

Treatment

Primary treatment is hysterectomy. Small studies and analysis of the National Cancer Institute's Surveillance, Epidemiology and End Results (SEER) database have examined if lymphadenectomy improved survival, since nodes are positive in 5–10% of patients with ESS. No survival advantage was noted, so it is difficult to

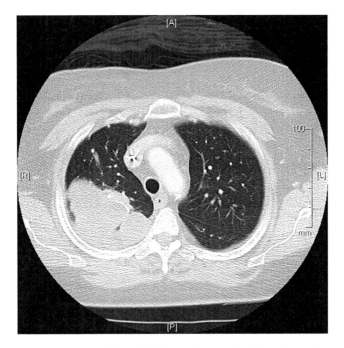

Fig. 21.3 Intravenous contrast-enhanced CT image of metastatic disease in a patient with undifferentiated endometrial sarcoma

routinely recommend the more extensive operation [7–10]. Radiation did not appear to affect clinical outcome and is generally not administered for patients with adequate primary surgery [7].

There are no randomized data to suggest the utility of hormonal therapy in the adjuvant setting for ESS [11–13], oophorectomy or GnRH agonists have activity as other means to affect estrogen levels in ESS, and patients who undergo total abdominal hysterectomy with bilateral salpingo-oophorectomy (TAH-BSO) as primary therapy may contaminate any benefit seen from adjuvant therapy.

For metastatic disease, progestins and antiestrogens are effective and usually relatively less toxic systemic therapy than chemotherapy, which also has activity [14–16]. It is also worth noting that given the slow evolution of disease in most patients, it is worthwhile considering surgery in the metastatic disease in selected patients (Table 21.1).

Outcome

Outcome for local recurrence and disease-specific survival for primary endometrial stromal tumors is shown in Figs. 21.4 and 21.5.

Table 21.1 Endometrial stromal sarcoma

Clinical scenario		Comments
Adjuvant systemic therapy		None; no clear benefit of adjuvant systemic therapy given long evolution of disease and effects of oophorectomy or other surgical procedures
Metastatic disease	1st line	Progestins, e.g., medroxyprogesterone, megestrol; oophorectomy or GnRH agonists in selected patients
	2nd line	Antiestrogens, e.g., aromatase inhibitors
	3rd line	Anthracyclines and/or ifosfamide; clinical trial

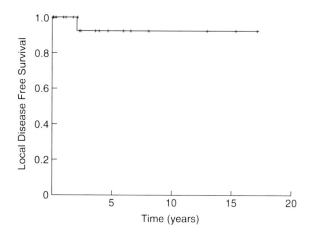

Fig. 21.4 Local disease-free survival for adult patients with primary uterine endometrial stromal sarcoma, all grades. MSKCC 7/1/1982 to 6/30/2010 n = 29

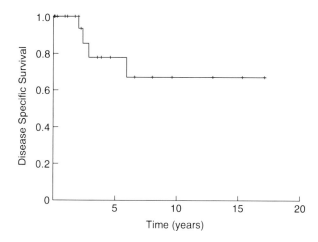

Fig. 21.5 Disease-specific survival for adult patients with primary uterine endometrial stromal sarcoma, all grades. MSKCC 7/1/1982 to 6/30/2010 n = 29

Undifferentiated Endometrial Sarcoma

Undifferentiated endometrial sarcoma (UES) increasingly is being accepted as a separate entity from endometrial stromal sarcoma and is termed by some undifferentiated uterine sarcoma. UES is usually estrogen receptor negative (ER-) and progesterone receptor negative (PR-), which differentiates UES from ESS (Fig. 21.6). Furthermore, UES does not appear to contain the translocations typically observed in ESS [17]. A collaborative effort has identified an entirely new translocation involving *YWHAE*, which hopefully will impact therapy for this aggressive sarcoma [18]. The t(10;17)(q22;p13), resulting in YWHAE-FAM22 fusion, was associated with a high-grade round cell morphology and aggressive clinical behavior compared to JAZF1-positive ESS [19]. However, in a subset of these high-grade lesions in addition to the undifferentiated round cell areas, there was a cytologically bland and mitotically weakly active spindle cell component, which was diffusely positive for ER, PR, and CD10, in contrast to the round cell areas, which were negative. This latter finding suggests the possibility of a histologic progression from an ESS to an UES. Of note, the same *YWHAE-FAM22* has been recently reported in the clear cell sarcoma of kidney [20].

Ifosfamide can be modestly active in this disease, but the response rate is low, making it difficult to recommend adjuvant chemotherapy for women with this diagnosis [16] (Table 21.2). We observed stable disease in one patient treated with an IGF1 receptor inhibitor, a finding we hope will be explored further, since YWHAE, a 14-3-3 protein, can interact with IGF1R-associated protein IRS1.

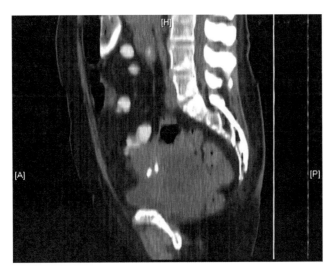

Fig. 21.6 CT image of a patient with a primary undifferentiated endometrial sarcoma, with extensive local extension

Table 21.2 Undifferentiated endometrial sarcoma, also called undifferentiated uterine sarcoma

Clinical scenario		Comments
Adjuvant chemotherapy		Not recommended, since the response rate in the metastatic setting is low
Metastatic disease	1st line	Ifosfamide-based therapy
	2nd line	Clinical trial; IGF1 receptor inhibitor or similar pathway inhibitor, if available

Outcome

An analysis utilizing the 2003 WHO classification of 3 endometrial stromal sarcoma (ESS) subtypes, including noninvasive, invasive low grade, and invasive undifferentiated [21], indicated that 5- and 10-year recurrence-free survival for 91 invasive ESS was 82% and 75%. Necrosis was an important prognostic predictor for overall survival, with 10-year survival of 89% in the absence of necrosis and 49% in those with prominent necrosis. By defining ESS low grade as mild atypia with no necrosis and undifferentiated as moderate/severe atypia present or necrosis present, disease-specific survivals were 98% versus 48%.

Uterine Carcinosarcomas and Other Malignant Mixed Müllerian Tumors

Age distribution for adult carcinosarcoma is shown in Fig. 21.7. Malignant mixed Müllerian tumors have elements of both stroma and epithelium and include adenofibroma, adenosarcoma, carcinofibroma, and carcinosarcoma. While adenofibroma is benign, the other tumors are malignancies. Carcinosarcoma, which presents in postmenopausal women as uterine bleeding, may represent a uterine carcinoma with divergent differentiation toward a sarcoma lineage. However, it is more aggressive overall compared to uterine carcinomas, with frequent metastasis to both peritoneum and lung, and thus appears to be clinically distinct from uterine carcinoma. CA125 is often elevated in patients with carcinosarcoma and may serve as a tumor marker.

No recurrent genetic event is observed in carcinosarcoma, and the tumors are generally aneuploid.

Primary therapy is TAH-BSO and proper gynecological staging with lymphadenectomy, omentectomy, and testing of peritoneal cytology. Both local-regional relapse and metastatic spread of carcinosarcoma are common, which has raised the question of the utility of abdominal radiation and systemic chemotherapy in the

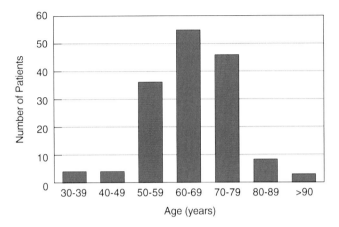

Fig. 21.7 Age distribution of adult patients with uterine carcinosarcoma (malignant mixed Müllerian tumors). MSKCC 7/1/1982 to 6/30/2010 n = 156

adjuvant setting. A randomized study of adjuvant radiation for uterine sarcomas and carcinosarcomas showed better local control but no improvement in overall survival and is not routinely recommended. Conversely, a retrospective analysis of a large number of patients treated with radiation, written by a radiation oncologist, suggested possible clinical benefit from adjuvant irradiation [22, 23].

A phase III GOG study showed that adjusting for stage and age, the recurrence rate was 21% lower for patients who received ifosfamide-cisplatin adjuvant therapy over whole abdominal radiation for stage I–IV carcinosarcoma, although the crude data showed no significant difference in the recurrence rate [24]. While thus a reasonable standard of care in the adjuvant setting, cisplatin-ifosfamide is obviously a toxic regimen, and careful patient selection for such treatment is necessary.

Other agents active in carcinosarcoma include carboplatin and taxanes. The combination of carboplatin and paclitaxel was examined in a retrospective series at MSKCC and showed activity compared to (nonrandomized) patients who receive radiation alone. Carboplatin-paclitaxel is undergoing evaluation in a phase III clinical trial through the GOG as of 2013.

For metastatic disease, agents not used in the adjuvant setting can be considered. Cisplatin, ifosfamide, carboplatin, and paclitaxel all appear to have some activity. Topotecan has activity in metastatic disease [25], as may doxorubicin. The combination of gemcitabine and docetaxel [26] has minor activity. Imatinib, sorafenib, and thalidomide are all inactive against carcinosarcoma from phase II studies (Table 21.3).

Table 21.3 Uterine carcinosarcomas and other malignant mixed Müllerian tumors

Clinical scenario		Comments
Primary therapy		For completely resected disease, cisplatin-ifosfamide is superior to whole abdominal radiation therapy, but risk is still high for relapse; carboplatin-paclitaxel is reasonable in the adjuvant setting as well
Metastatic disease	1st line	Topotecan, platinum agents, taxanes, combinations
	2nd line	Gemcitabine or combinations, clinical trial

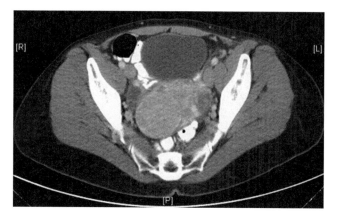

Fig. 21.8 Intravenous-enhanced contrast CT scan of a patient with a 6-cm PEComa of the uterus

PEComas

Perivascular epithelioid cell tumors (PEComas) are a relatively newly coined diagnostic category of tumors having hybrid smooth muscle and melanocytic differentiation. The uterus is among the most common sites of origin of this rare tumor (Fig. 21.8), and those tumors are described in a separate chapter.

Outcome

Outcome for primary adult carcinosarcoma by local and disease-specific survival is shown in Figs. 21.9 and 21.10. Outcome, as with other uterine malignancy, is highly stage dependent, with curative surgery with or without adjuvant therapy, and poor long-term prognosis in advanced or metastatic disease.

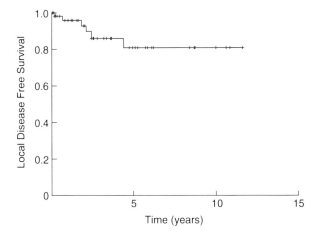

Fig. 21.9 Local disease-free survival for adult patients with primary uterine carcinosarcoma (malignant mixed Müllerian tumor). MSKCC 7/1/1982 to 6/30/2010 n = 56

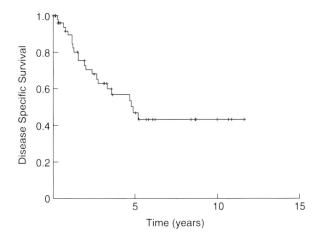

Fig. 21.10 Disease-specific survival for adult patients with primary uterine carcinosarcoma (malignant mixed Müllerian tumor). MSKCC 7/1/1982 to 6/30/2010 n = 56

References

1. Abrams J, Talcott J, Corson JM. Pulmonary metastases in patients with low-grade endometrial stromal sarcoma. Clinicopathologic findings with immunohistochemical characterization. Am J Surg Pathol. 1989;13(2):133–40.
2. Aubry MC, Myers JL, Colby TV, et al. Endometrial stromal sarcoma metastatic to the lung: a detailed analysis of 16 patients. Am J Surg Pathol. 2002;26(4):440–9.

3. Dal Cin P, Aly MS, De Wever I, et al. Endometrial stromal sarcoma t(7;17)(p15-21;q12-21) is a nonrandom chromosome change. Cancer Genet Cytogenet. 1992;63(1):43–6.

4. Koontz JI, Soreng AL, Nucci M, et al. Frequent fusion of the JAZF1 and JJAZ1 genes in endometrial stromal tumors. Proc Natl Acad Sci USA. 2001;98(11):6348–53.

5. Nucci MR, Harburger D, Koontz J, et al. Molecular analysis of the JAZF1-JJAZ1 gene fusion by RT-PCR and fluorescence in situ hybridization in endometrial stromal neoplasms. Am J Surg Pathol. 2007;31(1):65–70.

6. Oliva E, de Leval L, Soslow RA, et al. High frequency of JAZF1-JJAZ1 gene fusion in endometrial stromal tumors with smooth muscle differentiation by interphase FISH detection. Am J Surg Pathol. 2007;31(8):1277–84.

7. Barney B, Tward JD, Skidmore T, et al. Does radiotherapy or lymphadenectomy improve survival in endometrial stromal sarcoma? Int J Gynecol Cancer. 2009;19(7):1232–8.

8. Thomas MB, Keeney GL, Podratz KC, et al. Endometrial stromal sarcoma: treatment and patterns of recurrence. Int J Gynecol Cancer. 2009;19(2):253–6.

9. Shah JP, Bryant CS, Kumar S, et al. Lymphadenectomy and ovarian preservation in low-grade endometrial stromal sarcoma. Obstet Gynecol. 2008;112(5):1102–8.

10. Gadducci A, Sartori E, Landoni F, et al. Endometrial stromal sarcoma: analysis of treatment failures and survival. Gynecol Oncol. 1996;63(2):247–53.

11. Garrett A, Quinn MA. Hormonal therapies and gynaecological cancers. Best Pract Res Clin Obstet Gynaecol. 2008;22(2):407–21.

12. Reich O, Regauer S. Survey of adjuvant hormone therapy in patients after endometrial stromal sarcoma. Eur J Gynaecol Oncol. 2006;27(2):150–2.

13. Katz L, Merino MJ, Sakamoto H, et al. Endometrial stromal sarcoma: a clinicopathologic study of 11 cases with determination of estrogen and progestin receptor levels in three tumors. Gynecol Oncol. 1987;26(1):87–97.

14. Dahhan T, Fons G, Buist MR, et al. The efficacy of hormonal treatment for residual or recurrent low-grade endometrial stromal sarcoma. A retrospective study. Eur J Obstet Gynecol Reprod Biol. 2009;144(1):80–4.

15. Pink D, Lindner T, Mrozek A, et al. Harm or benefit of hormonal treatment in metastatic low-grade endometrial stromal sarcoma: single center experience with 10 cases and review of the literature. Gynecol Oncol. 2006;101(3):464–9.

16. Sutton G, Blessing JA, Park R, et al. Ifosfamide treatment of recurrent or metastatic endometrial stromal sarcomas previously unexposed to chemotherapy: a study of the Gynecologic Oncology Group. Obstet Gynecol. 1996;87(5 Pt 1):747–50.

17. Kurihara S, Oda Y, Ohishi Y, et al. Endometrial stromal sarcomas and related high-grade sarcomas: immunohistochemical and molecular genetic study of 31 cases. Am J Surg Pathol. 2008;32(8):1228–38.

18. Lee CH, Ou WB, Marino-Enriquez A, et al. 14-3-3 fusion oncogenes in high-grade endometrial stromal sarcoma. Proc Natl Acad Sci USA. 2012;109(3):929–34.

19. Lee C-HMDP, Marino-Enriquez AMD, Ou WP, et al. The Clinicopathologic Features of YWHAE-FAM22 Endometrial Stromal Sarcomas: a histologically high-grade and clinically aggressive tumor. Am J Surg Pathol. 2012;36(5):641–53.

20. O'Meara E, Stack D, Lee CH, et al. Characterization of the chromosomal translocation t(10;17)(q22;p13) in clear cell sarcoma of kidney. J Pathol. 2012;227(1):72–80.

21. Feng W, Malpica A, Robboy SJ, et al. Prognostic value of the diagnostic criteria distinguishing endometrial stromal sarcoma, low grade from undifferentiated endometrial sarcoma, 2 entities within the invasive endometrial stromal neoplasia family. Int J Gynecol Pathol. 2012;31(2):151–8.

22. Reed NS, Mangioni C, Malmstrom H, et al. Phase III randomised study to evaluate the role of adjuvant pelvic radiotherapy in the treatment of uterine sarcomas stages I and II: an European Organisation for Research and Treatment of Cancer Gynaecological Cancer Group Study (protocol 55874). Eur J Cancer. 2008;44(6):808–18.

23. Sampath S, Schultheiss TE, Ryu JK, et al. The role of adjuvant radiation in uterine sarcomas. Int J Radiat Oncol Biol Phys. 2010;76(3):728–34.
24. Wolfson AH, Brady MF, Rocereto T, et al. A gynecologic oncology group randomized phase III trial of whole abdominal irradiation (WAI) vs. cisplatin-ifosfamide and mesna (CIM) as post-surgical therapy in stage I-IV carcinosarcoma (CS) of the uterus. Gynecol Oncol. 2007;107(2):177–85.
25. Miller DS, Blessing JA, Schilder J, et al. Phase II evaluation of topotecan in carcinosarcoma of the uterus: a Gynecologic Oncology Group study. Gynecol Oncol. 2005;98(2):217–21.
26. Miller BE, Blessing JA, Stehman FB, et al. A phase II evaluation of weekly gemcitabine and docetaxel for second-line treatment of recurrent carcinosarcoma of the uterus: a Gynecologic Oncology Group Study. Gynecol Oncol. 2010;118(2):139–44.

Chapter 22
Extraskeletal Osteogenic Sarcoma

Osteogenic sarcoma can arise in soft tissue, although it is much more commonly observed as a primary bone tumor. There is debate as to whether extraskeletal osteogenic sarcoma (ESOS) should be managed as a soft tissue or a bone tumor. Biologically, the tumor is typically the osteoblastic subtype and can arise spontaneously or after irradiation.

Age distribution for adult patients over age 16 is shown in Fig. 22.1 and site distribution in Fig. 22.2. The lower extremity is the dominant site.

Imaging

Primary ESOS is often multilobulated in appearance and has evidence of calcification, as the tumor name implies (Figs. 22.3, 22.4, and 22.5). Bone invasion occurs (Fig. 22.6). Satellite lesions and soft tissue metastatic spread may be more common than with other soft tissue sarcoma subtypes, in our own experience.

Diagnosis

Microscopic pathology of ESOS lesions shows highly pleomorphic cells in a background of lacelike osteoid matrix, which is the basis for the calcification seen in masses radiographically (Fig. 22.7). As with other osteosarcomas, ESOS is aneuploid without defining molecular changes saved for mutations in DNA repair genes such as *TP53*.

M.F. Brennan et al., *Management of Soft Tissue Sarcoma*,
DOI 10.1007/978-1-4614-5004-7_22, © Springer Science+Business Media New York 2013

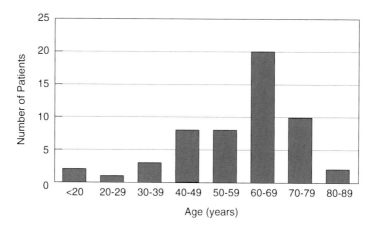

Fig. 22.1 Age distribution of adult patients with extraskeletal osteosarcoma. MSKCC 7/1/1982 to 6/30/2010 n = 54

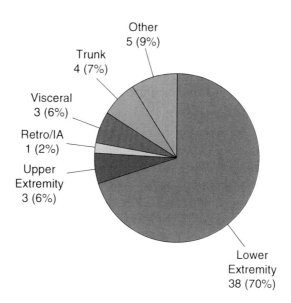

Fig. 22.2 Primary site distribution of adult patients with extraskeletal osteosarcoma. MSKCC 7/1/1982 to 6/30/2010 n = 54 *Retro/IA* retroperitoneal/intra-abdominal

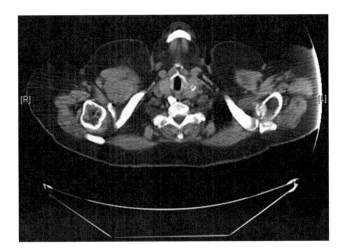

Fig. 22.3 Noncontrast CT image of a right subpectoral extraskeletal osteosarcoma

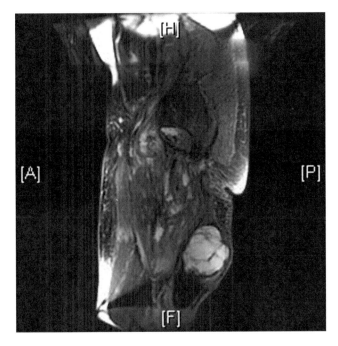

Fig. 22.4 T1-weighted MRI image of a left thigh extraskeletal osteosarcoma

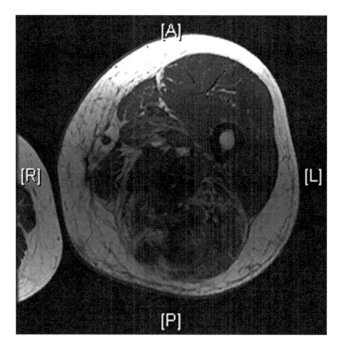

Fig. 22.5 T1-weighted MRI image of a left thigh extraskeletal osteosarcoma

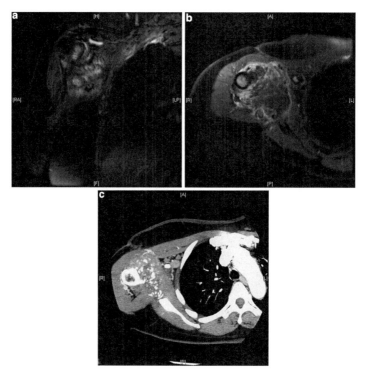

Fig. 22.6 Extraskeletal osteosarcoma bone invasion

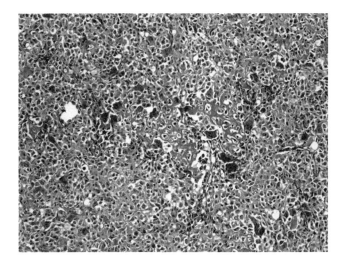

Fig. 22.7 Microscopic H&E image of high-grade extraskeletal osteosarcoma showing lacelike osteoid matrix deposition by highly pleomorphic sarcoma cells

Treatment

As with osteogenic sarcoma of bone, primary resection of ESOS is paramount. It is not clear if adjuvant irradiation or chemotherapy is helpful to improve the poor cure rate in adults. A number of patients in one of the few series published in adults received chemotherapy for metastatic disease with a low response rate, suggesting that adjuvant chemotherapy is not helpful for people with this diagnosis [1]. However, a summary of patients treated with ESOS on a pediatric clinical trial of osteogenic sarcoma of bone fared better than historical controls. [2] The topic remains unsettled as the long term event-free survival for the patients in these two studies was 56% in the German study (who received adjuvant chemotherapy) and 47% in the MD Anderson series (who did not receive adjuvant chemotherapy).

In the metastatic setting, agents active in osteosarcoma or soft tissue sarcoma can be utilized, but the response rate is low (Table 22.1).

Outcome

Most reports of this rare tumor consist of single case series. Local recurrence for adult patients treated primarily at MSKCC is shown in Fig. 22.8 and for those patients disease-specific survival in Fig. 22.9, with all disease-specific deaths occurring before 4 years and 5–10 year disease-specific survival of 50%. These data are consistent with the findings from the MD Anderson and European series and

Table 22.1 Systemic therapy recommendations for patients with extraskeletal osteogenic sarcoma

Clinical scenario		Comments
Adjuvant chemotherapy		Controversial; one study indicated patients fare better compared to historical controls with use of regimens used for osteosarcoma of bone
Metastatic disease	1st line	Ifosfamide-based therapy, if not given previously
	2nd line and greater	Gemcitabine or combinations; pazopanib; clinical trial

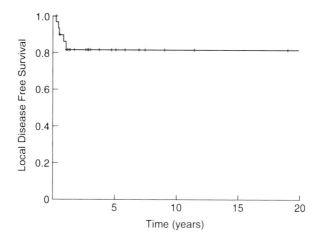

Fig. 22.8 Local disease-free survival of adult patients with primary extraskeletal osteosarcoma. MSKCC 7/1/1982 to 6/30/2010 n = 33

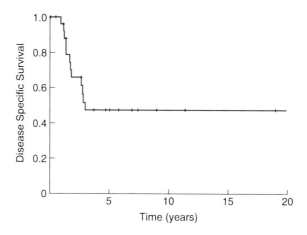

Fig. 22.9 Disease-specific survival of adult patients with primary extraskeletal osteosarcoma. MSKCC 7/1/1982 to 6/30/2010 n = 33

involved a group of patients who largely did not receive adjuvant chemotherapy. These data continue to call into question any benefit of adjuvant chemotherapy for this aggressive sarcoma subtype.

References

1. Ahmad SA, Patel SR, Ballo MT, Baker TP, Yasko AW, Wang X, et al. Extraosseous osteosarcoma: response to treatment and long-term outcome. J Clin Oncol. 2002;20(2):521–7.
2. Goldstein-Jackson SY, Gosheger G, Delling G, Berdel WE, Exner GU, Jundt G, et al. Extraskeletal osteosarcoma has a favourable prognosis when treated like conventional osteosarcoma. J Cancer Res Clin Oncol. 2005;131(8):520–6.

Chapter 23
Sustentacular Tumors of Lymph Tissue

As proof that cancers can occur in essentially any cell type, antigen-presenting cells (e.g., dendritic cells or Langerhans cells) can form cancers. Since these tumors can arise from lymph nodes, but do not arise from lymphocytes themselves, they are sometimes termed sarcomas. Other pathologists use the more noncommittal term "tumor" instead of "sarcoma" in this context. If anything, sustentacular tumors of lymphatic tissue represent the correct use of the term "histiocytic sarcoma," as opposed to malignant fibrous histiocytoma (MFH, now termed undifferentiated pleomorphic sarcoma [UPS]), which are not composed of histiocytes, as are these tumors.

Dendritic cell tumors, also termed reticulum cell tumors, can arise in either lymph nodes or extranodal lymphatic tissue. Follicular dendritic cell tumor (FDCT)/ dendritic reticulum cell tumors are tumors that affect the follicular dendritic cells that present antigens to B cells and as a result arise in germinal centers of lymph nodes. Conversely, interdigitating reticulum cell tumors (IDRCT) are conventional dendritic cells derived from Langerhans cells that migrate to lymph nodes, where they present antigen to T cells and thus arise in the cortex of the lymph node. Langerhans cell histiocytoses (LCH) can arise in skin, lung, and bone and represent a separate class of tumors associated with a variety of pathologies, such as lung infiltrates and pituitary dysfunction.

Characteristic markers of these rare tumors are indicated below for reference purposes (Table 23.1). Age and site distribution for these rare tumors presenting as primary lesions in adults is shown in Figs 23.1 and 23.2.

M.F. Brennan et al., *Management of Soft Tissue Sarcoma*,
DOI 10.1007/978-1-4614-5004-7_23, © Springer Science+Business Media New York 2013

Table 23.1 Immunohistochemical characteristics of sustentacular tumors of lymph tissue

Tumor type	CD21	CD35	S100	CD1a	Clusterin	CD11c	CD68	Desmin
FDCT	(+)	(+)	Occasionally (+)	(−)	(+)	(−)	(−)	(−)
IDRCT	(−)	(−)	(+)	Variable, usually (−)	(−)	(+)	(−)	(−)
LCH	(−)	(−)	Varies	(+)	(−)	(+)	(−)	(−)
True histiocytic sarcoma	(−)	(−)	Varies	(−)	(−)	(+)	(+)	(−)

FDCT follicular dendritic cell tumor, *IDRCT* interdigitating reticulum cell tumors, *LCH* Langerhans cell histiocytoses

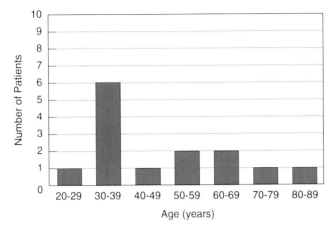

Fig. 23.1 Age distribution of adult patients with primary sustentacular malignancies of lymph nodes. MSKCC 7/1/1982 to 6/30/2010 n = 14

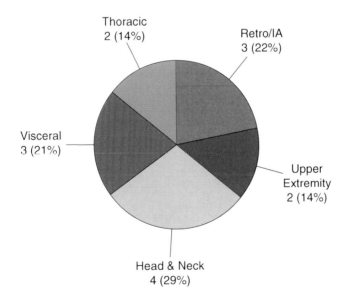

Fig. 23.2 Site distribution of adult patients with sustentacular malignancies of lymph nodes. MSKCC 7/1/1982 to 6/30/2010 n = 14 *Retro/IA* retroperitoneal/intra-abdominal

Follicular Dendritic Cell Tumor (Dendritic Reticulum Cell Tumor [FDCT]) and Interdigitating Reticulum Cell Tumor (IDRCT)

Reviews of series of these patients are helpful guides to FDCT and IDRCT [1–3]. Of the two diagnoses, IDRCT is the more aggressive. FDCT arise in neck lymph nodes more than in other sites such as abdomen; if limited in size, surgery can render patients disease-free. PET scan can be helpful in delineating other sites of tumor as these tumors demonstrate some features of Hodgkin lymphoma and some features of sarcomas, with spread to other local-regional lymph nodes as well as to lung and other sites. There is presently no characteristic genetic change known for FDCT or IDRCT, unlike Langerhans cell histiocytosis, in which *BRAF* mutations are common [3]. Clusterin, gamma-synuclein, CXCL13, and podoplanin may be markers for FDCT [3–6].

Since they are confused with non-Hodgkin lymphomas (NHL), it is not surprising that anthracycline-based regimens such as CHOP (cyclophosphamide-doxorubicin-vincristine-prednisone) have been used for both FDCT and IDRCT, with some success. In our experience, responses have been modest and much less pronounced than that seen for NHL or Hodgkin lymphoma. Nonetheless, given the high-risk nature of these tumors, adjuvant chemotherapy or chemotherapy and radiation therapy are considerations for patients with primary disease as one would treat some forms of lymphoma. For recurrent disease therapy, other NHL regimens are utilized. The role of high-dose therapy with stem cell support for patients with these diagnoses is unknown. We have also observed anecdotes of patients with responses to sorafenib and other multitargeted tyrosine kinase inhibitors. The target in FDCT and IDRCT is unknown but could be CSF1, M-CSF, FLT3, or others (Table 23.2).

True Histiocytic Sarcoma

Like FDCT and IDRCT, true histiocytic sarcoma is a tumor of antigen-presenting cells, in this case a monocyte-derived cell. It tends to occur in the skin and bowel, where in the former case Langerhans cell tumor is in the differential diagnosis, while

Table 23.2 Systemic therapy recommendations for patients with follicular dendritic cell tumor (dendritic reticulum cell tumor [FDCT]) and interdigitating reticulum cell tumor (IDRCT)

Clinical scenario		Comments
Adjuvant therapy		Consider vincristine-doxorubicin-cyclophosphamide-based therapy, local-regional radiation
Metastatic disease	1st line	Anthracycline-based therapy, if not given previously
	2nd line	Clinical trial; multitargeted kinase inhibitors of CSF1, M-CSF, FLT3, or BRAF may have activity

Table 23.3 Systemic therapy recommendations for patients with true histiocytic sarcoma

Clinical scenario		Comments
Adjuvant chemotherapy		Consider vincristine-doxorubicin-cyclophosphamide-based therapy
Metastatic disease	1st line	Anthracycline-based therapy, if not given before
	2nd line	Clinical trial; the activity of multitargeted tyrosine kinase inhibitors as discussed for FDCT and IDRCT is unknown

in the latter case FDCT and IDRCT are both in the differential diagnosis [7–9]. In this respect, we are concerned that M5 monocytic leukemia has to be considered in the differential diagnosis as well, and more complete evaluation for leukemia is warranted (e.g., bone marrow analysis). For these rare diagnoses with uncertain outcome (certainly some patients with recurrence and death from tumor), chemotherapy can be considered in the adjuvant or recurrent setting (Table 23.3).

Langerhans Cell Tumors

A large medical literature exists around conditions involving excessive Langerhans cells, including description of histiocytosis X (now termed Langerhans cell histiocytosis [LCH]), Letterer-Siwe syndrome (disseminated histiocytosis of children), and Hand-Schüller-Christian disease (osseous and skull base histiocytosis and diabetes insipidus), among others. Mortality in children was significant before the development of effective chemotherapy that forms a standard of care for children with LCH. The therapy for LCH is a function of organ involvement and is beyond the scope of this review. Good references regarding treatment were published in 2008 and 2010 [10, 11]. Comments regarding adult versus pediatric patients [11] and web sites help keep the community updated on expert centers and available treatment protocols [12] (Table 23.4).

Outcome

It is presently impossible to meaningfully predict outcomes from these rare lesions; however, for the primary presentation to our institution, local recurrence and disease-free survivals are shown in Figs. 23.3 and 23.4. Rare events such as spontaneous regression [13] have been reported. In a combined retrospective review of a Chinese series of 50 patients, much more favorable results were suggested, with as many as 80% alive and disease-free [14]; however, that has not been our experience. Any number of reasons, such as variances in pathology interpretation or stage at presentation, makes it difficult to compare across studies.

Table 23.4 Systemic therapy recommendations for patients with Langerhans cell tumors

Clinical scenario		Comments
Systemic chemotherapy		Depends on degree of organ involvement, usually vinblastine and/or methotrexate based; treatment will likely change with the finding of V600E BRAF mutations in over half of tumors
Recurrent disease	1st line	Salvage protocols
		See web site: www.histiocytesociety.org

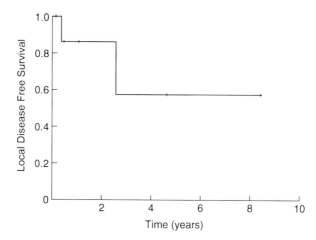

Fig. 23.3 Local recurrence-free survival of adult patients with primary sustentacular malignancies of lymph nodes. MSKCC 7/1/1982 to 6/30/2010 n = 8

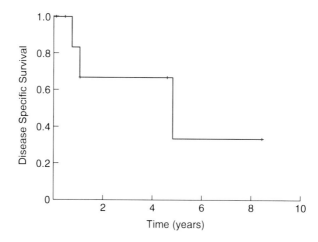

Fig. 23.4 Disease-specific survival of adult patients with primary sustentacular malignancies of lymph nodes. MSKCC 7/1/1982 to 6/30/2010 n = 8

References

1. Fonseca R, Yamakawa M, Nakamura S, et al. Follicular dendritic cell sarcoma and interdigitating reticulum cell sarcoma: a review. Am J Hematol. 1998;59(2):161–7.
2. Pileri SA, Grogan TM, Harris NL, et al. Tumours of histiocytes and accessory dendritic cells: an immunohistochemical approach to classification from the International Lymphoma Study Group based on 61 cases. Histopathology. 2002;41(1):1–29.
3. Grogg KL, Lae ME, Kurtin PJ, et al. Clusterin expression distinguishes follicular dendritic cell tumors from other dendritic cell neoplasms: report of a novel follicular dendritic cell marker and clinicopathologic data on 12 additional follicular dendritic cell tumors and 6 additional interdigitating dendritic cell tumors. Am J Surg Pathol. 2004;28(8):988–98.
4. Zhang H, Maitta RW, Bhattacharyya PK, et al. gamma-Synuclein is a promising new marker for staining reactive follicular dendritic cells, follicular dendritic cell sarcoma, Kaposi sarcoma, and benign and malignant vascular tumors. Am J Surg Pathol. 2011;35(12):1857–65.
5. Vermi W, Lonardi S, Bosisio D, et al. Identification of CXCL13 as a new marker for follicular dendritic cell sarcoma. J Pathol. 2008;216(3):356–64.
6. Xie Q, Chen L, Fu K, et al. Podoplanin (d2-40): a new immunohistochemical marker for reactive follicular dendritic cells and follicular dendritic cell sarcomas. Int J Clin Exp Pathol. 2008;1(3):276–84.
7. Mongkonsritragoon W, Li CY, Phyliky RL. True malignant histiocytosis. Mayo Clin Proc. 1998;73(6):520–8.
8. Elghetany MT. True histiocytic lymphoma: is it an entity? Leukemia. 1997;11(5):762–4.
9. Soria C, Orradre JL, Garcia-Almagro D, et al. True histiocytic lymphoma (monocytic sarcoma). Am J Dermatopathol. 1992;14(6):511–7.
10. Gadner H, Grois N, Potschger U, et al. Improved outcome in multisystem Langerhans cell histiocytosis is associated with therapy intensification. Blood. 2008;111(5):2556–62.
11. Gadner H. Treatment of adult-onset Langerhans cell histiocytosis–is it different from the pediatric approach? Ann Oncol. 2010;21(6):1141–2.
12. Histiocyte Society. The Histiocyte Society--home page. 2009. http://www.histiocytesociety.org/. Accessed 12 Aug 2010.
13. De Leon Caces DB, Daniel S, Paredes-Tejada JM, et al. Spontaneous regression of follicular dendritic cell sarcoma. J Clin Oncol. 2012;30(3):e24–6.
14. Wang H, Su Z, Hu Z, et al. Follicular dendritic cell sarcoma: a report of six cases and a review of the Chinese literature. Diagn Pathol. 2010;5:67.

Chapter 24
Uncommon/Unique Sites

Heart and Great Vessels

The heart and great vessels are rare sites of primary sarcoma but are more commonly observed as the site of metastatic disease [1]. While the clinical presentation is varied from an incidental finding to peripheral emboli to congestive cardiac failure, cardiac sarcomas should be suspected in patients who have undergone prior mediastinal radiation. As a metastatic site, various histologies can be seen, whereas primary lesions tend to be either angiosarcoma, leiomyosarcoma, or undifferentiated. A diagnosis unique to this site is intimal sarcoma. Other histologies may rarely include synovial sarcoma (Fig. 24.1) and hemangioendothelioma (Fig. 24.2). Histologies of sarcomas of the mediastinum are indicated in Fig. 24.3 and represent a subset of sarcomas of heart and great vessels. The second most common histology is high-grade undifferentiated pleomorphic sarcoma (UPS). A recent update [2] suggests that primary cardiac sarcomas represent 20% of all primary cardiac tumors and diagnosis is predominantly made by transthoracic echocardiography and subsequent sampling.

Primary treatment is surgical, and increasingly with the opportunities for cardiopulmonary bypass and arrest, this is possible. In selective situations, cardiac transplantation can be utilized [3]. There is consideration that cardiac transplantation should be reserved for patients with low-grade tumors as the risk for metastatic disease in high-grade tumors is so high and the consequences of transplantation and immunosuppression are significantly detrimental to question the value of such an approach. Chemotherapy can be utilized, but it is only of palliative value.

M.F. Brennan et al., *Management of Soft Tissue Sarcoma*,
DOI 10.1007/978-1-4614-5004-7_24, © Springer Science+Business Media New York 2013

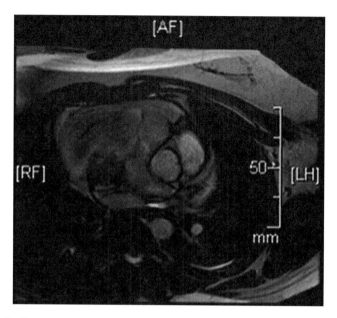

Fig. 24.1 Cardiac-gated T1-weighted MRI image of a synovial sarcoma arising in the great vessels

The therapeutic options are suggested to be those containing anthracyclines, ifosfamide, or taxanes. Median survival is approximately 9–16 months with patients with left atrial lesions apparently having an improved prognosis, but this would appear to be predominantly due to the fact that they are more commonly of low histological grade and often are technically resectable. Myxomas are common in comparison to primary cardiac sarcoma and only rarely present with metastatic lesions. Systemic therapy for such metastases is undefined.

Primary Sarcomas of the Breast

Primary sarcomas of the breast constitute <5% of all soft tissue sarcomas and <1% of all breast tumors. At Memorial Sloan-Kettering Cancer Center between July 1982 and June 2010, the types of tumors seen in the breast are shown in Fig. 24.4. One of the more common lesions is cystosarcoma phyllodes, also termed phyllodes tumor (see below). Angiosarcoma is commonly seen in the breast usually postradiation with or without chemotherapy, but other sarcomatous types can be seen with these radiation-associated tumors (see Predisposing and Genetic Factors in Chap. 1). Primary angiosarcoma of breast is less common and occurs in younger patients, typically in their third decade of life, and shows an infiltrative growth

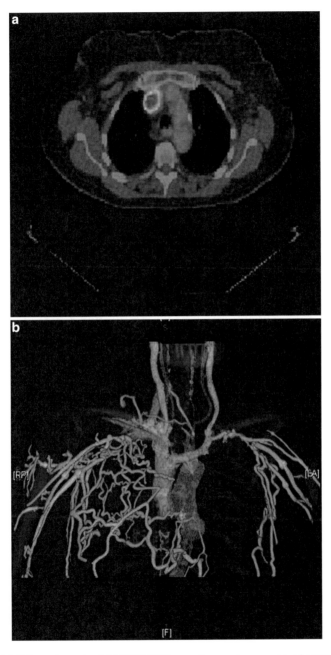

Fig. 24.2 (a) Color-enhanced axial 18FDE-PET scan of a superior vena cava hemangioendothelioma. (b) Color-enhanced 3-dimensional reconstructed computed tomography of the same superior vena cava hemangioendothelioma

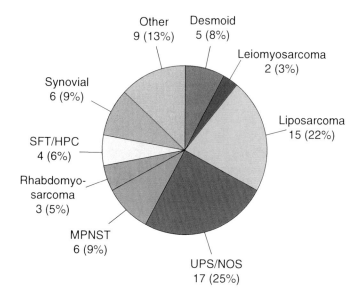

Fig. 24.3 Distribution of histologies of adult primary soft tissue malignancies of the mediastinum. *MSKCC* 7/1/1982 to 6/30/2010 n=67 *SFT* solitary fibrous tumor, *HPC* hemangiopericytoma, *MPNST* malignant peripheral nerve sheath tumor, *UPS* undifferentiated pleomorphic sarcoma, *NOS* not otherwise specified

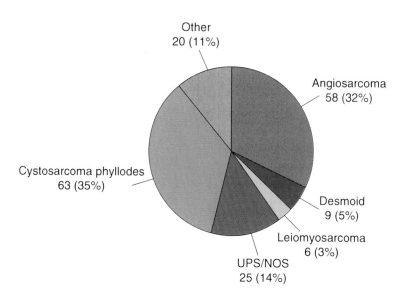

Fig. 24.4 Distribution of histologies of adult primary soft tissue malignancies of the breast. MSKCC 7/1/1982 to 6/30/2010 n=181 *UPS* undifferentiated pleomorphic sarcoma, *NOS* not otherwise specified

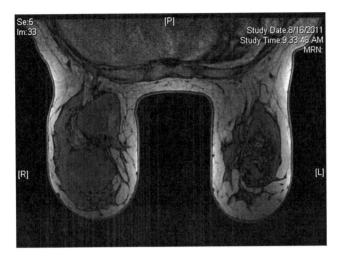

Fig. 24.5 T1-weighted MRI image of a patient with a right breast phyllodes tumor (cystosarcoma phyllodes)

pattern within breast parenchyma. In contrast, secondary postradiation breast/chest wall angiosarcomas involve the skin, as multifocal lesions, in elderly patients (see angiosarcoma, Chap. 13.) Treatment is similar to that of other sarcomas, i.e., complete operative excision with or without radiation and subsequent chemotherapy. As with other sarcomas, ancillary nodal dissection is rarely indicated as these tumors rarely spread to lymph nodes [4].

Phyllodes Tumor

Phyllodes tumor is a rare entity thought to arise from predisposing fibroadenoma. This lesion, often considered benign, does have a malignant subtype. The majority of patients are premenopausal, and a retrospective study of 84 patients [5] suggests the median age as 34 years for benign lesions compared to 52 years for those with malignant change. In another review of 124 patients, tumors were benign in 49%, borderline in 35%, and malignant in 16%. It was suggested that malignancy may be more common in patients of Hispanic origin, but referral bias is likely [6].

Patients present with a large painless breast mass which can reach a very large size. The tumor is variegated in color often with cystic areas. Myxoid degeneration is common (Fig. 24.5).

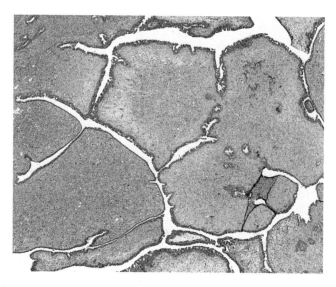

Fig. 24.6 Low-power H&E image of a phyllodes tumor of the breast, demonstrating the clefts seen in the gross tumor specimen

Diagnosis

The challenge to define benign from malignant is difficult [7]. The malignant type is described as being similar to adult-type fibrosarcoma. Imaging studies are similar, although on occasion MRI or CT evidence of neoplastic dystrophic tissue containing cartilage or bone can be identified.

Grossly, these tumors are firm and lobulated and on cut surface have a leaflike architecture (phyllos means leaf in Greek). They are well circumscribed grossly, and the cut surface shows a whirling pattern with visible clefts. Larger tumors will present with cystic spaces and areas of necrosis and/or hemorrhage. Microscopically, these tumors have two elements, like fibroadenomas, having clefts with epithelial cell lining as well as a cellular stromal component (Fig. 24.6). The appearance of the stromal element can vary from relatively benign appearing to frank sarcomatous change with stromal overgrowth, nuclear atypia, higher mitotic rate, and stromal overgrowth of the glandular component. There are now criteria to help predict the risk of recurrence based on clinical and pathologic factors [8]. These tumors are aneuploid, and research is underway to identify specific molecular defects.

Simple mastectomy is usually the primary treatment of choice as lymph node metastasis is uncommon. Breast-conserving surgery could be considered in an appropriate patient, but given the local recurrence risk, immediate reconstruction seems inadvisable.

Phyllodes tumors are largely unresponsive to chemotherapy or hormonal therapy. Adjuvant chemotherapy is not administered to patients, and patients should be considered for clinical trials even in first line for metastatic disease. Ifosfamide-based therapy is a reasonable option for patients without clinical trial options.

Outcome

In one series with limited follow-up, local recurrence of 6% was associated with tumor size, grade, mitotic rate, and margin status, similar to other sarcomas [6].

Head and Neck

Head and neck sarcomas are rare. They usually present as a mass lesion, and the histology is widely diverse (Fig. 24.7). Because of utilization of radiation therapy for lymphoma and other head and neck diseases, sarcoma that is radiation associated is a particularly difficult problem.

As with other sites, imaging predominantly utilizes CT and MRI to determine the extent of the lesion, particularly the involvement of vital structures. Diagnosis is

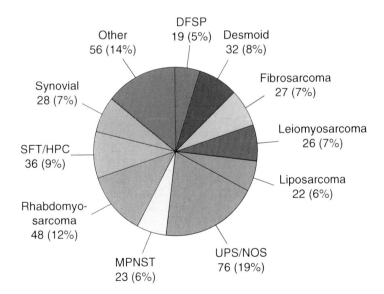

Fig. 24.7 Distribution of histologies of adult primary soft tissue malignancies of the head and neck. MSKCC 7/1/1982 to 6/30/2010 n=393 *DFSP* dermatofibrosarcoma protuberans, *MPNST* malignant peripheral nerve sheath tumor, *UPS* undifferentiated pleomorphic sarcoma, *NOS* not otherwise specified, *SFT* solitary fibrous tumor, *HPC* hemangiopericytoma

consistent with other sites based on molecular histopathology. Often, given the rarity of sarcomas, they are confused with primary epithelial neoplasms of the head and neck and oropharynx. Identification can often focus on the presence or absence of lymph node metastasis, which, while common in epithelial lesions, is very uncommon in soft tissue sarcoma. Diagnosis is usually made by core needle biopsy, and it is important to establish that a sarcoma is suspected when there is a mass lesion without a primary identified.

Treatment

Treatment is absolutely constrained because of the close juxtaposition of tumors to major arterial, venous, and neurological structures. The consequence is that, while complete surgical resection remains the primary form of therapy, radiation is more commonly used given the limitations of resection and margin. Preoperative treatment, particularly chemotherapy or radiation in high-grade lesions, can be considered even when the lesions are <5 cm. In similar fashion, adjuvant radiation therapy is perhaps more commonly used than in other sites owing to the morbidity of procedures in the head and neck. Very few valuable studies exist. However, Glenn et al. [9] showed that chemotherapy was utilized in 31 patients in a randomized trial. Patients in this group who had complete resection received between 60 and 63 Gy over 8 weeks and adjuvant chemotherapy with doxorubicin, cyclophosphamide, and methotrexate. That study, which has not been reproduced, was at a time when the amount of doxorubicin given was considerably in excess of what would be considered appropriate now. Three-year actuarial survival in the chemotherapy arm was 77% compared to 49% in the no-chemotherapy arm ($p = 0.075$). Actuarial overall survival was not different, being 68% in both arms. The high probability is that despite the small numbers, no proven benefit of adjuvant chemoradiation therapy is established.

A review of our experience has been published [10]. In that study, 60 patients over a 7-year period were identified. The most common site was on the face, and the majority of patients presented having had previous treatment. Again, as with other sites of disease, control was improved in low-grade tumors compared to high-grade tumors. Despite close or positive margins, 50% of those patients did not recur locally. Overall survival was 70%, and disease-free survival was 60%. Further information is best provided by referring to the relevant histopathology section.

Primary Sarcomas of the Mediastinum

The wide variation in histopathology for this anatomic site is demonstrated in Fig. 24.3. We have previously reported our limited experience with this particularly rare entity [11]. Forty-seven patients with a median age of 39 years were treated, and all varieties of sarcoma were identified. As with other sites, primary treatment is operation, but only 22 of 47 of those patients were able to undergo complete resection. As a consequence, local recurrence is very high, over 60% in the reported study by Burt. Because of poor local control, overall survival is poor, approximately 30%, and as with other sites, high-grade lesions fair worse than low-grade lesions. Sarcomas arising from mediastinal (and other) germ cell tumors present a unique problem in management. Like nonseminomas, both surgery and chemotherapy are typically employed, as may be radiation on a case-by-case basis. Over time a standard of using chemotherapy directed both against the germ cell tumor as well as the specific sarcoma subtype is generally employed, be it rhabdomyosarcoma, angiosarcoma, or other specific diagnoses. Sarcomas in this setting will be i12p positive, confirming their germ cell origin. Their outcome is poor in comparison to patients with primary germ cell tumors (of both testis and mediastinum) alone [12–14]. Further information is available under the relevant section based on histopathology.

Liver

Certain histopathologies are relatively common or specific to the liver. Epithelioid hemangioendothelioma is a vascular sarcoma that frequently presents with multifocal disease in the liver, lungs, and pleura, described further in Chap. 14, Fig. 14.4. Unique to the liver is embryonal sarcoma, a primitive small round blue cell tumor treated much like Ewing sarcoma. More information on this rare diagnosis is found in Chap. 15 on sarcomas more common in children. Rhabdomyosarcoma is occasionally found in the biliary tree in children and must be distinguished from embryonal sarcoma in children. GIST abutting the liver or metastatic to liver is more common in older adults.

Even rarer is desmoplastic nested spindle cell tumor, also described briefly in Chap. 15. Far more common is the liver as a metastatic site from sarcoma, frequently from GIST or visceral leiomyosarcoma.

References

1. Putnam Jr JB, Sweeney MS, Colon R, et al. Primary cardiac sarcomas. Ann Thorac Surg. 1991;51(6):906–10.
2. Orlandi A, Ferlosio A, Roselli M, et al. Cardiac sarcomas: an update. J Thorac Oncol. 2010;5(9):1483–9.
3. Michler RE, Goldstein DJ. Treatment of cardiac tumors by orthotopic cardiac transplantation. Semin Oncol. 1997;24(5):534–9.
4. Moore MP, Kinne DW. Breast sarcoma. Surg Clin North Am. 1996;76(2):383–92.
5. Zissis C, Apostolikas N, Konstantinidou A, et al. The extent of surgery and prognosis of patients with phyllodes tumor of the breast. Breast Cancer Res Treat. 1998;48(3):205–10.
6. Pimiento JM, Gadgil PV, Santillan AA, et al. Phyllodes tumors: race-related differences. J Am Coll Surg. 2011;213(4):537–42.

7. Rajan PB, Cranor ML, Rosen PP. Cystosarcoma phyllodes in adolescent girls and young women: a study of 45 patients. Am J Surg Pathol. 1998;22(1):64–9.

8. Taira N, Takabatake D, Aogi K, et al. Phyllodes tumor of the breast: stromal overgrowth and histological classification are useful prognosis-predictive factors for local recurrence in patients with a positive surgical margin. Jpn J Clin Oncol. 2007;37(10):730–6.

9. Glenn J, Kinsella T, Glatstein E, et al. A randomized, prospective trial of adjuvant chemotherapy in adults with soft tissue sarcomas of the head and neck, breast, and trunk. Cancer. 1985;55(6):1206–14.

10. Kraus DH, Dubner S, Harrison LB, et al. Prognostic factors for recurrence and survival in head and neck soft tissue sarcomas. Cancer. 1994;74(2):697–702.

11. Burt M, Ihde JK, Hajdu SI, et al. Primary sarcomas of the mediastinum: results of therapy. J Thorac Cardiovasc Surg. 1998;115(3):671–80.

12. Contreras AL, Punar M, Tamboli P, et al. Mediastinal germ cell tumors with an angiosarcomatous component: a report of 12 cases. Hum Pathol. 2010;41(6):832–7.

13. Ehrlich Y, Beck SD, Ulbright TM, et al. Outcome analysis of patients with transformed teratoma to primitive neuroectodermal tumor. Ann Oncol. 2010;21(9):1846–50.

14. Donadio AC, Motzer RJ, Bajorin DF, et al. Chemotherapy for teratoma with malignant transformation. J Clin Oncol. 2003;21(23):4285–91.

Part II
Benign and Less
Aggressive Lesions: Introduction

In contrast to the soft tissue sarcomas and other tumors mentioned in the prior section, in these sections diagnoses that are generally benign are outlined. Some of these lesions can present a significant local-regional recurrence risk, while occasional higher grade or familial versions of the lesions noted in Chap. 25 can indeed be multifocal or metastasize and be responsible for patient deaths. Chapter 26 discusses common benign lesions, which are at least 100 fold more common than soft tissue sarcomas. Chapter 27 briefly discusses reactive lesions that can be confused from time to time with sarcomas. The link between these less aggressive lesions and more aggressive soft tissue or bone sarcomas remains largely mysterious. Attention to the less aggressive lesions may give us insights into the more aggressive lesions described in the sections of Part I.

Chapter 25
Mostly Benign/Rarely Metastasizing Soft Tissue Tumor

Ossifying Fibromyxoid Tumor

Ossifying fibromyxoid tumor (OFMT) is a very uncommon soft tissue lesion that can occur anywhere in the body but most commonly in the lower extremity. While most tumors are benign, malignant examples may metastasize in more than half of cases [1]. The largest series to date included only typical cases, excluding tumors with other morphologies, and in that series there were no patients who developed metastatic disease. In the few patients that we have observed recurrences, metastases are observed, typically to lung, and local-regional recurrence can be observed in a multifocal "shotgun" pattern around the area of the tumor, as has been observed in patients with epithelioid sarcoma.

The cell of origin of these tumors is unknown, and there is no specific genetic alteration known to occur in OFMT. Radiographically, scattered calcifications can be found throughout the lesion. Primary treatment of these tumors mirrors that of other soft tissue tumors, surgery and radiation for larger tumors, but adjuvant chemotherapy is difficult to recommend as the response rate to standard agents is very low. Given the relatively slow growth rate of the tumor, sustained exposure with lower doses of an agent continuously would appear a better means to treat these tumors than high-dose therapy over the short term. The few patients we have treated have not responded durably to standard agents, so new options for care are needed (Fig. 25.1) (Table 25.1).

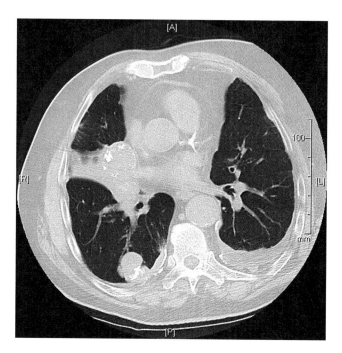

Fig. 25.1 Noncontrast CT image of metastatic ossifying fibromyxoid tumor featuring pleural effusions, lung and pleural-based metastases, and speckled calcification of the metastatic deposits

Table 25.1 Systemic therapeutic recommendations for ossifying fibromyxoid tumor

Clinical scenario		Comments
Adjuvant chemotherapy		Not administered outside the setting of a clinical trial, given the poor response rate in the metastatic setting
Metastatic disease	1st line	Clinical trial; standard agents (doxorubicin, ifosfamide) appear largely inactive

Perivascular Epithelioid Cell Tumor (PEComa) and Related Entities: Lymphangioleiomyomatosis, Angiomyolipoma, and Sugar Cell Tumor

The PEComa family of tumors includes a variety of tumors that express markers of both smooth muscle and melanocytes [2]. Thus, they are positive for SMA (smooth muscle actin) as well as for melanocytes markers such as HMB45 and melan-A. A variety of names for these tumors have been developed before the concept of PEComa was recognized as a distinct biological entity, on the basis of all lesions containing perivascular epithelioid cells, an unusual cell with no recognized normal counterpart. As a result, the PEComa family of tumors encompasses a variety of diagnoses such as angiomyolipoma, clear cell "sugar" tumors of the lung and other sites, lymphangioleiomyomatosis, and tumors with a similar morphology at a variety of other sites. At least a subset of these tumors, perhaps best demonstrated by angiomyolipoma, show inactivation of *TSC2* (tuberin). Tuberin is one of the genes associated with tuberous sclerosis, as is *TSC1*, also called hamartin [3, 4].

By virtue of their *TSC2* loss, angiomyolipomas and other PEComas show activation of the mammalian target of rapamycin (mTOR) and activate a program of transcription and translation with the cell as a result [5, 6]. mTOR exists with other proteins in two complexes, mTORC1 and mTORC2. First-generation TOR inhibitors such as sirolimus only block mTORC1 but do not affect mTORC2 signaling, providing a bypass pathway for signaling when mTORC1 is blocked.

Therapy

Primary treatment is surgical, when feasible; radiation plays little role in the primary treatment of these tumors since they tend to be visceral (Fig. 25.2). For patients with unresectable or recurrent disease, mTORC1 inhibitors, such as sirolimus, have been proven clinically useful in patients with recurrent angiomyolipoma [7], lymphangioleiomyomatosis [7], and recently in recurrent/metastatic PEComas [8, 9]. We have observed that responses to mTORC1 inhibitors are not as robust as that of imatinib in GIST, with median duration of response on the order of 6–12 months. It is not clear if mTOR inhibitors beyond sirolimus are useful for this diagnosis, but it is the opinion of the authors that the near equivalence of most of the first-generation mTOR inhibitors speaks to their interchangeability and lack of activity of the others if one of them fails. We have not observed activity of anthracyclines or of ifosfamide in the small number of patients we have treated with standard agents, arguing that such patients are appropriate for clinical trials. Less investigated agents such as combinations containing gemcitabine, or agents yielding greater "area under the curve," may be worth examining (Table 25.2).

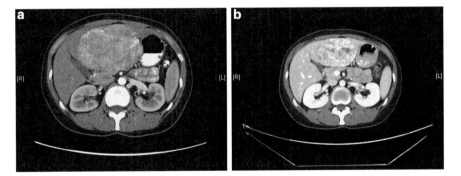

Fig. 25.2 CT response of a recurrent angiomyolipoma (PEComa family of tumors) to sirolimus 4 mg oral daily. (**a**) Pretreatment, 12.6×7.6 cm mass; (**b**) after 3 months, mass size 9.1×5.6 cm

Table 25.2 Systemic therapeutic recommendations for perivascular epithelial cell tumor (PEComa) and related entities, lymphangioleiomyomatosis, angiomyolipoma, and sugar cell tumor of the pancreas

Clinical scenario		Comments
Adjuvant chemotherapy		Not administered due to low risk of relapse and lack of long-term efficacy of systemic agents in the recurrent setting
Metastatic disease	1st line	Sirolimus or other mTOR inhibitors
	2nd line	Gemcitabine-based therapy; clinical trial; standard anthracyclines and ifosfamide appear inactive

Giant Cell Tumor of Tendon Sheath/ Pigmented Villonodular Synovitis

Giant cell tumor of tendon sheath (TGCT), also termed pigmented villonodular synovitis (PVNS), is an uncommon neoplasm of the synovium of joints that can occur in any joint but most commonly affects fingers. Unlike synovial sarcoma, which does not appear to be related nor resemble synovium microscopically, TGCT/PVNS is a true tumor of the synovium. The tumor comes in several forms: a localized variety most common in small joints, a diffuse type more common in large joints like the knee, and an extra-articular variety.

The key finding that has changed treatment for TGCT/PVNS is the consistent translocation t(1;2)(p11;q36-37) (*COL6A3-CSF1*) found in a minority of the cells of the lesion, which leads to the production of CSF-1 and presumed activation of FMS (the M-CSF receptor), and local cytokine production that leads to the characteristic inflammatory changes in the lesion [10].

The tumor presents as an inflammatory mass and/or effusion. Primary therapy consists of primary resection, but recurrence is common within several years of primary diagnosis, typically with the diffuse variety of the tumor (Fig. 25.3). Rare cases of metastatic disease to lung are reported. In the past, postoperative intra-articular radioactive phosphate (labeled with ^{32}P) or ^{90}Y (yttrium) has been used as an antiproliferative measure for recurrence of disease [11], though there is significant toxicity in treating at least certain anatomic sites with intra-articular radionuclides [12, 13]. Postoperative external beam radiation (~35 Gy) has been used successfully in some patients with recurrence of disease [11, 13]. The long-term effects of moderate-dose radiation in terms of joint function and secondary cancers are unknown.

As a coincidence, imatinib blocks FMS (as well as BCR-ABL, KIT, PDGFRs, and other targets), owing to their structural similarity, and there are anecdotes of patient responses to imatinib [14]. In the index case study, a responding patient stopped therapy and the lesion recurred rapidly but then responded again to another course of imatinib [15]. Other anecdotes support this finding; thus, FMS-directed therapy appears to be one option for care for TGCT/PVNS, although it does not

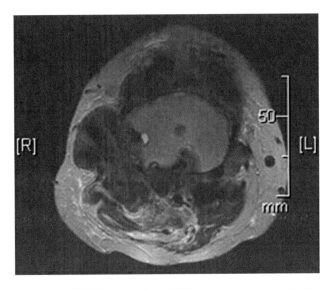

Fig. 25.3 T1-weighted axial MRI image of a multiply recurrent tenosynovial giant cell tumor of the knee

Table 25.3 Systemic therapeutic recommendations for giant cell tumor of tendon sheath/pigmented villonodular synovitis

Clinical scenario		Comments
Adjuvant chemotherapy		Not administered due to low risk of relapse
Recurrent/metastatic disease	1st line	Reoperation; imatinib
	2nd line	Alternative tyrosine kinase inhibitor; surgery and external beam radiation; surgery and intra-articular radionuclide; clinical trial

appear to represent definitive therapy like repeat resection and external beam radiation. A recent experience collecting anecdotes from several centers demonstrated that there was significant activity of imatinib in TGCT/PVNS, but given the concern of recall bias, these data may represent an upper estimate of activity [16] (Table 25.3).

Giant cell tumors of soft tissue can rarely be seen in other sites. They usually occur subcutaneously but can be seen in deep muscle tissue. The cytological characteristics are often clear and can be identified by aspiration cytology. The majority behave in a benign fashion although rare malignant counterparts occur. Surgical excision is usually curative.

Myoepithelioma of Soft Tissue

Myoepithelioma of soft tissue is a distinct entity from the pleomorphic adenoma arising in salivary glands, from which myoepithelial carcinoma can develop. Myoepithelioma of soft tissue is an extremely rare benign neoplasm which typically occurs in the superficial or deep soft tissue of the limbs or head and neck of both children and adults (Fig. 25.4). However, as in the salivary glands, transition to myoepithelial carcinoma has been reported, along with an unusual fusion gene, *EWSR1-ZNF444* [17]. Recently other fusion partners have been described, in particular *POU5F1* and *PBX1* [18]. Soft tissue myoepithelial tumors are defined by the coexpression of cytokeratin, vimentin, S100 protein, and smooth muscle actin. In a recent review [19], treatment is standard surgical resection and the majority of the lesions behave in a benign or indolent fashion such that surgery is curative. As mentioned, malignant examples can occur, often with a virulent course.

Chemotherapy is not well defined for patients with such recurrences. It is difficult to more than speculate on treatment given the few cases of this family of tumors treated in the literature [20].

Glomus Tumor

Glomus tumors must not be confused with paragangliomas (e.g., glomus faciale, glomus jugulare, glomus tympanicum, glomus vagale, or carotid body tumors) as pertains to anatomy and terminology [21]. While paragangliomas can occur associated

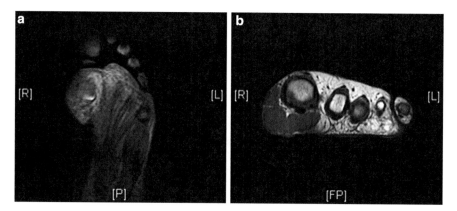

Fig. 25.4 Coronal (**a**) and axial (**b**) T1-weighted MRI images of a left foot low-grade myoepithelioma involving flexor hallucis longus and subcutaneous tissue

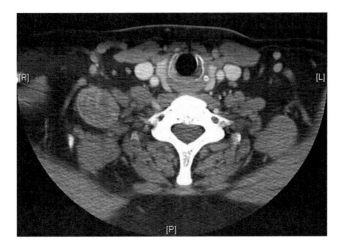

Fig. 25.5 Axial contrast-enhanced CT image of a malignant glomus tumor of the right neck

with the carotid body, for example, glomus tumors are tumors of the cells that give rise to glomus bodies, the specialized smooth muscle that controls blood flow to the periphery/skin. Glomus tumors have histology that can be classified by their predominant components, for example, glomangioma, glomangiomyoma, and rare malignant counterparts called malignant glomus tumor or glomangiosarcoma, among other varieties.

Benign glomus tumors, which have a broad age distribution among adults, classically present as painful lesions in a subungual location on the fingers or on the skin of the distal extremities. Treatment is surgical for what are typically small tumors [22–24]. They are also occasionally found in the wall of the stomach and less commonly in other visceral locations, and again surgery is typically curative (Fig. 25.5). These lesions are positive for smooth muscle actin, like leiomyomas and leiomyosarcomas.

Remarkably, there is a familial condition involving familial glomus tumors, which are called glomangiomas or glomangiovenous malformations, mimicking arteriovenous malformations [25–29]. Multiple discolored lesions are found in the skin in this condition, in which their germ line mutations are found in the glomulin gene on chromosome 1p.

For the rare person with a malignant glomus tumor (in which there is evidence of mitotic activity or atypical mitotic figures), metastatic spread to lungs is common (similar to leiomyosarcomas) or to peritoneum or bowel. Chemotherapy is undefined for such rare lesions, but agents typically used for leiomyosarcoma for the rare patient requiring chemotherapy can be suggested based on histology alone, although there are no reports of therapy in the literature (Table 25.4).

Table 25.4 Treatment recommendations for malignant glomus tumor

Primary disease	Surgical resection; no adjuvant chemotherapy or radiation is employed
Recurrent/metastatic disease	Clinical trials; we speculate that doxorubicin, dacarbazine, or gemcitabine-based therapy is reasonable if there are no clinical trial options

References

1. Folpe AL, Weiss SW. Ossifying fibromyxoid tumor of soft parts: a clinicopathologic study of 70 cases with emphasis on atypical and malignant variants. Am J Surg Pathol. 2003;27(4):421–31.
2. Folpe AL, Mentzel T, Lehr HA, et al. Perivascular epithelioid cell neoplasms of soft tissue and gynecologic origin: a clinicopathologic study of 26 cases and review of the literature. Am J Surg Pathol. 2005;29(12):1558–75.
3. Kenerson H, Folpe AL, Takayama TK, et al. Activation of the mTOR pathway in sporadic angiomyolipomas and other perivascular epithelioid cell neoplasms. Hum Pathol. 2007;38(9): 1361–71.
4. El-Hashemite N, Zhang H, Henske EP, et al. Mutation in TSC2 and activation of mammalian target of rapamycin signalling pathway in renal angiomyolipoma. Lancet. 2003;361(9366): 1348–9.
5. Kwiatkowski DJ. Animal models of lymphangioleiomyomatosis (LAM) and tuberous sclerosis complex (TSC). Lymphat Res Biol. 2010;8(1):51–7.
6. Martignoni G, Pea M, Reghellin D, et al. Molecular pathology of lymphangioleiomyomatosis and other perivascular epithelioid cell tumors. Arch Pathol Lab Med. 2010;134(1):33–40.
7. Lee JS, Fetsch JF, Wasdhal DA, et al. A review of 40 patients with extraskeletal osteosarcoma. Cancer. 1995;76(11):2253–9.
8. Italiano A, Delcambre C, Hostein I, et al. Treatment with the mTOR inhibitor temsirolimus in patients with malignant PEComa. Ann Oncol. 2010;21(5):1135–7.
9. Wagner AJ, Malinowska-Kolodziej I, Morgan JA, et al. Clinical activity of mTOR inhibition with sirolimus in malignant perivascular epithelioid cell tumors: targeting the pathogenic activation of mTORC1 in tumors. J Clin Oncol. 2010;28(5):835–40.
10. West RB, Rubin BP, Miller MA, et al. A landscape effect in tenosynovial giant-cell tumor from activation of CSF1 expression by a translocation in a minority of tumor cells. Proc Natl Acad Sci USA. 2006;103(3):690–5.
11. O'Sullivan C. The psychosocial determinants of depression: a lifespan perspective. J Nerv Ment Dis. 2004;192(9):585–94.
12. Overbeek SE, O'Sullivan S, Leman K, et al. Effect of montelukast compared with inhaled fluticasone on airway inflammation. Clin Exp Allergy. 2004;34(9):1388–94.
13. Riad S, Griffin AM, Liberman B, et al. Lymph node metastasis in soft tissue sarcoma in an extremity. Clin Orthop Relat Res. 2004;426:129–34.
14. Ghert MA, Abudu A, Driver N, et al. The indications for and the prognostic significance of amputation as the primary surgical procedure for localized soft tissue sarcoma of the extremity. Ann Surg Oncol. 2005;12(1):10–7.
15. Blay JY, El Sayadi H, Thiesse P, et al. Complete response to imatinib in relapsing pigmented villonodular synovitis/tenosynovial giant cell tumor (PVNS/TGCT). Ann Oncol. 2008;19(4): 821–2.
16. Cassier PA, Gelderblom H, Stacchiotti S, et al. Efficacy of imatinib mesylate for the treatment of locally advanced and/or metastatic tenosynovial giant cell tumor/pigmented villonodular synovitis. Cancer 2012;118(6):1649–55.
17. Brandal P, Panagopoulos I, Bjerkehagen B, et al. t(19;22)(q13;q12) translocation leading to the novel fusion gene EWSR1-ZNF444 in soft tissue myoepithelial carcinoma. Genes Chromosomes Cancer. 2009;48(12):1051–6.

18. Antonescu CR, Zhang L, Chang NE, et al. EWSR1-POU5F1 fusion in soft tissue myoepithelial tumors. A molecular analysis of sixty-six cases, including soft tissue, bone, and visceral lesions, showing common involvement of the EWSR1 gene. Genes Chromosomes Cancer. 2010; 49(12):1114–24.

19. Sasaguri T, Tanimoto A, Arima N, et al. Myoepithelioma of soft tissue. Pathol Int. 1999;49(6):571–6.

20. Noronha V, Cooper DL, Higgins SA, et al. Metastatic myoepithelial carcinoma of the vulva treated with carboplatin and paclitaxel. Lancet Oncol. 2006;7(3):270–1.

21. Strauchen JA. Germ-line mutations in nonsyndromic pheochromocytoma. N Engl J Med. 2002;347(11):854–5. author reply 854-855.

22. Lee IJ, Park DH, Park MC, et al. Subungual glomus tumours of the hand: diagnosis and outcome of the transungual approach. J Hand Surg Eur Vol. 2009;34(5):685–8.

23. Ozdemir O, Coskunol E, Ozalp T, et al. Glomus tumors of the finger: a report on 60 cases. Acta Orthop Traumatol Turc. 2003;37(3):244–8.

24. Van Geertruyden J, Lorea P, Goldschmidt D, et al. Glomus tumours of the hand. A retrospective study of 51 cases. J Hand Surg Br. 1996;21(2):257–60.

25. McCusick VA. Online Mendelian Inheritance in Man. Glomulovenous malformations; GVM. MIM ID #138000. 2010. http://www.ncbi.nlm.nih.gov/omim/138000. Accessed 25 Nov 2010.

26. Gorlin RJ, Fusaro RM, Benton JW. Multiple glomus tumor of the pseudocavernous hemangioma type; report of case manifesting a dominant inheritance pattern. Arch Dermatol. 1960;82:776–8.

27. Happle R, Konig A. Type 2 segmental manifestation of multiple glomus tumors: a review and reclassification of 5 case reports. Dermatology. 1999;198(3):270–2.

28. Keefer CJ, Brantley B, DeLozier 3rd JB. Familial infiltrative glomangiomas: diagnosis and treatment. J Craniofac Surg. 1996;7(2):145–7.

29. Magliulo G, Parnasi E, Savastano V, et al. Multiple familial facial glomus: case report and review of the literature. Ann Otol Rhinol Laryngol. 2003;112(3):287–92.

Chapter 26
Benign Soft Tissue Tumors

Lipoma

Lipomas are the most common benign neoplasm and usually arise in subcutaneous tissue. The trunk and proximal limbs are the most frequent sites. Although deep-seated benign lipomas do occur in the mediastinum or retroperitoneum, seemingly mature fatty neoplasms in the retroperitoneum should be considered well-differentiated (WD) liposarcoma. Most lipomas are solitary, soft, and painless and grow slowly; 2–3% of patients have multiple lesions that are occasionally seen in a familial pattern.

Solitary lipomas are well-circumscribed, lobulated lesions composed of fat cells, demarcated from surrounding fat by a thin fibrous capsule. Most subcutaneous, solitary lipomas show reproducible cytogenetic aberrations: translocations involving 12q13-15, rearrangements of 13q, or rearrangements involving 6p21-33 [1].

In spindle cell lipoma, mature fat is replaced by collagen-forming spindle cells; this lesion typically arises in the posterior neck and shoulder in men between the ages of 45 and 65. Spindle cell lipomas show consistent chromosomal aberrations of 13q and 16q [2].

Pleomorphic lipoma is closely related to spindle cell lipoma and is classified as a single family of lesions in the World Health Organization of soft tissue tumors. Local excision of lipoma and these variants is generally curative, with a local recurrence after simple excision in no more than 1–2% of cases.

Intramuscular lipomas differ by usually being poorly circumscribed and infiltrative (Fig. 26.1). These typically present in mid-adult life as a slow-growing, deep-seated mass most often located in the thigh or trunk. Approximately 10% of intramuscular lipomas are noninfiltrative and well circumscribed. In a patient with a deep-seated fatty tumor, it is important to exclude an atypical lipomatous tumor, the lowest grade version of well-differentiated liposarcoma (ALT; see Liposarcoma), which tends to be more common than an intramuscular lipoma. As a form of well-differentiated liposarcoma, ALT has a known risk of local recurrence.

Surgical resection of symptomatic lesions or lesions ≥5 cm is usually recommended and often curative.

M.F. Brennan et al., *Management of Soft Tissue Sarcoma*,
DOI 10.1007/978-1-4614-5004-7_26, © Springer Science+Business Media New York 2013

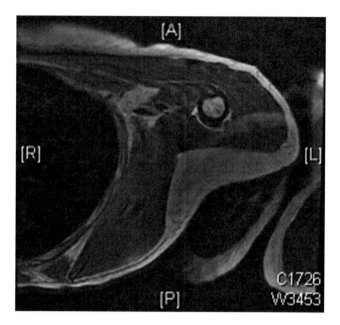

Fig. 26.1 T1-weighted axial MRI image of an intramuscular lipoma of the trunk

Lipomatosis

Lipomatosis is a term applied to poorly circumscribed overgrowth of mature adipose tissue growing in a somewhat infiltrative pattern. It can occur in the intraperitoneal area, in the retroperitoneum, and in multiple other sites. A relationship to mutations in HMGA2 is suggested [3]. Rarely, it has been considered an unusual side effect of cytotoxic chemotherapy. Lipodystrophy is a form of redistribution of body fat more commonly seen than lipomatosis as a complication of antiretroviral agents, among other medications.

An entity considered benign symmetric lipomatosis is described usually in the sub-cutaneous tissues around the neck. A usual association with alcoholism and the presence of glucose intolerance have been described. This lesion should be considered a lipodystrophy when associated with alcoholism or administration of HIV protease inhibitors. Other unusual sites have resulted in spinal cord compression. There is a variant of congenital type which involves infiltration of the fascial subcutaneous tissue.

Lipoblastoma/Lipoblastomatosis

Lipoblastoma has been reported to occur in the head and neck in children as a rare, benign encapsulated tumor usually arising from embryonic white fat. It is rare to see such tumors over the age of 20. They usually present as a growing mass in children under the age of 5 with many occurring before age 1. Clinically the lesions are commonly mistaken for a benign lipoma or hemangioma.

More commonly seen in the extremities and trunk, there is no sex preselection, but tumor can grow quite rapidly. Very rarely do they obtain a size to become symptomatic.

Histological appearance usually contains primitive mesenchymal cells, myxoid and fibrous bands, and variably differentiated adipocytes. They differ from lipoma by their cellular immaturity and their close resemblance to the myxoid liposarcoma.

Confirmation by cytogenetics involves identification of a break point involving chromosome 8q11.2.

Lipoblastoma has an excellent prognosis, and surgical excision is the treatment of choice. Inadequate surgical resection is accompanied by recurrence. In surgical treatment, it is important to preserve neurovascular bundles even in the presence of large tumors, since these tumors typically do not recur.

Lipoblastomatosis is a multifocal variant of lipoblastoma.

Angiolipoma

Angiolipomas present as subcutaneous nodules, usually in young adults, and in more than 50% of cases are multiple. The most common site is the upper extremity. Angiolipomas rarely reach more than 2 cm in size, but they often are painful, especially during their initial growth period. Microscopically, these tumors consist of adipocytes with interspersed vascular structures. Myxoid and fibroblastic angiolipomas are recognized. Treatment is surgical excision (Fig. 26.2).

Angiomyolipoma

The term *angiomyolipoma* is used for a nonmetastasizing renal or hepatic tumor that is composed of fat, smooth muscle, and blood vessels. Angiomyolipoma is more common in women than in men and renal angiomyolipoma is seen in association with tuberous sclerosis (see more on the section on PEComa). Although angiomyolipoma is usually well demarcated from normal kidney, it may extend into the surrounding retroperitoneum (Fig. 26.3). Angiomyolipomas may be solitary or multicentric and may produce abdominal pain, hematuria, or intraperitoneal hemorrhage. Wide excision is curative.

In the presence of tubular sclerosis, tumors are often multiple. These are associated with loss of *TSC2* encoding tuberin. Rare cutaneous angiomyolipomas have been reported.

Angiomyolipomas of the liver have been described and may be difficult to differentiate from hepatocellular carcinoma. In a recent publication of 74 hepatic angiomyolipomas [4], there was a strong female predominance and mean age was 42. As opposed to in the kidney, tuberous sclerosis is only rarely seen. The majority were, as in the kidney, asymptomatic. Only one patient developed metastatic disease.

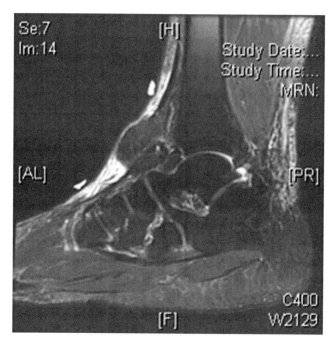

Fig. 26.2 T2-weighted sagittal MRI image of an angiolipoma of the distal ankle and forefoot

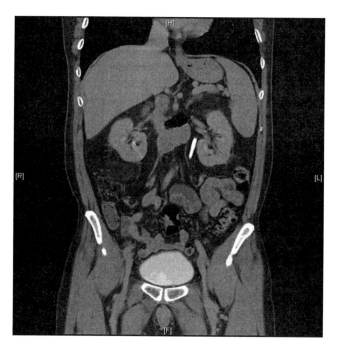

Fig. 26.3 Coronal reconstruction of late contrast-enhanced CT images of right kidney angiomyolipoma

Imaging is classical and can often make the diagnosis with vascular and fatty components readily identified on CT or MRI.

Rare extrarenal angiomyolipomas are uncommon although, in addition to liver, have been reported in bone, colon, and other structures. They are rare in the adrenal where the lesion is usually angiomyelolipoma (see below).

The usual treatment of angiomyolipoma is surgical resection, although many patients have been treated with selective arterial embolization. In many patients, especially those with large hepatic tumors, expectant observation is an acceptable approach.

Tumor rupture with hemorrhage is a severe complication of renal angiomyolipoma and is an indication for selective embolization. The goal in treatment is to perform as much nephron-sparing procedure as is possible. Rarely, extensive angiomyolipoma can include inferior vena caval thrombosis.

Radio-frequency ablation has been reported for angiomyolipoma, with uncertain results.

For systemic therapy of recurrent angiomyolipomas, see Chap. 25, Table 25.2.

Angiomyelolipoma

Angiomyelolipomas are lesions that commonly occur in the adrenal gland and can be confused with adrenal tumors. They have been reported in association with Carney's complex (pigmented nodular cortical hyperplasia, intra- and extracardiac myxoma, blue nevi, peripheral nerve tumors). A patient may be followed if a diagnosis can be made, although in large size lesions, excision is usually recommended. Spontaneous rupture has rarely been seen, especially in patients on long-term anticoagulation (Figs. 26.4 and 26.5)

Hibernoma

Hibernomas are rare tumors that are slow growing and benign. They resemble the glandular fat found in hibernating animals. The tumor is usually well vascularized with some poorly differentiated cells resembling brown adipocyte precursors. Brown adipocytes express the marker protein UCP1 and are thought to arise in close association with vessel walls. These tumors commonly occur in young adult males and usually in the posterior thorax. They are well defined by imaging with intermediate T1 and T2 signaling and are PET avid, as is normal brown fat [5].

Surgical resection is usually curative and rarely the lesions have been identified within the thorax and even within the pericardium (Figs. 26.6 and 26.7). Lesions have been described in the buttock and thigh and may show intense FDG-PET uptake.

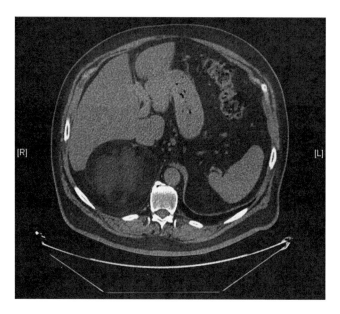

Fig. 26.4 Noncontrast axial CT image of a myelolipoma of the right adrenal gland

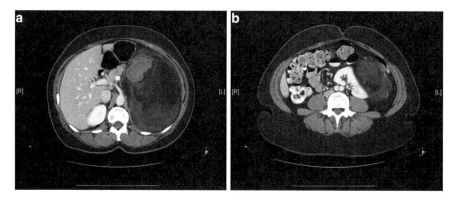

Fig. 26.5 Contrast-enhanced axial CT images (**a** and **b**) of a left adrenal myelolipoma

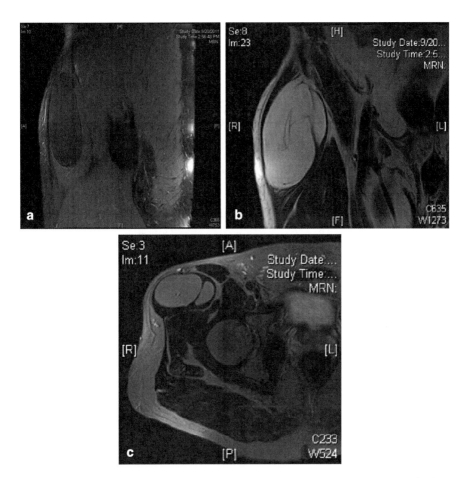

Fig. 26.6 T2 coronal (**a**) and T1 (**b, c**)-weighted coronal (**b**) and axial (**c**) MRI images of a right thigh hibernoma

Elastofibroma

Elastofibroma is an uncommon, benign, very slow-growing soft tissue tumor. The cause is unknown and it usually presents at the inferior pole of the scapula (Figs. 26.8 and 26.9). They can be bilateral, often familial, and will often have limited symptoms. MRI and CT are excellent imaging modalities and treatment is primarily surgical, although there is no real indication for operation in the absence of symptoms. This is particularly true if the lesions are extensive beneath the scapula where resection would have some significant morbidity.

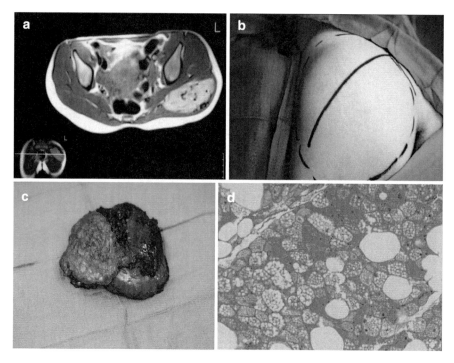

Fig. 26.7 (**a**) Axial T1-weighted image MRI of a left buttock hibernoma. (**b**) Preoperative and (**c**) specimen images of hibernoma. (**d**) High-power microscopic image of a hibernoma (H&E, 400X)

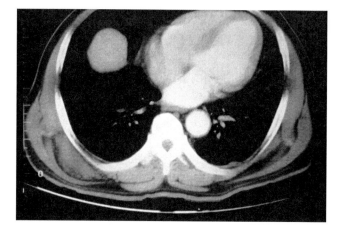

Fig. 26.8 Contrast-enhanced axial CT image of an elastofibroma of inferior right periscapular soft tissue (Used with permission from: Brennan and Lewis [6])

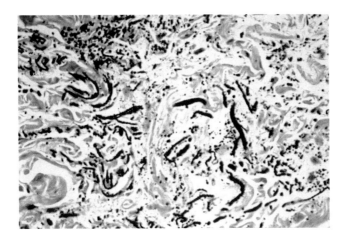

Fig. 26.9 Elastin-stained microscopic image of an elastofibroma (400 magnification) (Used with permission from: Brennan and Lewis [6])

Chromosome analyses have been performed showing variable losses of 1p,13q;19p and 22q and gains in *APC* (5q21) and *PAH* (12q23). The significance of these findings is uncertain. The increased preponderance of lesions on the right side suggests that they may be associated with a response to shoulder motion.

Granular Cell Tumor

Granular cell tumors are neural tumors of Schwann cell derivation with abundant lysosomal content and diffuse S-100 protein reactivity. Many behave in benign fashion but malignant forms have certainly been described.

Granular cell tumors can occur in the most unusual locations. Because of their origin from Schwann cells, they have been seen in the skin, soft tissue, and brain and can occur in synchronous sites. They have also been reported in the tongue and in the brain, but they are seen in any site where Schwann cells can be expected.

Hemangioma

Hemangiomas are benign proliferations of blood vessels. They represent one end of a spectrum of tumors of endothelium that extends to borderline tumors with intermediate prognosis such as epithelioid hemangioendothelioma to the frankly malignant and often fatal angiosarcoma, as well as many relatively rare diagnoses along this spectrum. Other benign lesions of vasculature include vascular malformations, reactive proliferations, telangiectasias, and lymphangiomas.

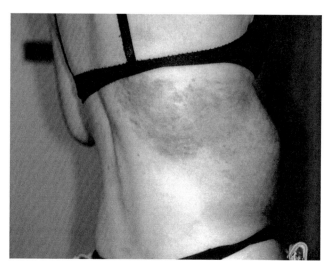

Fig. 26.10 Hemangioma of the entire right lateral chest and abdominal wall (Used with permission from: Brennan and Lewis [6])

Hemangiomas, which are among the most common soft tissue tumors, are broken down by a number of descriptors. Hemangiomas are typically described as cutaneous, subcutaneous, synovial, osseous, or intramuscular; by type of blood vessel (capillary, venous, cavernous); and/or by cell type (e.g., epithelioid, spindle cell). Hemangiomas are distinguished from vascular malformations as hemangiomas grow over time in excess to the growth of the normal structure, can regress spontaneously, and have a proliferative endothelial component. They also need to be distinguished from reactive lesions such as the lesions of bacillary angiomatosis (*Bartonella* sp. infection) or similar lesions found in Oroya fever (*B. bacilliformis* infection) [7].

Hemangiomas can be managed surgically, but have a wide variety of patterns of change over time, from indolent and slow growing to aggressive and destructive (Figs. 26.10, 26.11, and 26.12). Interestingly, pediatric hemangiomas go through phases of growth and involution and often can be observed. Pediatric hemangiomas are the diagnosis in which Judah Folkman's angiogenesis theories of cancer [8] were first tested, in the form of interferon [9]. It is rather remarkable that involution of hemangiomas can be triggered with the use of beta blockers such as propranolol [10], which may have effects on β2 adrenergic receptors which then have effect on vasoconstriction, angiogenesis, and apoptosis [11]. Glucocorticoids have also been employed and can be used for a brief (2–3-week) course before tapering if there are no beneficial effects observed.

For superficial pediatric hemangiomas in the proliferative stage, pulsed dye lasers (585–590 nm) can treat lesions less than 2–3 mm in thickness [12]. For thicker lesions, laser treatments are not nearly as effective. Radio-frequency ablation can be considered for deep, smaller lesions. There are other situations where more

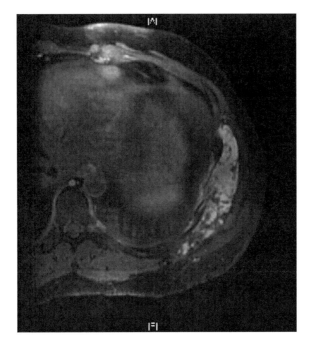

Fig. 26.11 T1-weighted axial MRI image of a chest wall hemangioma

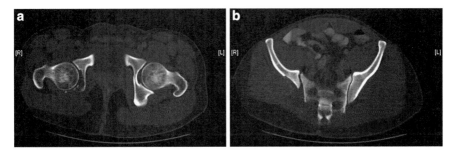

Fig. 26.12 Noncontrast CT images (**a** and **b**) using bone windows demonstrating a soft tissue hemangioma causing bony destruction of the acetabulum, ilium, and sacrum

traditional surgical techniques can be employed for treatment of hemangiomas, for example, partial hepatectomy for giant hemangiomas of the liver causing abdominal pain [13]. The concern for some lesions is the anatomical restrictions of an anatomical site to resect such a lesion completely, for example, in the mediastinum, which not surprisingly is associated with recurrence. In other cases, attempts must be made to resect or at least embolize the primary tumor, given the consumptive coagulopathy observed with some benign vascular lesions, termed Kasabach-Merritt syndrome [14].

Other systemic agents such as vincristine can be employed in symptomatic lesions. Antiangiogenic therapy with bevacizumab has been shown effective in case reports of bevacizumab in choroidal hemangiomas (sometimes in combination with photo-dynamic therapy), while the use of oral VEGF receptor inhibitors has yielded mixed results in the few patients we have treated. The treatment of hemangiomas remains an area open to research and innovation both on local and systemic therapy fronts.

Leiomyoma

Benign tumors of smooth muscle are much more common in the uterus, but they can occur in the gastrointestinal tract and among some mucosal sites but rarely deep in the extremity or retroperitoneum. In the uterus, leiomyomas are far more common than leiomyosarcomas. Uterine leiomyomas may have an increased mitotic rate, which makes such tumors difficult to distinguish from a very low-grade leiomyosar-coma. Those tumors in the gray zone regarding malignancy are termed smooth muscle tumors of uncertain malignant potential, or STUMP [15]. PEComas, which can also mark positive for smooth muscle markers (and melanoma markers), are part of the differential diagnosis.

Schwannoma

Schwannomas are benign lesions most commonly identified in the 20–50 year-old age group. Common sites include the retroperitoneum and neck. These lesions are slow growing, and when the diagnosis can be made, symptomatic patients can be followed. Given the characteristics and histological picture, the diagnosis is readily made even on a core needle biopsy. Retroperitoneal paravertebral schwannomas are more likely to contain a cellular schwannoma, more cellular variant of the classical schwannoma (Fig. 26.13). On occasions, the schwannoma can mimic a malignant tumor with extensive bone invasion

Rarely, malignant transformation has been described ex-schwannoma, typically presenting as epithelioid malignant peripheral nerve sheath tumors, in the absence of familial syndromes (neurofibromatosis type I) [16]. If the diagnosis is firm and the patient is symptomatic, schwannomas may be removed with minimally invasive surgery to limit morbidity.

Neurofibroma

Neurofibromas are common and can occur either in the presence or absence of neurofibromatosis. Those occurring as solitary lesions are usually small, slow-growing cutaneous or subcutaneous nodules (Fig. 26.14). Those occurring in

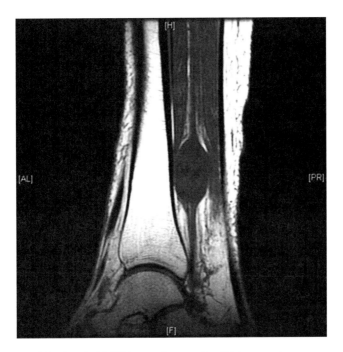

Fig. 26.13 T1-weighted sagittal MRI image of a posterior tibial nerve schwannoma

neurofibromatosis have an autosomal dominant mutation at the 17q11.2 locus and are associated with other finds such as café au lait spots, multiple cutaneous neurofibromas, and hamartomas of the iris. Patients with neurofibromatosis are at risk of malignant transformation (i.e., malignant peripheral nerve sheath tumors) in their preexistent plexiform or intraneural neurofibromas as well as other malignant lesions in the brain or adrenal gland.

Myxoma

Intramuscular myxoma is a rare tumor that occurs in adults, usually in the extremities within the larger muscles. Diagnosis is made by histological examination of a lesion characterized with abundant mucoid material but very few cells. The lesions are often less than 10 cm and behave in a clinically benign fashion [17].

Myxomas can essentially occur in any muscular area of the body and are a common primary cardiac tumor, most commonly arising in the left atrium [18]. They present slow-growing, deep-seeded lesions, which show on CT as an area with thin septation and mild to zero PET image uptake. They have been characterized by content of glucosamine glycans, and the challenge is to separate them from the grade one

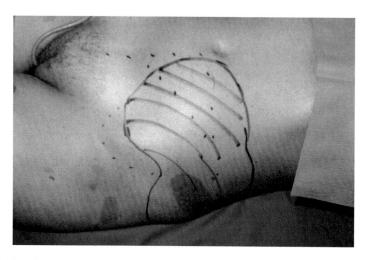

Fig. 26.14 Café au lait spot and large left hip malignant peripheral nerve tumor (Used with permission from: Brennan and Lewis [6])

myxofibrosarcomas. Albumin content has also been used for further characterization [19]. A recurrent GNAS1 activating mutation has been shown to be present in most intramuscular myxomas, which can serve as a very useful molecular test in excluding the look-alike myxoid lesions (i.e., low-grade myxofibrosarcomas) [20]. Furthermore, myxomas lack the characteristic chromosomal translocations, as seen in myxoid liposarcoma, low-grade fibromyxoid sarcomas, and myxoid chondrosarcomas.

Angiomyxoma

Angiomyxomas, particularly of the genital, pelvic, or perineal areas, have been confused with scrotal masses, hydroceles, and inguinal hernia and are thought to be more common in females but also be seen in males (Fig. 26.15). They are usually immunoreactive for estrogen and progesterone receptors. Histologically, they are characterized by oval to spindle cell tumor cells in a myxoid stroma along with hyalinized vessels and a characteristic immunophenotype. Local recurrence can result in very significant morbidity, but distant metastases do not occur [21]. The primary management remains surgical resection, although gonadotropin-releasing hormone agonists and antiestrogens have been utilized for recurrent disease [22] (Fig. 26.16)

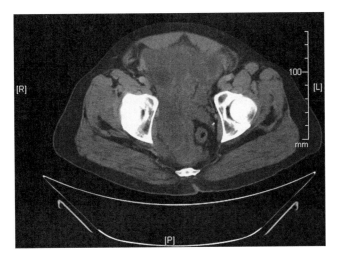

Fig. 26.15 Axial contrast-enhanced CT image of a recurrent pelvic angiomyxoma

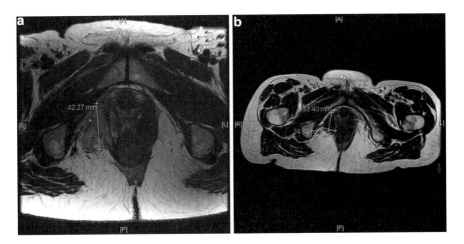

Fig. 26.16 Axial T1-weighted MRI images of a paravaginal angiomyxoma before (**a**) and after (**b**) leuprolide therapy

References

1. Willen H, Akerman M, Dal Cin P, et al. Comparison of chromosomal patterns with clinical features in 165 lipomas: a report of the CHAMP study group. Cancer Genet Cytogenet. 1998;102(1):46–9.
2. Dal Cin P, Sciot R, Polito P, et al. Lesions of 13q may occur independently of deletion of 16q in spindle cell/pleomorphic lipomas. Histopathology. 1997;31(3):222–5.
3. Prontera P, Stangoni G, Manes I, et al. Encephalocraniocutaneous lipomatosis (ECCL) in a patient with history of familial multiple lipomatosis (FML). Am J Med Genet A. 2009;149A(3):543–5.

4. Hu WG, Lai EC, Liu H, et al. Diagnostic difficulties and treatment strategy of hepatic angiomyolipoma. Asian J Surg. 2011;34(4):158–62.
5. Cypess AM, Lehman S, Williams G, et al. Identification and importance of brown adipose tissue in adult humans. N Engl J Med. 2009;360(15):1509–17.
6. Brennan MF, Lewis JJ. Diagnosis and management of soft tissue sarcoma. London: Martin Dunitz; 1998.
7. Dehio C. Molecular and cellular basis of bartonella pathogenesis. Annu Rev Microbiol. 2004;58:365–90.
8. Folkman J. Tumor angiogenesis: therapeutic implications. N Engl J Med. 1971;285(21): 1182–6.
9. Ezekowitz RA, Mulliken JB, Folkman J. Interferon alfa-2a therapy for life-threatening hemangiomas of infancy. N Engl J Med. 1992;326(22):1456–63.
10. Buckmiller LM, Munson PD, Dyamenahalli U, et al. Propranolol for infantile hemangiomas: early experience at a tertiary vascular anomalies center. Laryngoscope. 2010;120(4):676–81.
11. Lawley LP, Siegfried E, Todd JL. Propranolol treatment for hemangioma of infancy: risks and recommendations. Pediatr Dermatol. 2009;26(5):610–4.
12. Leonardi-Bee J, Batta K, O'Brien C, et al. Interventions for infantile haemangiomas (strawberry birthmarks) of the skin. Cochrane Database Syst Rev. 2011;5:CD006545.
13. Kammula US, Buell JF, Labow DM, et al. Surgical management of benign tumors of the liver. Int J Gastrointest Cancer. 2001;30(3):141–6.
14. Hall GW. Kasabach-Merritt syndrome: pathogenesis and management. Br J Haematol. 2001;112(4):851–62.
15. Ip PP, Tse KY, Tam KF. Uterine smooth muscle tumors other than the ordinary leiomyomas and leiomyosarcomas: a review of selected variants with emphasis on recent advances and unusual morphology that may cause concern for malignancy. Adv Anat Pathol. 2010;17(2): 91–112.
16. Carter JM, O'Hara C, Dundas G, et al. Epithelioid malignant peripheral nerve sheath tumor arising in a schwannoma, in a patient With "Neuroblastoma-like" schwannomatosis and a novel germline SMARCB1 mutation. Am J Surg Pathol 2012;36(1):154–60.
17. Enzinger FM. Intramuscular Myxoma; a review and follow-up study of 34 cases. Am J Clin Pathol. 1965;43:104–13.
18. Bossert T, Gummert JF, Battellini R, Richter M, Barten M, Walther T, Falk V, Mohr FW. Surgical experience with 77 primary cardiac tumors. Interact Cardiovasc Thorac Surg 2005;4(4):311–5.
19. Willems SM, Schrage YM, Baelde JJ, et al. Myxoid tumours of soft tissue: the so-called myxoid extracellular matrix is heterogeneous in composition. Histopathology. 2008;52(4): 465–74.
20. Willems SM, Mohseny AB, Balog C, et al. Cellular/intramuscular myxoma and grade I myxofibrosarcoma are characterized by distinct genetic alterations and specific composition of their extracellular matrix. J Cell Mol Med. 2009;13(7):1291–301.
21. Steeper TA, Rosai J. Aggressive angiomyxoma of the female pelvis and perineum. Report of nine cases of a distinctive type of gynecologic soft-tissue neoplasm. Am J Surg Pathol. 1983;7(5):463–75.
22. Fine BA, Munoz AK, Litz CE, et al. Primary medical management of recurrent aggressive angiomyxoma of the vulva with a gonadotropin-releasing hormone agonist. Gynecol Oncol. 2001;81(1):120–2.

Chapter 27
Reactive Lesions

Myositis Ossificans

Myositis ossificans usually occurs in the extremity following an episode of trauma. This diagnosis can usually be excluded in late presentation by a plain film showing soft tissue calcification or an MRI showing the classic infiltration of soft tissues rather than discrete tumor masses (Fig. 27.1). Calcifications are not specific and may occur in synovial sarcoma or osteogenic sarcoma and should always be considered. Resolution of the lesion is to be expected in myositis ossificans, in particular, when the diagnosis is made early. The diagnosis can be difficult and lesions are often hemorrhagic on biopsy; given that other entities including dedifferentiated liposarcoma can calcify, caution should be made before casually giving a diagnosis.

Nodular Fasciitis

Nodular fasciitis, also termed pseudosarcomatous fasciitis, is a benign lesion usually seen in middle-aged adults but has been reported in older and young patients. The lesion often grows rapidly but is usually self-limited, and pain and tenderness are common features of presentation. Most commonly seen in the upper extremity

M.F. Brennan et al., *Management of Soft Tissue Sarcoma*,
DOI 10.1007/978-1-4614-5004-7_27, © Springer Science+Business Media New York 2013

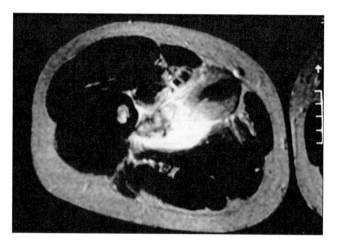

Fig. 27.1 Myositis ossificans: T1-weighted MRI showing absence of discrete mass and intermuscular extension (Used with permission from Brennan and Lewis [1])

around the elbow joint, the lesion arises in subcutaneous fascia. Diagnosis can be difficult as the lesions are often nodular and nonencapsulated, consisting predominantly of myofibroblasts arranged in irregular bundles or fascicles. More recently, a recurrent MYH9-USP6 gene fusion has been described suggesting a novel model of transient neoplasia [2]. Simple excision is usually curative.

Sarcoma Masquerade

Unilateral hypertrophy of the tensor fascia lata can be confused with a soft tissue tumor [3]. The patient presents with a palpable mass, but it is not discrete. However, it is clearly different from the contralateral side. Although cases are limited, it appears to be more common in females but can be readily distinguished on CT or MRI (Fig. 27.2).

A further masquerade is the Morel-Lavallée lesion. This lesion commonly occurs in the proximal thigh and is has characteristic features on MRI. Morel-Lavallée lesions are unusual effusions, usually the result of skin and subcutaneous fatty tissue separating from the underlying fascia. They are common in the trochanteric region because of the rich vascular plexus that pierces the fascia lata. The disrupted capillaries continuously drain into the perifascial plane filling the cavity with blood, lymph, and debris. Because the inflammatory reaction occurs, they can appear encapsulated and be suggestive of sarcoma [4]. An example is shown in Fig. 27.3, where following a resection of a synovial sarcoma recurrence was expected, but instead the sarcoma masquerade demonstrated (see MRI).

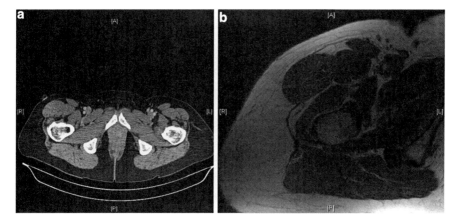

Fig. 27.2 (a) CT image and (b) T1-weighted MRI image of a patient with unilateral tensor fascia lata hypertrophy

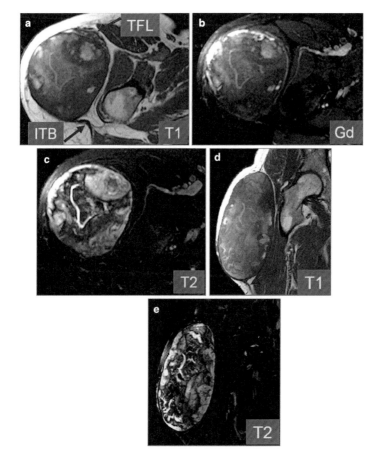

Fig. 27.3 (a–e) MRI images (T1- or T2-weighted) of a Morel-Lavallée lesion of the proximal right thigh. *TFL* tensor fascia lata, *ITB* iliotibial band, *Gd* gadolinium enhancement

References

1. Brennan MF, Lewis JJ. Diagnosis and management of soft tissue sarcoma. London: Martin Dunitz; 1998.
2. Erickson-Johnson MR, Chou MM, Evers BR, et al. Nodular fasciitis: a novel model of transient neoplasia induced by MYH9-USP6 gene fusion. Lab Invest. 2011;91(10):1427–33.
3. Ilaslan H, Wenger DE, Shives TC, et al. Unilateral hypertrophy of tensor fascia lata: a soft tissue tumor simulator. Skeletal Radiol. 2003;32(11):628–32.
4. Mellado JM, Perez del Palomar L, Diaz L, et al. Long-standing Morel-Lavallee lesions of the trochanteric region and proximal thigh: MRI features in five patients. AJR Am J Roentgenol. 2004;182(5):1289–94.

Suggested Keywords

Chapter 1

Etiology
    Distribution
    Histopathology
    Carcinogens
    Lymphedema
    Genetic syndromes
    Li-Fraumeni syndrome
    Gardner syndrome
    Neurofibromatosis type I
    Familial GIST
    Rb
    Retinoblastoma
    Chromosomal translocation

Chapter 2

Natural history
    Outcome predictions
    Local recurrence
    Disease free survival
    Overall survival
    Nomogram
    Endpoint
    Bayesian Belief Model
    Staging system
    AJCC American Joint Committee on Cancer

M.F. Brennan et al., *Management of Soft Tissue Sarcoma*,
DOI 10.1007/978-1-4614-5004-7, © Springer Science+Business Media New York 2013

Chapter 3

Treatment
  Surgery
  Chemotherapy
  Radiation
  Primary surgery
  Metastasis surgery
  Adjuvant radiation
  Adjuvant chemotherapy
  Neoadjuvant therapy
  Intra-arterial therapy

Part I

Histological subtypes

Chapter 4

GIST
  Gastrointestinal stromal tumor
  KIT
  imatinib
  sunitinib
  regorafenib (I have a new reference when we get feedback)
  adjuvant therapy

Chapter 5

Liposarcoma
  Well differentiated liposarcoma
  Dedifferentiated liposarcoma
  Myxoid liposarcoma
  Round cell liposarcoma
  Pleomorphic liposarcoma
  MDM2
  CDK4

Chapter 6

Leiomyosarcoma
    Uterine leiomyosarcoma
    Inferior vena cava leiomyosarcoma
    Adjuvant therapy
    Metastatic disease

Chapter 7

UPS
    Undifferentiated pleomorphic sarcoma
    Malignant fibrous histiocytoma; see undifferentiated pleomorphic sarcoma
    Myxofibrosarcoma
    local recurrence
    metastatic disease

Chapter 8

Synovial
    SS18
    SSX
    Ifosfamide
    Immunotherapy
    NY-ESO-1

Chapter 9

MPNST
    Malignant peripheral nerve sheath tumor
    NF1
    Neurofibromatosis type I
    Plexiform neurofibroma
    Triton tumor

Chapter 10

Desmoid
  Gardner syndrome
  FAP
  Familial adenomatous polyposis
  Pregnancy
  APC
  Adenomatous polyposis coli
  Beta-catenin
  Wnt

Chapter 11

SFT HPC
  Solitary fibrous tumor
  Doege-Potter syndrome
  IGF2
  IGF1 receptor
  hemangiopericytoma

Chapter 12

Fibrosarcoma
  Dermatofibrosarcoma protuberans
  Low grade fibromyxoid sarcoma (of Evans) : Evans tumor
  Sclerosing epithelioid fibrosarcoma
  Inflammatory myofibroblastic tumor
  Infantile fibrosarcoma
  Myxoinflammatory fibroblastic sarcoma
  Adult fibrosarcoma
  translocation
  PDGF
  ALK
  INI1

Chapter 13

<u>Vascular sarcomas</u>
    Epithelioid hemangioendothelioma
    Angiosarcoma
    Kaposi sarcoma
    VEGF
    VEGF receptors
    TIE-1, TIE-2
    bevacizumab
    tyrosine kinase inhibitor

Chapter 14

<u>Epithelioid sarcoma</u>
    Proximal type
    Distal type
    INI1
    lymph node

Chapter 15

<u>Pediatric sarcoma</u>
    Ewing sarcoma
    Ewing sarcoma-like small round blue cell tumor
    Rhabdomyosarcoma
    Embryonal sarcoma
    Calcifying nested stromal and epithelial tumor
    translocations
    IGF1 receptor
    IGF2
    ETS
    FOXO1

Chapter 16

<u>Radiation induced sarcoma</u>
    UPS undifferentiated pleomorphic sarcoma

osteogenic sarcoma
angiosarcoma
local control

Chapter 17

ASPS
Alveolar soft part sarcoma
VEGF inhibitor
papillary renal cancer
MCT1
CD147
cediranib

Chapter 18

Clear cell sarcoma
MiTF
microphthalmia transcription factor
melanoma of soft parts

Chapter 19

DSRCT
Desmoplastic small round cell tumor
P6 chemotherapy regimen
VEGF inhibitor
intraperitoneal chemotherapy
gender
ethnicity

Chapter 20

EMC
Extraskeletal myxoid chondrosarcoma
orphan nuclear receptor
EWSR1 oncogene

NR4A3
TAF15

Chapter 21

Uterine
    Endometrial stromal sarcoma
    Undifferentiated endometrial sarcoma
    Uterine carcinosarcoma
    Malignant mixed Müllerian tumors
    estrogen
    tamoxifen
    megesterol
    IGF1 receptor
    translocation
    cisplatin

Chapter 22

ESOS
    Extraskeletal osteogenic sarcoma
    skeletal osteosarcoma
    adjuvant chemotherapy

Chapter 23

Sustentacular tumors
    Follicular dendritic cell tumor (FDCT)
    Interdigitating reticular cell tumor (IDRCT)
    Histiocytic sarcoma
    Langerhans cell tumor
    CD35
    BRAF
    histiocytosis X
    hemophagocytic histiocytosis
    monocyte

Chapter 24

Uncommon unique
    Heart
    Breast
    Head & neck
    Mediastinum
    Liver
    phyllodes tumor
    intimal sarcoma
    embryonal sarcoma

Part II

Benign lesions
    Lesions of unknown malignant potential

Chapter 25

Benign or less aggressive
    Perivascular epithelial cell tumor (PEComa)
    Giant cell tumor tendon sheath
    Pigmented villonodular synovitis
    Myoepithelioma
    Glomus tumor
    Ossifying fibromyxoid tumor
    Myopericytoma
    TOR
    mTOR
    lymphangioleiomyomatosis
    clear cell sugar tumor

Chapter 26

Benign tumors
    Lipoma & variants
    Lipomatosis
    Lipoblastoma

Lipoblastomatosis
Angiolipoma
Angiomyolipoma
Angiomyelolipoma
Hibernoma
Elastofibroma
Granular cell tumor
Hemangioma
Leiomyoma
Schwannoma
Neurofibroma
Myxoma
Angiomyxoma

Chapter 27

Reactive lesions
Myositis ossificans
Nodular fascitis
Sarcoma masquerade
Tensor fascia lata
Morel-Lavallee lesion

Index

M.F. Brennan et al., *Management of Soft Tissue Sarcoma*,
DOI 10.1007/978-1-4614-5004-7, © Springer Science+Business Media New York 2013